Your Pregnancy and Childbirth

Month to Month

FIFTH EDITION

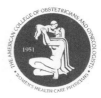

The American College of
Obstetricians and Gynecologists

Women's Health Care Physicians

Your Pregnancy and Childbirth: Month to Month, Fifth Edition, was developed by a panel of experts working in consultation with staff of the American College of Obstetricians and Gynecologists:

Editorial Task Force Members
Bonnie J. Dattel, MD, *Chair*
Ann Brown, CNM
Nancy Chescheir, MD
Mark S. DeFrancesco, MD
Rajiv B. Gala, MD
Paul A. Gluck, MD
Brian Mercer, MD
Susan M. Ramin, MD

ACOG Staff
Hal Lawrence III, MD, *Vice President, Practice Activities*
Thomas Dineen, *Senior Director, Publications*
Deirdre Allen, MPS, *Editorial Director*
Kathleen Scogna, MA, *Managing Editor, Patient Education*

The contributions of the following people are gratefully acknowledged:
Glenda Fauntleroy, *Writer*
Naylor Design, Inc., *Book Design*
Steven Freeman 2010, *Cover photograph*
Dragonfly Media Group, *Illustration*
John Yanson, *Illustration*
Lightbox Visual Communications, Inc., *Illustration*

Library of Congress Cataloging-in-Publication Data
Your pregnancy and childbirth : month to month / American College of
Obstetricians and Gynecologists, Women's Health Care Physicians. — 5th ed.
   p. cm.
  Rev. ed. of: Your pregnancy & birth. 4th ed. c2005.
  Includes index.
  ISBN 978-1-934946-89-3
  I. American College of Obstetricians and Gynecologists. Women's Health Care
Physicians. II. Your pregnancy & birth.
  RG525.A26 2010
  618.2—dc22

                         2009049226

Designed as an aid to patients, *Your Pregnancy and Childbirth: Month to Month* sets forth current information and opinions on subjects related to women's health and reproduction. The information does not dictate an exclusive course of treatment or procedure to be followed and should not be construed as excluding other acceptable methods of practice. Variations, taking into account the needs of the individual patient, resources, and limitations unique to the institution or type of practice, may be appropriate. The mention of a product, device, or drug in this publication does not constitute a guarantee or endorsement of the quality or value of such product, device, or drug or of the claims made for it by the manufacturer.

5/4

Contents

Preface

Your *Pregnancy and Childbirth: Month to Month* is written by the experts at the American College of Obstetricians and Gynecologists —the preeminent authority on women's health. For more than 50 years, this distinguished group of more than 52,000 leading health professionals has provided leadership and guidance on all aspects of women's health. The companion organization, called the American Congress of Obstetricians and Gynecologists, focuses on the economic and political aspects of women's health care. *Your Pregnancy and Childbirth* draws on this vast body of knowledge and experience to provide an authoritative pregnancy resource that you can trust. Because it presents this information in a reassuring, straightforward, and easy-to-understand way, *Your Pregnancy and Childbirth* encourages you to be informed about your pregnancy and empowers you to work with your health care provider as an active participant in one of the most fulfilling times in your life.

Now in its fifth edition, the book has undergone extensive revision and reorganization. Some of the new features in this edition are listed as follows:

- New month-to-month chapters cover the developmental milestones that your baby has reached that month, the changes taking place in your body, advice on exercise and nutrition appropriate for that particular month, a description of the month's prenatal visit, and a discussion of issues and decisions that you may want to think about at this point in your pregnancy.

- The second half of the book includes a section on labor, delivery, and the postpartum period, from the first few days up to 6 weeks and beyond. A chapter on designing the optimal pregnancy diet and a chapter on feeding your baby, which covers both breastfeeding and bottle-feeding, also are included. Separate chapters deal with the most common medical conditions that can affect pregnancy, such as diabetes mellitus, hypertension, and obesity. Multiple pregnancy has its own chapter, as does pregnancy the second (or third) time around.

• Confused about all of the options for prenatal testing? The birth defects chapter (Chapter 22) answers all of your questions, gives the latest guidelines, and includes a useful table that compares the options.

• Pregnancy complications are covered in detail in several chapters that include the signs and symptoms to watch for, as well as diagnosis and treatment for each condition.

• Up-to-date information is offered on the topics of most concern to pregnant women, such as vaginal birth after cesarean delivery, weight gain during pregnancy, how to handle labor, breastfeeding tips for working moms, and the various tests that are used to monitor the baby's well-being.

• Expert advice is included about many of the important decisions facing parents-to-be, such as how to choose a health care provider for your pregnancy (and for your baby), how to plan your birth experience, and when to tell your other children about your pregnancy.

• New illustrations—including a full-color section that shows fetal development and the changes that take place in the mother's body—are featured in this edition. Other illustrations show you various positions to use for breastfeeding, what genes are, and the events that happen during each stage of labor, to name a few.

• A complete glossary is included that defines important terms used throughout the book, which are highlighted in boldface and italics.

• *Your Pregnancy and Childbirth: Month to Month* also has a web site, which can be accessed at www.yourpregnancyandchildbirth.com. This web site offers additional information, interactive calculators and forms, and links to various resources.

What has not changed in this new edition is the College's commitment to providing a complete, factual guide to pregnancy and childbirth. We sincerely hope that *Your Pregnancy and Childbirth** becomes a trusted resource and a comforting presence that you can turn to throughout your pregnancy.

---

*A note about the gender pronouns used in the book: Alternate chapters in Your Pregnancy and Childbirth: Month to Month *use one gender pronoun to refer to the baby. For example, Chapter 4 uses all female pronouns, while Chapter 5 uses all male pronouns.*

Part I
Pregnancy Month by Month

The following full-color illustrations show fetal development and the changes that occur in a woman's body throughout the 9 months of pregnancy. These illustrations are also found in each month-to-month chapter. Seeing them all together, however, gives an idea of how a woman's body adjusts to accommodate the growth of a baby.

Mother and baby: Weeks 1–8.

Fingers and toes are present

Eyelids are forming

Heart is beating

The first 8 weeks of pregnancy are a time of rapid growth for your baby. At the end of 8 weeks, most of the organ systems have begun to form.

Mother and baby: Weeks 9–12.

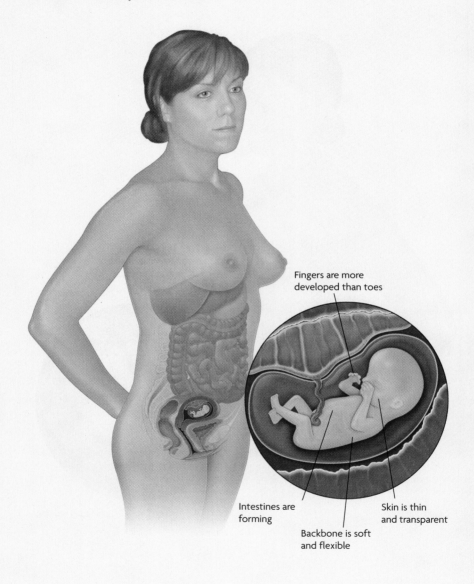

Fingers are more developed than toes

Intestines are forming

Backbone is soft and flexible

Skin is thin and transparent

At this point, your baby weighs just more than 1 ounce and is about 3½ inches long.

Mother and baby: Weeks 13–16.

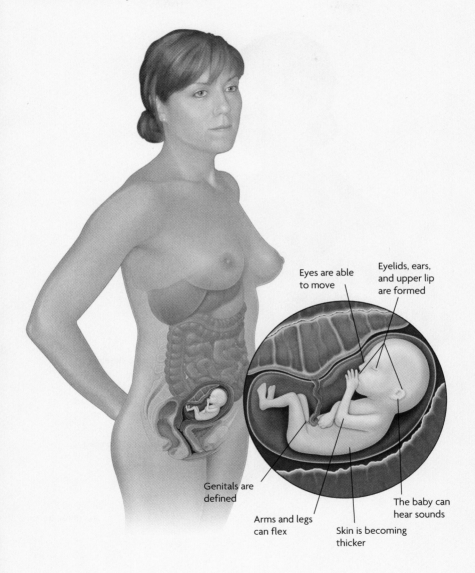

Eyes are able to move

Eyelids, ears, and upper lip are formed

Genitals are defined

Arms and legs can flex

Skin is becoming thicker

The baby can hear sounds

Your baby weighs about 5 ounces and is now about 6–7 inches long.

Mother and baby: Weeks 17–20.

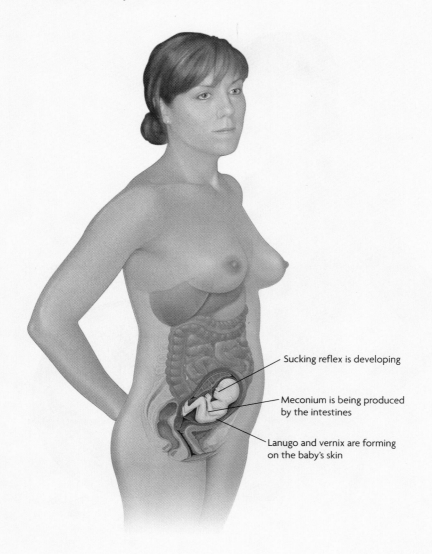

Sucking reflex is developing

Meconium is being produced by the intestines

Lanugo and vernix are forming on the baby's skin

The baby may weigh as much as a pound and is about 10 inches long. You may be able to feel your baby move this month.

Mother and baby: Weeks 21–24.

The brain is very active

Tear ducts are developing

The baby moves in response to sounds

This month, your baby has fingerprints, and you may feel her hiccuping.

Mother and baby: Weeks 25–28.

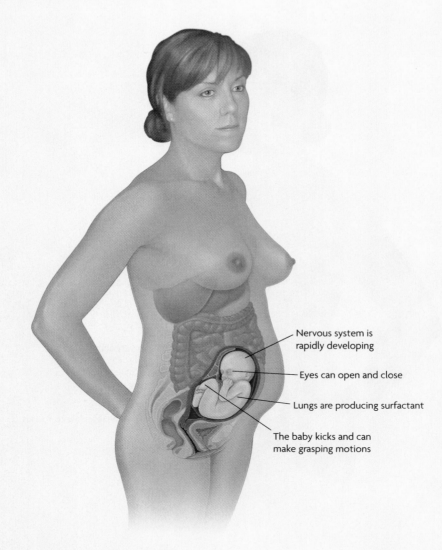

Nervous system is rapidly developing

Eyes can open and close

Lungs are producing surfactant

The baby kicks and can make grasping motions

By the end of this month, your baby will weigh about 2 ½ pounds and will be 14 inches long.

Mother and baby: Weeks 29–32.

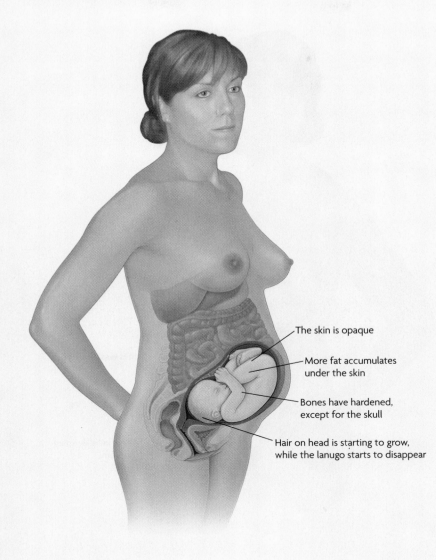

The skin is opaque

More fat accumulates under the skin

Bones have hardened, except for the skull

Hair on head is starting to grow, while the lanugo starts to disappear

With major development now complete, your baby will put on weight rapidly in the last 2 months.

Mother and baby: Weeks 33–36.

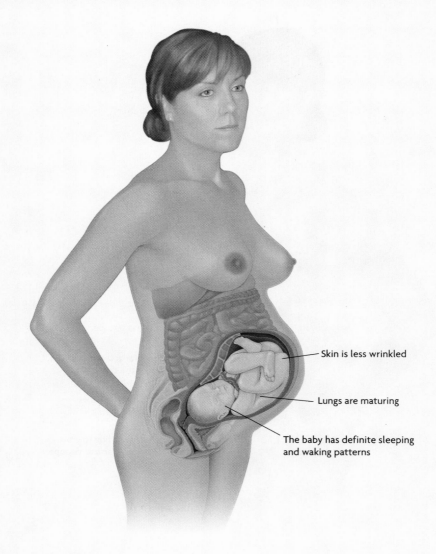

Skin is less wrinkled

Lungs are maturing

The baby has definite sleeping and waking patterns

This month, your baby will most likely gain about 2 pounds in weight but won't get much longer than 20 inches.

Mother and baby: Term (Weeks 37–40).

There is very little room for the baby to move

The baby drops lower into the pelvis

More fat accumulates, especially around the elbows, knees, and shoulders

Your baby is now ready to be born.

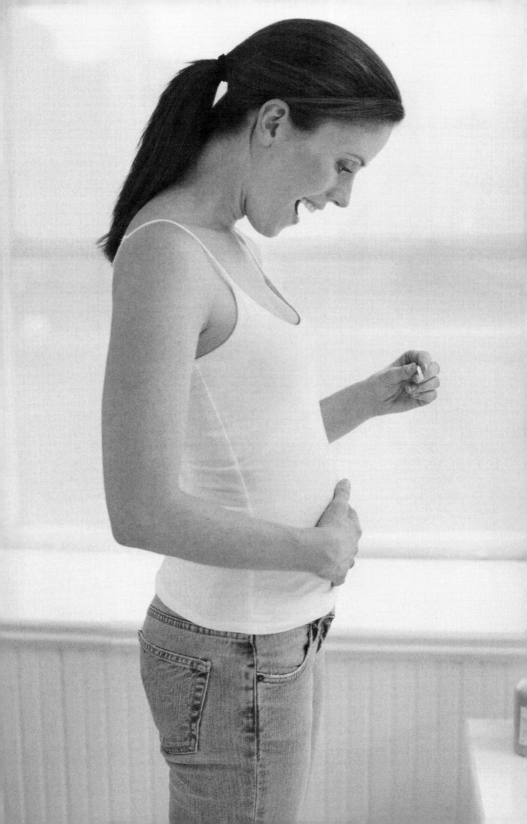

Chapter 1

Months 1 and 2

(Weeks 1–8)

YOUR GROWING BABY

Week 1

Fertilization, the union of an *egg* and a *sperm*, is the first step in a complex series of events that leads to pregnancy. When the egg and sperm unite, they form a single *cell* called a zygote. Fertilization takes place in the woman's *fallopian tube*. After fertilization, the zygote divides, forming two cells. These cells then divide, forming four cells, and then eight cells, and so on. At the same time, the mass of dividing cells moves down the fallopian tube toward the *uterus*.

Week 2

Approximately 7 days after fertilization, the rapidly dividing ball of cells, now called a blastocyst, enters the uterus. The *endometrium*, or uterine lining, has prepared itself for potential pregnancy. The blastocyst burrows deep into the uterine lining, a process called implantation.

Week 3

Once the blastocyst has implanted in the uterine lining, the part that will develop into the placenta starts producing a *hormone* called *human chorionic gonadotropin (hCG).* This hormone signals your *ovaries* to stop releasing eggs and triggers your body to produce more of the hormones *estrogen* and *progesterone*. The increased levels of these hormones stop your menstrual period and start the growth of the *placenta*. Once fully

13

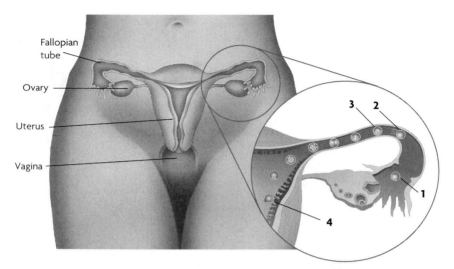

Fertilization. Each month during ovulation, an egg is released (1) and moves into one of the fallopian tubes. If a woman has sex around this time, and if the egg and sperm meet in the fallopian tube (2), the two may join. If they join (3), the fertilized egg begins dividing as it moves through the fallopian tube into the uterus (4), where it becomes attached to the uterine lining.

formed, the placenta functions as the life support system for the baby, delivering oxygen, nutrients, and hormones from the mother and removing waste products. It also provides a pathway for harmful substances, such as drugs and viruses, to reach the baby. As the placenta takes shape, small finger-like projections grow out of it. In these projections, called ***chorionic villi***, blood vessels form. The tips of these vessels burrow into the uterine wall and connect to the mother's blood supply. On the side of the placenta nearest the baby, the umbilical cord forms. The ***umbilical cord*** bridges the connection between the mother's bloodstream and the baby. This tube-like structure is attached to your baby in the center of the belly. After birth, this cord is cut. The remnants become the baby's navel.

Week 4

The neural tube, from which the brain, spinal cord, and backbone will form, is completing its development during the fourth week of pregnancy. Balls of cells called somites start to appear along the neural tube. They eventually will develop into the bones of the spine and muscles of the back. Other major organs, such as the heart and lungs, are developing during this period. Although the heart is not yet fully formed, it has started to beat. Also present are the ***amniotic sac***, which contains the baby during the pregnancy, and ***amniotic fluid***, which cushions the baby as it grows.

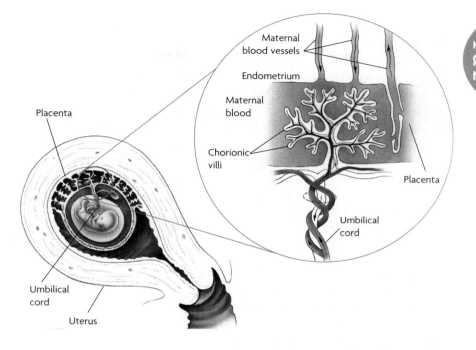

The placenta. The placenta is composed of chorionic villi. Chorionic villi contain fetal cells.

Week 5

At this stage, the baby looks like a curled tube and is approximately ½ inch long—about the size of a pumpkin seed. Arm and leg buds appear. The long tube that will become your baby's digestive tract has taken shape.

Week 6

Your baby's heart is beating approximately 80 times per minute. The nose, mouth, and ears are beginning to form, and webbed fingers and toes are poking out from your baby's hands and feet. The inner ear begins to develop.

Week 7

Bones are forming but won't begin to harden for a few weeks. Fingers and toes are present. Your baby's external *genitals* are starting to develop. Eyelids form but remain closed.

Week 8

At 8 weeks, your baby is now 1 inch long. By the end of the second month, all major organs and body systems have begun to develop. Breathing tubes extend from the throat to the developing lungs. In the brain, nerve cells are branching out to connect with one another. Up until the eighth week of development, the baby is known as an **embryo**. This week marks the end of the embryonic phase of development. After the end of week 8, the baby is called a **fetus**.

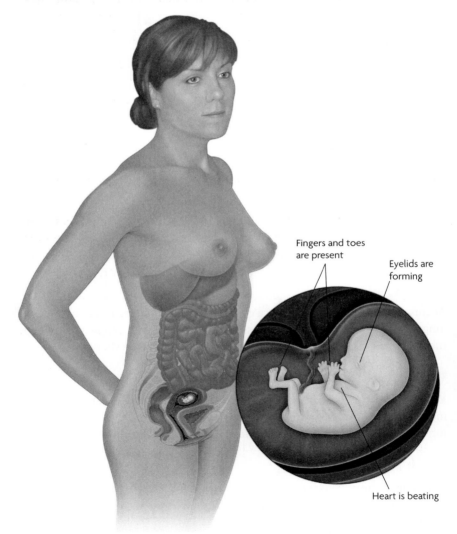

Fingers and toes are present

Eyelids are forming

Heart is beating

Mother and baby: Weeks 1–8. The first 8 weeks of pregnancy are a time of rapid growth for your baby. At the end of 8 weeks, most of the organ systems have begun to form.

YOUR PREGNANCY

❱ Your Changing Body

By the end of week 2, you probably don't know that you are pregnant, but you may notice a little spotting. Known as implantation bleeding, this spotting can occur when the fertilized egg becomes attached to the lining of the uterus. The spotting is very light, and not all women have it. Some women mistake it for menstrual bleeding. Implantation bleeding is normal and doesn't signal a problem.

Many signs and symptoms of pregnancy are thought to be caused by changing hormone levels. Some women are not aware of the early signs and symptoms, while others notice the sometimes subtle changes right away.

Hormones

Hormones are the chemical messengers that orchestrate the body's functions. The following hormones play a leading role in reproduction, pregnancy, and birth:

- *Estrogen* and *progesterone*—Initially produced by the ovaries, these hormones trigger the lining of the uterus to thicken during each menstrual cycle and to be shed if pregnancy doesn't occur. After an egg is fertilized, an increase in estrogen and progesterone levels prevents further ovulation.

- *Follicle-stimulating hormone (FSH)* and *luteinizing hormone (LH)*— These hormones are made by the pituitary gland, a small organ at the base of the brain. FSH causes an egg to ripen in one of the ovaries. LH triggers the egg's release.

- *Gonadotropin-releasing hormone (GnRH)*—This hormone, also made in the pituitary gland, is the signal to produce FSH and LH.

- *hCG*—Made by certain cells from the fertilized and dividing egg, hCG spurs increased estrogen and progesterone production during pregnancy. It's the hormone that pregnancy tests detect.

Signs and Symptoms of Pregnancy

Could you be pregnant? Most likely you will not have symptoms until about the time you've missed your menstrual period or even about 1 week or 2 weeks later. Some women notice symptoms earlier than others.

A missed menstrual period is the most obvious sign of pregnancy. If your menstrual cycles are regular and your menstrual period does not arrive on time, you may suspect that you are pregnant long before you notice any signs or symptoms. Here are the six most common:

1. *Tender, swollen breasts*—One of the early signs of pregnancy is sensitive, sore breasts caused by increasing levels of hormones. The soreness may feel like a more intense version of how your breasts feel before your menstrual period. The pain and discomfort should decrease after the first few weeks, as your body adjusts to the hormonal changes.

2. *Frequent urination*—Soon after you become pregnant, you may find yourself rushing to the bathroom all the time. During pregnancy, the amount of blood and other fluids in your body increases, which leads to extra fluid being processed by your kidneys and ending up in your bladder. This symptom usually continues as your pregnancy progresses and your growing baby puts more pressure on your bladder.

3. *Nausea or vomiting*—Most women do not experience a queasy stomach and vomiting until about 1 month after becoming pregnant. However, some women do start to feel nausea a bit earlier, and some women never experience nausea or vomiting.

4. *Fatigue*—Fatigue is a common symptom of early pregnancy. No one knows for sure what causes early pregnancy fatigue, but rapidly increasing levels of the hormone progesterone may be contributing to your sleepiness. You should start to feel more energetic once you enter your second trimester. Fatigue usually returns late in pregnancy when you're carrying around a lot more weight and some of the common discomforts of pregnancy make it more difficult to get a good night's sleep.

5. *Moodiness*—You may notice that your emotions are up one moment and down the next. Having mood swings during this time is normal.

6. *Bloating*—Hormonal changes in early pregnancy may leave you feeling bloated, similar to the feeling some women have just before their menstrual periods start. The bloating may cause your clothes to fit tighter around the waistline, even early on when your uterus is still quite small.

Pregnancy Tests

If you've missed your menstrual period and are experiencing some of the previously mentioned symptoms, it's time to take a pregnancy test or see your health care provider. There are several brands of home pregnancy tests you can buy. All of them are easy to use and can be done in the privacy of your own home.

With home pregnancy tests, you urinate on a stick that detects the presence of hCG in your *urine*. Human chorionic gonadotropin is made in the placenta and first enters your bloodstream and urine when the fertilized egg implants in your uterus. As soon as hCG enters your urine (approximately 6–12 days after fertilization), a home pregnancy test can detect it.

Home pregnancy tests are highly accurate. Many tests claim to be approximately 99% accurate on the day you miss your menstrual period. However, results of some research has shown that most brands of tests do not consistently detect pregnancy that early. You may want to wait to take the test when your menstrual period is at least 1 week late, when the accuracy of the test is highest. Also, make sure that you follow the directions for taking the test exactly as indicated. Doing so may yield more accurate results. For example, most tests advise you to take the test with the first urine of the day, when hCG levels are highest.

If your results are positive, you are probably pregnant. If you have not already done so, contact your health care provider right away for an appointment. Your health care provider may want to give you a blood test to confirm your results. You and your health care provider also will start to plan your prenatal care.

If your results are negative and you still have some pregnancy symptoms, you may want to wait a few days and take the test again. Home pregnancy tests sometimes give a false-negative result even if you are pregnant. If you really want to be sure, see your health care provider for a blood test. This test detects the presence of hCG in the blood. It is more sensitive than the urine tests and is not as likely to give a false-negative result.

Your Due Date

The day your baby is due is called the estimated date of delivery (EDD), also known as the due date. Although only approximately 1 in 20 women give birth on their exact due dates, the EDD is useful for a number of reasons. It is used as a guide for checking the baby's growth and your pregnancy's progress. Your due date also affects the timing of prenatal tests. In some cases, the test result depends on the stage of your pregnancy.

Your due date is most often calculated from the first day of your last menstrual period. Some women know the exact date they became pregnant—either by ovulation symptoms or by using an ovulation prediction kit. But most women do not know this date. For this reason, the menstrual dating method is used.

> ## Estimating Your Due Date
>
> 1. Take the date that your last normal menstrual period started.
> 2. Add 7 days.
> 3. Count back 3 months.
>
> **Example:** The first day of your last menstrual period was January 1. Add 7 days to get January 8. Then count back 3 months. Your due date is October 8.

You may notice that, according to this method, your last menstrual period is included even though you were not actually pregnant yet. Pregnancy is assumed to occur 2 weeks after your menstrual period. Therefore, an extra 2 weeks is counted at the beginning of your pregnancy when you aren't actually pregnant. Many women are surprised to learn that pregnancy "officially" lasts 10—not 9—months (40 weeks) because of these extra weeks. Also, this dating technique is based on a 28-day cycle, which does not apply to all women. It's important to realize that the EDD gives only a rough idea of when your baby will be born. Most women go into labor within approximately 2 weeks of their due dates—either before or after.

The 40 weeks of pregnancy are divided into three **trimesters**. Each trimester lasts about 12–13 weeks (or about 3 months):

1st trimester: 0–13 weeks (Months 1–3)
2nd trimester: 14–27 weeks (Months 4–7)
3rd trimester: 28–40 weeks (Months 7–9)

▶ Discomforts and How to Manage Them

The signs and symptoms of early pregnancy are mere annoyances for some women; for others, they can be severe. It's not possible to predict which women will have more severe symptoms. A woman may have different symptoms during each of her pregnancies. Whether mild or severe, there are ways to manage these discomforts safely and effectively.

Morning Sickness

Morning sickness is not just a feeling that happens before noon. The nausea and vomiting that define morning sickness can strike at any time of day—morning, noon, or night—and may last all day long.

No one knows for sure what causes the nausea and vomiting, but the increasing levels of hormones during pregnancy may play a role. Between 70% and 85% of pregnant women experience morning sickness during their first trimester. The nausea usually starts around the sixth week of pregnancy. It tends to get worse over the next month or so.

About one half of the women who experience nausea and vomiting usually feel complete relief by approximately 14 weeks. For most of the rest, it takes another month or so for the queasiness to ease up. It may return later, though, and come and go throughout pregnancy. Until the nausea and vomiting go away, there are a few things you can do to ease them:

- *Take a supplement*—Vitamin B_6 is known to help relieve nausea in some women. Your health care provider may recommend a combination of vitamin B_6 and an over-the-counter medication called doxylamine. Remember to talk to your health care provider first before taking any medication, including vitamins.

- *Keep snacks by the bed*—Try eating dry toast or crackers in the morning before you get out of bed to avoid moving around on an empty stomach.

- *Drink fluids*—Your body needs more water in these early months so aim to drink fluids often during the day.

- *Avoid smells that bother you*—Foods or odors that may have never bothered you before may now trigger nausea. Do your best to stay away from them.

- *Eat small and often*—Make sure your stomach is never empty by eating five or six small meals each day. Try the "BRATT" diet (bananas, rice, applesauce, toast, and tea), which is low in fat and easy to digest.

- *Try ginger*—Ginger ale made with real ginger, ginger tea made from fresh grated ginger, and ginger candies can help settle your queasy stomach.

Up to 2% of women who have morning sickness have a severe form called **hyperemesis gravidarum**. No one knows what causes this condition. It has been suggested that women carrying more than one baby (twins, triplets, or more) are more likely to have severe nausea and vomiting than women carrying a single baby.

If you can't keep any food or fluids down for more than a day or are becoming dehydrated, call your health care provider. You may be given medication to help control your nausea and vomiting. If you have a severe case of hyperemesis gravidarum, you may need to stay in the hospital for a short time and receive fluids intravenously.

Don't worry if you haven't had any morning sickness. At least 70% of pregnant women will have morning sickness, which means that 30% of women won't have it.

Fatigue

The days during your first trimester will probably have you feeling totally exhausted and wiped out. You may find it hard to even get out of bed in the morning. This is normal. Being pregnant puts a strain on your entire body, which can make you feel very tired. Your body is supporting a developing new life. Your hormone levels have increased and your metabolism is running high and burning energy (even while you sleep). Women may experience even more fatigue during subsequent pregnancies than during their first pregnancy because of the need to take care of other children, as well as other demands on their time.

To help alleviate fatigue, listen to the signals your body is sending you. Slow down and get the rest you need. Try going to bed earlier than usual or take a 15-minute nap during lunchtime. Don't forget that during these first couple of months, getting enough rest is important—more important than finishing everything on your "to do" list. So, if need be, let some things go undone until you have the energy, or enlist some help from your partner, friends, or family members. A healthy diet and exercise also may help boost your energy.

Fatigue usually begins to go away after the first trimester. By your fourth month, most of your energy will come back. However, most women begin to feel tired again in the last months of pregnancy.

Smells and Your Appetite

You might notice that your sense of smell has increased since you became pregnant. The main downside of this is that it can make nausea and a queasy stomach worse. It can become so bad that on some days you can't even think about taking a bite of anything. Try your best to pinpoint what odors (like certain foods or perfume) make you lose your appetite and avoid them as much as possible. Learn what foods you are able to keep down, and keep your refrigerator stocked with them.

▶ Nutrition

For some women, pregnancy is a planned event. They've been exercising, eating healthy foods, and taking vitamins for months beforehand. For others, pregnancy is a surprise. Many women need to make lifestyle changes after they become pregnant. Although it's best to make these changes before pregnancy, it's also okay to adjust your lifestyle when you first find out you're pregnant.

Chapter 13, "Nutrition During Pregnancy," provides comprehensive information about planning a healthy pregnancy diet. One of the most important things you need to do in early pregnancy (and ideally, before pregnancy) is to make sure that you are getting enough *folic acid*, a vitamin that helps reduce the risk of certain birth defects.

Focus on Folic Acid

Folic acid is a B vitamin also known as folate. Before pregnancy and during the first 12 weeks of pregnancy, you need to take 400 micrograms of folic acid daily in order to reduce the risk of *neural tube defects*, such as *spina bifida* and *anencephaly*. Neural tube defects occur when the coverings of the spinal cord do not close completely during prenatal development. If you have had a previous child with one of these defects, if you take certain medications (such as antiseizure medications), or if you have certain health conditions (such as sickle cell disease), you will need to take 10 times this amount—4 milligrams daily—as a separate vitamin supplement. Your health care provider will base this decision on your health history.

Although folic acid is found in many foods and is also added as a supplement to breads, cereals, and pastas, it is difficult to get the recommended amount from diet alone. For this reason, all women of childbearing age should take a daily vitamin supplement containing folic acid. Taking folic acid before pregnancy ensures that you are getting the recommended amount even if an unplanned pregnancy occurs, or if you don't realize that you are pregnant until you are several weeks along. Prenatal vitamin supplements usually contain 600–800 micrograms of folic acid, so if you are taking a prenatal vitamin before pregnancy, you don't need to take an extra daily vitamin supplement as well.

Prenatal Vitamin Supplements

It's a good idea to start taking a prenatal vitamin as soon as you find out you are pregnant, ideally before pregnancy. These vitamin supplements are available without a prescription. They contain all the recommended daily vitamins and minerals you will need during your pregnancy such as vitamins A, C, and D; folic acid; and minerals such as zinc and copper. During pregnancy, taking prenatal vitamins can ensure that you're getting all of the important nutrients, especially if you're battling nausea and finding it hard to eat all of the foods you should.

At your first prenatal care visit, tell your health care provider if you have been taking prenatal vitamins; you may want to bring the bottle with you. It's important to tell your health care provider that you're taking vitamins because excess amounts of some vitamins can be harmful.

If the smell of your vitamins makes you queasy or if you find it difficult to keep them down, you can take two children's chewable vitamins. Be sure to tell your health care provider that you're taking children's vitamins.

Weight Gain

A healthy diet is crucial during pregnancy. The details of how to eat well, what to eat, and how much to eat are covered in Chapter 13, "Nutrition During Pregnancy." During the next 8 months, while you're paying close attention to how well you're eating, it's also important to watch how much weight you gain. A certain amount of weight gain is normal during pregnancy. However, too much weight gained too quickly can be a problem.

How much weight you should gain while you're pregnant depends on what you weighed before your pregnancy. To figure this out, your health care provider will calculate your body mass index (BMI) based on both your height and weight (Appendix A). Your BMI is an indication of whether you are at a healthy weight for your height. According to the Centers for Disease Control and Prevention, if your BMI falls between 18.5 and 24.9, you are at a normal, healthy weight. However, a BMI more than 25 is considered overweight.

If you are a normal weight before pregnancy, you need only about 300 extra calories per day to provide all of the necessary nutrients to keep your body running efficiently and to fuel the extra growth and development of your baby. It may sound like a lot, but 300 extra calories adds up fast; it's the

Where Does the Weight Come From?

The average newborn weighs approximately 7.5 pounds. Yet, most mothers-to-be are advised to gain 25–35 pounds when they are pregnant. Where do the other pounds come from? Here's a breakdown of the weight gain for a normal-weight woman who gains 30 pounds during pregnancy:

- Baby—7.5 pounds
- Amniotic fluid—2 pounds
- Placenta—1.5 pound
- Uterus—2 pounds
- Breasts—2 pounds
- Body fluids—4 pounds
- Blood—4 pounds
- Maternal stores of fat, protein, and other nutrients—7 pounds

TABLE 1-1 Amount of Weight You Should Gain During Pregnancy

Prepregnancy Body Mass Index	Recommended Total Weight Gain During Pregnancy	Recommended Rate of Weight Gain per Week in the Second and Third Trimesters*
Underweight (BMI less than 18.5)	28–40 lb	1–1.3 lb
Normal weight (BMI 18.5–24.9)	25–35 lb	0.8–1 lb
Overweight (BMI 25–29.9)	15–25 lb	0.5–0.7 lb
Obese (BMI more than 30)	11–20 lb	0.4–0.6 lb

*Assumes a first-trimester weight gain between 1.1 and 4.4 lb
BMI = body mass index
Data from Institutes of Medicine (US). Weight gain during pregnancy: reexamining the guidelines. Washington, DC: National Academies Press; 2009.

amount in a bowl of cereal with fruit and low-fat milk, a whole-wheat bagel with cream cheese, or two ounces of potato chips. If you are overweight to begin with, you may need less than 300 extra calories.

Keep in mind that you will gain weight differently throughout the different months of your pregnancy. During the first 3 months, you may see little gain. In fact, some women lose a few pounds because of morning sickness. You will gain most of your weight during the second and third trimesters, when your baby is growing at a faster pace. However, your rate of weight gain should stay within a certain range (see Table 1-1).

Do not worry about how much weight other pregnant women gain. Also, if you are pregnant for the second time, you may gain weight differently. Your health care provider will check your weight gain at each of your prenatal care visits and will let you know whether you are on a healthy track.

▶ Exercise

You're tired. You're gaining weight. For many pregnant women, exercise is the last thing they want to do. But exercise actually can boost your energy levels. Being active and exercising—or even just walking—at least 30 minutes on most days of the week can benefit your pregnancy in many ways:

- Reduces backaches, constipation, bloating, and swelling
- Boosts your mood
- Promotes muscle tone, strength, and endurance
- Helps you sleep better

The ideal exercise routine gets your heart pumping, keeps you limber, and controls your weight gain without causing too much physical stress for you or the baby. Exercising now also will make it easier for you to get back in shape after the baby is born. Some exercise routines can help you relieve pregnancy-related aches and pains. For instance, the extra weight you are carrying affects your posture and can be hard on your back. Exercise may help ease back pain by toning muscles and making them stronger.

Before you start your exercise program, talk with your health care provider to make sure you do not have any health conditions that may limit your activity. If you have heart disease, are at risk for preterm labor, or have vaginal bleeding, your health care provider may advise you not to exercise. Women with any of the following conditions are advised to not exercise during pregnancy:

- Some forms of heart and lung disease
- Cervical problems
- Multiple pregnancy that is at risk for preterm labor
- Vaginal bleeding
- Preterm labor during the current pregnancy
- *Premature rupture of membranes*
- *Preeclampsia* or high blood pressure caused by pregnancy

Unless your health care provider tells you not to, you should do moderate exercise for 30 minutes or more on most days, if not every day. The 30 minutes do not have to be all at one time; it can be a total of different exercise periods. If you have not been active, start with a few minutes each day and build up to 30 minutes or more.

Pregnancy Changes That Can Affect Your Exercise Routine

Some of the changes in your body during pregnancy affect the kinds of activities you can do safely. Consider the following things when choosing an exercise program that will be safe for you during pregnancy:

- *Joints*—Some pregnancy hormones cause the ligaments that support your joints to stretch. This makes them more prone to injury.

- *Balance*—The weight you gain in the front of your body shifts your center of gravity. This puts stress on your joints and muscles—mostly those in the lower back and pelvis. It also can make you less stable and more likely to fall.

- *Heart rate*—Extra weight also makes your body work harder than it did before you were pregnant. This is true even if you are working out at a slower pace. Intense exercise boosts oxygen and blood flow to the muscles and away from other parts of your body—such as your uterus. If you can't talk at a normal level during exercise, then you are working too hard.

Starting an Exercise Program During Pregnancy

If you've never exercised, pregnancy is a great time to start. Discuss your plan to start exercising with your health care provider. Also, remember to start slowly. Begin with as little as 5 minutes of exercise a day and add 5 minutes each week until you can stay active for 30 minutes per day.

Many sports are safe during pregnancy, even for beginners:

• Walking is a good exercise for anyone. Brisk walking gives a total body workout and is easy on the joints and muscles. If you were not active before getting pregnant, walking is a great way to start an exercise program.

• Swimming is great for your body because it works so many muscles. The water supports your weight so you avoid injury and muscle strain. It also helps you stay cool and may prevent your legs from swelling.

• Cycling provides a good aerobic workout. However, your growing belly can affect your balance and make you more prone to falls. You may want to stick with stationary or recumbent biking later in pregnancy.

• Aerobics is a good way to keep your heart and lungs strong. There are even aerobics classes designed just for pregnant women. Low-impact aerobics and water aerobics also are good exercise. However, if you have certain con-

Warning Signs to Stop Exercise

Whether you're a seasoned athlete or a beginner, watch for the following warning signs during exercise. If you have any of them, stop exercising and call your health care provider.

• Dizziness or faintness
• Increased shortness of breath
• Uneven or rapid heartbeat
• Chest pain
• Trouble walking
• Calf pain or swelling
• Headache
• Vaginal bleeding
• Uterine contractions that continue after rest
• Fluid gushing or leaking from your vagina
• Decreased fetal movement

ditions, including heart disease, preeclampsia, or preterm labor, you should avoid aerobic exercise. Talk to your health care provider if you are unsure.

Continuing an Exercise Program During Pregnancy

Many women are dedicated exercisers and maintain a high level of activity during pregnancy. There are a few things that you need to remember while continuing an exercise program during pregnancy. First, avoid any exercise or sport that could injure your abdomen. For instance, while playing soccer, you are at risk of a ball directly hitting your abdomen at a high speed. Contact sports are also off-limits. Also, don't start a new sport during pregnancy. The following exercises are safe for women who have done them for a while before pregnancy:

- *Running*—If you were a runner before you became pregnant, you often can keep running during pregnancy, although you may have to modify your routine. Talk to your health care provider about whether running during pregnancy is safe for you.

- *Racquet sports*—In some racquet sports, such as badminton, tennis, and racquetball, your changing balance may affect rapid movements, which can increase your risk of falling. You may want to avoid some racquet sports.

- *Strength training*—Strength training will make your muscles stronger and may help prevent some of the aches and pains common in pregnancy.

The key is to discuss your exercise routine with your health care provider. Get your health care provider's okay regarding the type of activity that you plan to do throughout your pregnancy, as well as its intensity.

Exercise of the Month: Kegel Exercises

As your uterus grows in the coming months, it will put more pressure on your bladder. Even if your bladder is almost empty, it may still feel like it's full. The weight of your uterus on your bladder may even cause you to leak a little urine when you sneeze or cough. Doing **Kegel exercises** may help improve your bladder control. Kegel exercises strengthen the muscles that surround the opening of the vagina. Here's how they're done:

- Squeeze the muscles that you use to stop the flow of urine.
- Hold this position for 10 seconds, then release.

Do this 10–20 times in a row at least three times per day. You can do Kegel exercises anywhere—while working, driving in your car, or watching television.

❱ Healthy Decisions

In the first 2 months of pregnancy, you may have a lot of questions and decisions to make. The decisions facing you now may include making important lifestyle changes, picking a practitioner who will care for you during pregnancy, and deciding when to tell others your news.

Things to Avoid During Pregnancy

It's perfectly normal to be anxious about what you can and cannot do while you are pregnant. The list of "don'ts" may seem long, but most are easy to remember.

Smoking

If you smoke, it's best to quit before or as soon as you know that you are pregnant. Smoking cigarettes while you're pregnant is dangerous for you and your baby and raises your risk of the following complications:

- Vaginal bleeding
- *Preterm* birth
- A low-birth-weight baby (weighing less than 5 ½ pounds)
- A stillborn baby
- *Sudden infant death syndrome*

Why is smoking so dangerous? Cigarette smoke contains thousands of harmful chemicals, including lead, tar, nicotine, and carbon dioxide. When you smoke, these toxins go directly to your baby. These chemicals can cut off the flow of oxygen and nutrients to your baby.

Although you may be tempted to just cut down the number of cigarettes you smoke while you're pregnant, cutting down is not good enough. Every cigarette you smoke increases the risks to your pregnancy. Quitting altogether is the best thing to do for you and your baby.

Keep in mind that it's not just important for you to quit smoking while you're pregnant. Your partner, family members, co-workers, or friends who smoke should either quit or avoid smoking around you. Their secondhand smoke can harm you and your baby.

There are lots of ways to quit smoking. You may want to work with your health care provider to come up with a quitting plan that involves learning about quitting resources and setting a quit date. You may consider joining a stop-smoking group or getting individual counseling. Individual and group counseling can help smokers identify and cope with problems that come up during quitting. They also can help you keep from starting again. The American Cancer Society states that there is a strong link between how often and how long counseling lasts (its intensity) and the success rate of the counseling: the more intense the program, the greater the chance of success. To find out more about quitting programs in your area, to get information about quitting, or to find support, contact the American Cancer Society (see Resources).

Nicotine patches, gums, and sprays were designed to help ease withdrawal symptoms when you quit. The effects of these nicotine replacement aids on a developing baby and their potential to increase the smoking-related risk of complications is not known. However, cigarettes and cigarette smoke have many more harmful chemicals than these nicotine products. Some smokers find the prescription drugs bupropion (Wellbutrin) or varenicline (Chantix) to be helpful in quitting smoking. The safety of these drugs during pregnancy has not been adequately studied in humans.

Before using nicotine replacement or prescription medications to quit smoking, talk to your health care provider. It may be recommended that you try counseling first. If counseling doesn't work for you, you and your health care provider can decide whether the benefits of using these drugs or products to quit smoking outweigh any potential unknown risks to your pregnancy.

Drinking Alcohol
Alcohol can harm your baby's health. It's best to stop drinking before you become pregnant. If you did have some alcohol before you knew you were pregnant, most likely it will not harm your baby. The important thing is to avoid alcohol once you learn you're pregnant.

When a pregnant woman drinks alcohol, it quickly reaches her fetus. Alcohol is much more harmful to a fetus than it is to an adult. The more a pregnant woman drinks, the greater the danger to her baby. Alcohol abuse during pregnancy is a leading cause of developmental disabilities in children. Alcohol increases the chance of having a miscarriage or a preterm baby.

It is not known how much alcohol it takes to harm the fetus. The best course is not to drink at all during pregnancy. Also, there are no types of drinks that are safe. One beer, one shot of liquor, one mixed drink, or one glass of wine all contain approximately the same amount of alcohol. Thus, all forms of alcohol may be harmful.

It may be hard to stop drinking. If this is true for you, you may need help. Talk honestly to your health care provider about your drinking habits.

Using Illegal Drugs
Using illegal drugs, such as marijuana, cocaine, Ecstasy, methamphetamine, and heroin, while you're pregnant can increase the risk of many serious prob-

Do You Have a Drinking Problem?

Do you use alcohol or abuse it? Sometimes it's hard to tell. If you're not sure, ask yourself these questions:

T   How many drinks does it take to make you feel high? (TOLERANCE)

A   Have people ANNOYED you by criticizing your drinking?

C   Have you felt you ought to CUT DOWN on your drinking?

E   Have you ever had a drink first thing in the morning to steady your nerves or get rid of a hangover? (EYE OPENER)

Scoring:

• 2 points if your answer to the first question is more than two drinks.
• 1 point for every "yes" response to the other questions.

If your total score is 2 or more, you may have an alcohol problem.

Talk to your doctor about your drinking habits. He or she can help you decide if you have a problem. The doctor will refer you for counseling or treatment if needed. You also may want to think about contacting a substance abuse program. These groups can help you find someone to talk to about your problem and can give you needed support when you are trying to quit. Check your local yellow-page listings.

Modified from Sokol RJ, Martier SS, Ager JW. The T-ACE questions: practical prenatal detection of risk drinking. Am J Obstet Gynecol 1989;160:865.

lems. They may cause preterm birth, interfere with the baby's growth, or cause birth defects or learning and behavioral problems.

It has been difficult for researchers to link a particular problem to the use of a specific drug because women who use illegal drugs often use alcohol and tobacco, which also place pregnant women and their babies at risk. In addition, illegal drug users may have other unhealthy behaviors, such as poor nutrition, that are known to adversely affect pregnancy.

The bottom line is that you should make all illegal drugs off-limits while you are pregnant. If you are addicted to any of these drugs, seek help right away from a drug abuse treatment program in your area. Breaking a drug addiction is tough; don't try to do it alone. Tell your health care provider that you need help. Narcotics Anonymous is also a good resource (see Resources).

Medications and Herbal Supplements

Medications cross the placenta and enter the baby's bloodstream. In some cases, a medication could cause birth defects, addiction, or other problems in the baby. That doesn't mean you should throw out the contents of your medicine cabinet once you become pregnant. It means that you need to be careful.

Some medicines are safe to take during pregnancy. Also, the risks of taking some medicines may be outweighed by the effects of not taking them. For instance, certain diseases are more harmful to a fetus than the drugs used to treat them. Don't stop taking a medication prescribed for you. Ask your doctor about it first.

Tell anyone who prescribes medications for you that you are pregnant. That includes any doctors you see for nonpregnancy problems, your dentist, or a mental health care provider. Be sure that your pregnancy health care provider knows about any medical problems you may have. Tell him or her about all the medications you take and whether you have any drug allergies. If a medication you are taking poses a risk, your health care provider may recommend switching to a safer drug while you are pregnant.

Prescription medications also can be harmful if they are abused. Women who abuse prescription drugs risk overdose and addiction.

Over-the-counter medicines, including herbal medications and vitamin supplements, can cause problems during pregnancy too. Pain relievers such as aspirin and ibuprofen may be harmful to a fetus. Check with your health care provider before taking any over-the-counter drug. This includes pain relievers, laxatives, cold or allergy remedies, and skin treatments. But you don't have to have the discomfort of headaches or colds without relief. Your doctor can give you advice about medicines that are safe for use by pregnant women.

Choosing A Health Care Provider for Your Pregnancy

If you don't already have one, finding a health care provider for your pregnancy is probably one of the most important choices you'll make early on. Talk to your regular doctor for recommendations, or ask women you know to share their opinions about the health care providers who delivered their babies.

You also can find a pregnancy care provider through your health insurance provider list. All health plans offer a "find a doctor" service on their web sites, or you can call the plan directly. The American College of Obstetricians and Gynecologists' web site also provides a "Find a Physician" resource tool (see Resources).

Types of Providers

Four types of practitioners offer medical care for pregnancy and birth: *obstetrician–gynecologists* (ob-gyns), maternal–fetal medicine subspecialists (high-risk obstetricians), family physicians, certified nurse–midwives, and certified midwives.

1. *Ob-gyns*—Ob-gyns are doctors who specialize in the health care of women. After completing medical school, ob-gyns complete 4 years of specialized training in obstetrics and gynecology. To be certified, an ob-gyn must pass written tests and oral tests to show that he or she has obtained the knowledge and skills required for the medical and surgical care of women. A certified ob-gyn can then become a Fellow of the American College of Obstetricians and Gynecologists. This group helps doctors stay up-to-date on the latest medical advances.

2. *Maternal–fetal medicine subspecialists*—These doctors, who are also called perinatologists, have completed 4 years of training in obstetrics and gynecology and then received further training in high-risk obstetrics for 2–3 years. Maternal–fetal medicine subspecialists must pass written exams and oral exams to become certified. Women who have high-risk pregnancies may be referred to maternal–fetal medicine subspecialists for care.

3. *Family physicians*—Doctors in family practice provide general care for most conditions, including pregnancy. After completing medical school, family physicians complete 3 years of advanced training in family medicine (including obstetrics) and become certified by passing an exam. They are able to care for women with normal pregnancies and deliveries.

4. *Certified nurse–midwives and certified midwives*—Certified nurse–midwives (CNMs) and certified midwives are specially trained practitioners who provide care for women with low-risk pregnancies and their babies from early pregnancy through labor, delivery, and the weeks after birth. Certified nurse–midwives are registered nurses who have completed an accredited nursing program and have a graduate degree in midwifery. To be certified, they must pass a national written exam administered by the American Midwifery Certification Board and must maintain an active nursing license. Certified midwives have graduated from a midwifery education program accredited by the American College of Nurse-Midwives Division of Accreditation. They have successfully completed the same requirements, have passed the same American Midwifery Certification Board national certification exam, and adhere to the same professional standards as certified nurse–midwives. Both CNMs and certified midwives generally work with a qualified doctor who will provide backup support.

Types of Practices

Another factor to think about is whether a provider is in a solo practice, group practice, or collaborative practice. In a solo practice, one health care provider works alone but may have help from other providers to cover deliveries. In a group practice, two or more health care providers share duties for constant coverage of their patients' health care. A collaborative practice brings together a team of health care professionals—such as nurses, CNMs or certified midwives, laborists, nurse practitioners, physician assistants, and childbirth educators—with different knowledge and skills. The contributions of each member are key to the health care of the patient.

Questions to Ask
Once you find a health care provider who seems promising, it's a good idea to ask him or her questions that are important for you and your partner. Don't hesitate to write down a list of your concerns to take with you on your first prenatal care visit. Use this list as a guide for some questions you may want to ask:

- How does the office work? Are you in practice alone, or is there a group of doctors or providers?
- If it is a group, how often will I see the same health care provider when I come for my prenatal care visits?
- If you are in solo practice, who covers you when you are not available?
- Which hospital will I go to when I give birth?
- Do you have an after-hours office number I can call in case of an emergency or if I have questions?
- Who takes the after-hours calls?
- Who will deliver my baby?
- What are your views on anesthesia during labor, episiotomy, alternative birthing positions, cesarean delivery, and operative delivery?
- Who can be with me during delivery?

When to Spread the News

When to tell family and friends that you're pregnant is your personal choice. Many women choose to wait until after the first 12 weeks have passed. Others may decide to tell as soon as they get the positive pregnancy test result. Deciding when to deliver the news is a personal decision, but you may want to keep a few things in mind:

- The risk of miscarriage is highest in the first 3 months of pregnancy. You may want to wait until your second trimester to tell friends, co-workers, and extended family members that you're pregnant.

- Although discrimination against pregnant women is illegal, it may be better to wait to spread the news at work. Telling co-workers too early may make them anxious about who will do your work while you are on maternity leave.

Months 1 & 2

- Women who have had problems with past pregnancies, especially early problems, may feel more secure waiting until the second trimester to tell others. Your friends' and family members' concern about you may be heartfelt, but it may make your own anxiety about your pregnancy worse.

- When to tell your children depends on their ages. Tell your school-aged children before you tell anyone outside your family. If you don't, they might resent being the last to know. With young children, it's a good idea to wait until they ask about your changing body. The idea of a baby growing inside you may be too hard for small children to grasp before they can see your expanded belly.

▶ Other Considerations

Many pregnant women have jobs outside the home. Pregnant women often work right up until delivery and return to their jobs within weeks or months of the baby's birth. Women often can keep doing their normal jobs while they are pregnant. However, some jobs may not be safe for a pregnant woman. Also, the fatigue, nausea, and other discomforts can make working during early pregnancy a challenge.

A Safe Workplace

Some jobs may expose a woman to heavy duties. Jobs that involve a lot of heavy lifting, climbing, carrying, or standing may not be safe during pregnancy. That's because the dizziness, nausea, and fatigue common in early pregnancy can increase the chance of injury. Later on, the change in body shape can throw off your balance and can lead to falls. You may need to cut back on the hours you work, give up certain tasks, transfer to another position, or stop working until after the baby is born.

Some substances found in the workplace pose a risk during pregnancy. Although being exposed on the job to harmful substances is fairly rare, it makes sense to think about the things you come into contact with during the course of your workday. You also may come in contact with these agents through a hobby. Agents that pose a pregnancy risk are discussed in detail in Chapter 22, "Birth Defects."

If you think your job may bring you into contact with something harmful, find out for sure by asking your personnel office, employee clinic, or union. Let your health care provider know right away if you think you and your baby are at risk. Workplace safety hazards and tips can be found at the web sites of the Occupational Safety and Health Administration and the National

Institute for Occupational Safety and Health (see Resources). Also see "Your Workplace Rights" in Chapter 3, "Month 4 (Weeks 13–16)" on page 71.

Tips for Working During Early Pregnancy

Working when you are experiencing the nausea and fatigue of early pregnancy can be difficult. To cope, you may want to try the following:

- *Take advantage of flex time*—If your workplace has flex time, use this benefit to your advantage. What is the time of day when you feel the most energized? Consider coming in later if early morning is bad for you. If afternoons are a problem, arrive earlier so that you can leave earlier.

- *Bring snacks with you*—Healthy snacks throughout the day may help keep nausea at bay and supply a source of energy. Crackers; fresh, raw vegetables; or fruit and cheese are good choices.

- *Cat nap, if you can*—If you have an office, you can shut the door and rest during your lunch hour.

- *Stay hydrated*—Being dehydrated can make you feel worse. Make sure you are drinking enough fluids throughout the day.

▶ Prenatal Care Visits

As soon as you know you're pregnant, call your health care provider to schedule an appointment so you can start prenatal care right away. You'll have regular appointments throughout your pregnancy. At each visit, the health care provider will monitor your health as well as that of your growing baby.

Your first or second prenatal care visit will probably be one of your longest visits. Your health care provider will need to ask a lot of questions about your health and perform several tests. It's important to answer all the questions honestly and with as much detail as you can. A health history form is provided in Appendix B. You can fill out this form before your visit, or you can just read it through to see what questions will be asked. It may be helpful to bring a support person with you on your prenatal care visits. During these early visits, your health care provider may do the following:

- Ask about your health history, including your previous pregnancies, surgeries, or medical problems.

- Ask about any prescription or over-the-counter medications you're taking (bring them with you, if possible).

- Ask about your family's and the baby's father's health history.
- Do a complete physical exam with blood and urine tests.
- Do a **pelvic exam** with a **Pap test**.
- Measure your blood pressure, height, and weight.
- Calculate the baby's expected due date.

Some health problems are more likely to occur in certain families or in racial or ethnic groups. The more specific you and your partner can be about whether anyone in your families has had conditions such as sickle cell anemia, mental retardation, or cystic fibrosis, the better. If you have a family member or had a previous child with one of these conditions, the risk of your baby having the same condition may be higher. Your health care provider may suggest additional testing to look at your genetic backgrounds.

▶ Special Concerns

Although it's normal for pregnant women to worry about complications, most women have perfectly healthy pregnancies and give birth to healthy babies. However, it's best to be alert to signs and symptoms that may signal a problem. Often, the earlier you see your doctor, the more likely that the complication can be successfully managed.

Miscarriage

The loss of a pregnancy in the first 20 weeks is called a **miscarriage**. Nearly 15% of pregnancies end this way, and most occur in the first 13 weeks. Some miscarriages take place before a woman misses her menstrual period or even knows that she is pregnant.

The most common sign of a miscarriage is bleeding. Pay attention to the other warning signs and call your doctor if you have them:

- Spotting or bleeding without pain
- Heavy or persistent bleeding with abdominal pain or cramping
- A gush of fluid from your vagina but no pain or bleeding
- Passed fetal tissue

Most women who have gone through a miscarriage later go on to have healthy, successful pregnancies. Your health care provider will talk with you about when you and your partner can try to get pregnant again. Miscarriage is discussed in detail in Chapter 21 "Early Pregnancy Problems: Miscarriage, Ectopic Pregnancy, and Molar Pregnancy."

Ectopic Pregnancy

An *ectopic pregnancy* is one in which the fertilized egg attaches itself outside of the uterus. The egg usually implants in one of the fallopian tubes, but it can also implant in other locations, such as the cervix or abdomen. An ectopic pregnancy in a fallopian tube can cause serious health problems. The fallopian tube can burst (rupture), resulting in internal bleeding that can be life threatening. Approximately 2% of all pregnancies are ectopic.

An ectopic pregnancy may feel like a normal pregnancy, with some of the same symptoms, such as a missed menstrual period and nausea. If you have any vaginal bleeding, have pain in your pelvis, or feel dizzy or light-headed (caused by internal bleeding)—especially if you haven't yet had an *ultrasound* exam to confirm that your pregnancy is in your uterus—call your health care provider. Ectopic pregnancy is discussed in detail in Chapter 21.

YOUR QUESTIONS ANSWERED

I love coffee in the morning and caffeinated soft drinks at lunch. How much caffeine can I safely consume per day?

Many women have been told to limit their caffeine consumption during pregnancy because of a possible association with an increased risk of miscarriage, preterm birth, and low birth weight. However, recent research regarding caffeine consumption and miscarriage risk is conflicting. Some research suggests that women who consume 200 milligrams of caffeine (equal to one 12-ounce cup of coffee) or more a day are more than twice as likely as women who consume no caffeine to have a miscarriage. Yet other research found no relationship between caffeine consumption and the risk of miscarriage, regardless of the amount consumed. There also is no clear evidence that caffeine intake increases the risk of having a low-birth-weight baby. Because of these conflicting research results, it is not possible to give a recommendation about how much caffeine is safe to consume during pregnancy. As for the links between moderate caffeine intake and preterm birth, results from much of the research show that caffeine consumption does not appear to affect this complication.

Still, it may be a good idea to limit your caffeine intake for other reasons. Excess caffeine can interfere with much-needed sleep and can contribute to nausea and light-headedness. The diuretic effect of caffeine can increase urination and can lead to dehydration. If you do cut down on caffeine, don't just focus on coffee. Remember that caffeine also is found in tea, chocolate, energy drinks, and soft drinks.

I called my doctor as soon as I learned my home pregnancy test result was positive. She mentioned having an early ultrasound exam. What can I expect to see at this early date?

Some health care providers perform an ultrasound exam, which uses sound waves to show features inside the body, to confirm pregnancy. This exam may be done transvaginally, in which a special transducer (the instrument that transmits the sound waves) is placed in the vagina. If you are fewer than 5 weeks pregnant, the embryo may not be visible. If you are more than 5 weeks pregnant, don't expect to see much more than a small, circular shape that represents the amniotic sac in which the baby is growing. You will not be able to see arms or legs or any other distinct features until later in pregnancy.

Is it safe to douche during pregnancy?

No. It is best to avoid douching at all times, whether you're pregnant or not. Women do not need to douche to wash away blood, semen, or vaginal discharge. Most doctors say that it's better to let your vagina clean itself naturally. Douching can even increase your chances of getting a vaginal infection. Keep in mind that even healthy, clean vaginas may have a mild odor. Regular washing with warm water and soap during baths and showers will keep the outside of the vagina clean and healthy.

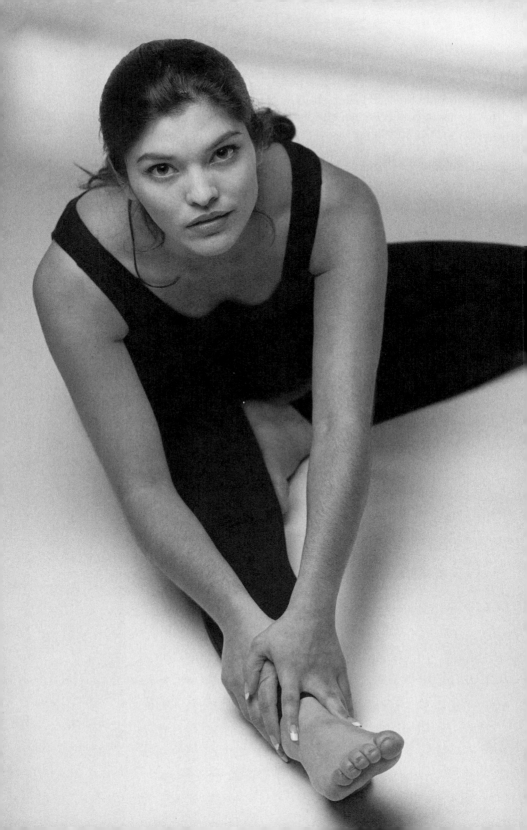

Chapter 2
Month 3
(Weeks 9–12)

YOUR GROWING BABY

Week 9

Your baby is about 2 inches in length now—about the same size as a strawberry. Buds for future teeth appear, and the intestines begin to form.

Week 10

Fingers and toes continue to grow, and soft nails begin to form. Although all of the organs are formed, they are not yet fully developed.

Week 11

Your baby is about 3 inches long now—about the same size as a lime. Bones are starting to harden, and muscles begin to develop. The backbone is soft and can flex. The skin is still thin and transparent but will soon start to thicken.

Week 12

At this point, your baby weighs just more than 1 ounce and is about 3½ inches long. The hands are more fully developed than the feet, and the arms are longer than the legs. Your baby moves on his own now but is still too small for you to feel his movements.

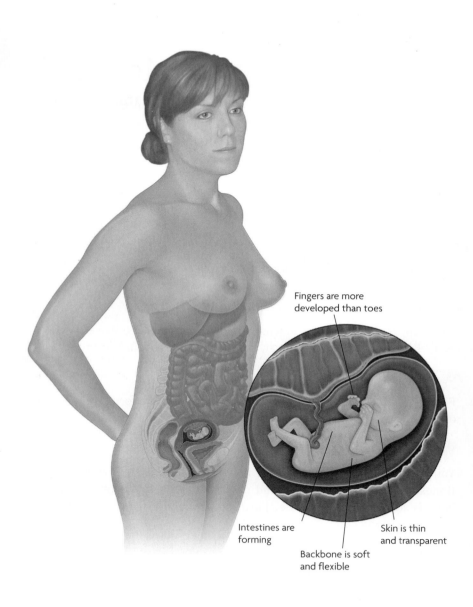

Fingers are more
developed than toes

Intestines are
forming

Backbone is soft
and flexible

Skin is thin
and transparent

Mother and baby: Weeks 9–12. At this point, your baby weighs just more than 1 ounce and is about 3½ inches long.

YOUR PREGNANCY

▶ Your Changing Body

You still may not look pregnant to others even though you may be able to tell your waist is getting a little thicker. When you are not pregnant, the *uterus* is about the size of a small pear. By around week 10, it is as big as a grapefruit.

▶ Discomforts and How to Manage Them

As you begin your third month of pregnancy, you may notice that your morning sickness is decreasing. At the same time, you may notice changes in your breasts, skin, and digestion. All of these changes are normal during pregnancy.

Nausea

Most women start to feel relief from nausea this month. While you wait for your symptoms to totally pass, remember to keep the remedies handy that help ease your queasiness and to drink as much fluids as you can during the day.

Fatigue and Sleep Problems

You probably are still feeling exhausted during the day from all the changes happening in your body. But, unfortunately, as these first few months pass, it may become more difficult to get a good night's sleep. As your abdomen grows larger, it will be harder to find a comfortable position. To help you get the rest you need, you may find the following suggestions helpful:

• Try sleeping on your side with a pillow under your abdomen and another pillow between your legs.

• Take a shower or warm bath at bedtime to help you relax.

• Exercise can promote good sleep. Try a relaxing exercise, like yoga, before bedtime to help initiate a restful sleep.

• Make sure your bedroom area is pleasant and relaxing. The bed should be comfortable, and the room should not be too hot or cold or too bright.

Acne

If you find that your skin is breaking out more now that you're pregnant, try washing a few times each day with mild cleanser. If your breakouts make you really uncomfortable, talk to your health care provider, who may prescribe a treatment. But don't use the acne products that contain isotretinoin or tetracycline—they are not safe to take during pregnancy because they can cause birth defects.

Breast Changes

Early in pregnancy, your breasts begin changing to get ready for feeding the baby. By now, your breasts may have even grown a whole bra-cup size. They may be very sore. Many changes are taking place:

- Fat builds up in the breasts, making your normal bra too tight.

- The number of milk glands increases as your body prepares for making milk.

- The nipples and areolas (the pink or brownish skin around your nipples) get darker.

- Your nipples may begin to stick out more, and the areolas will grow larger.

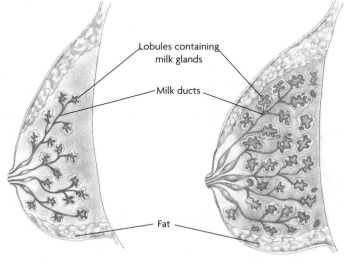

Lobules containing milk glands

Milk ducts

Fat

Before pregnancy   During pregnancy

Breast changes during pregnancy. During pregnancy, the fat layer of your breasts thickens, and the number of milk glands increases. Because of these changes, your breasts enlarge.

Your breasts may keep growing in size and weight during these first 3 months. If they are making you uncomfortable, now is the time to switch to a good maternity bra. These bras have wide straps, more coverage in the cups, and extra rows of hooks so you can adjust the band size. You also might want to buy a special sleep bra for nighttime support. If you regularly exercise, you may consider an athletic bra with good support.

By the end of your third trimester, your breasts may start leaking a thick, yellow fluid called **colostrum**. Colostrum contains proteins and antibodies that nourish your newborn until your breasts start making milk a few days after birth. Don't worry, however, if your breasts don't leak because it doesn't happen to all women.

Constipation

Increased levels of **hormones** cause your **digestive system** to work more slowly. This slower functioning of your gut may lead to constipation. To help ease constipation, drink plenty of liquids and increase your intake of fiber, which is found in fruits, vegetables, and whole grains. A side effect of increased fiber consumption, however, is gas formation. To combat this problem, try eating your meals more slowly, and avoid anything that causes you to swallow air, such as gum chewing and carbonated drinks. Your body will eventually adjust to the dietary changes. Discuss this with your health care provider if these measures don't ease constipation.

❱ Nutrition

This month, you may have started to put on a few extra pounds. Your health care provider will track your weight each month. As you plan your meals, make sure that you are getting enough iron—a key mineral that most women need more of during pregnancy.

Weight Gain

You may be noticing that your clothes are starting to fit a little snugly around the waist. By the end of your 12th week, most women commonly have gained between 1½ pound and 4½ pounds, although some women will have lost weight.

Month 3

Focus on Iron

Iron is used by your body to make the extra blood that you and your baby need during pregnancy. Pregnant women need 27 milligrams of iron a day, which is the amount in most prenatal vitamin supplements. Vitamin supplements with higher iron levels may cause digestion problems, such as constipation. Good dietary sources of iron are lean beef and pork, dried fruits and beans, sardines, and green leafy vegetables.

Sugar and Sugar Substitutes

Limit the amount of simple sugars you eat daily. Simple sugars are found in foods such as table sugar, honey, syrup, fruit juices, soft drinks, and many processed foods. Although they may give you a quick energy boost, they have more calories than other nutrients, and the energy they give is used up quickly. They also contribute to excess weight gain.

If you normally use some of the following artificial sweeteners, which are 200–600 times sweeter than sugar, they are still safe to use while you're pregnant as long as you use them in moderation:

- Saccharin (Sweet'n Low)
- Aspartame (Equal and NutraSweet)
- Sucralose (Splenda)
- Acesulfame-k (Sunett)

Another sweetener, called stevia, comes from an herb grown in South and Central America. It is sold in the United States under the product names Truvia and SweetLeaf. The U.S. Food and Drug Administration (FDA) recently has approved the use of stevia as a food additive and sweetener.

▌ Exercise

If you haven't been exercising regularly, try simple things—like taking the stairs instead of the elevator—to get more exercise into your life. If you have been exercising, this month's exercise can help you start toning strategic muscles in your hips and abdomen.

Month 3

Exercise of the Month: Diagonal Curl

This exercise strengthens your back, hips, and abdomen. Only attempt this exercise if you already have been exercising regularly:

1. Sit on the floor with your knees bent, feet on the floor, and hands clasped in front of you.

2. Twist your upper body to the left until your hands touch the floor. Do the same movement to the right. Repeat five times.

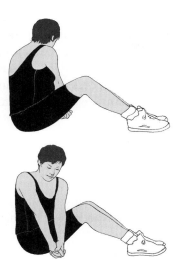

Diagonal curl. This exercise strengthens your back, hips, and abdomen. If you have not been exercising regularly, skip this one.

Get Moving

Ideally, pregnant women, as well as others, should get at least 30 minutes per day of exercise that increases heart rate and some strength exercises on most days of the week. However, it may be tough to get started if you're not used to exercising regularly. There are simple ways of adding additional movement into your daily life. Try going to your local shopping mall and walking to the farthest end and back. Or, while you're at the grocery store, do a couple of laps around the perimeter of the store—where the most healthy and least processed foods are found. Take the stairs instead of the elevator. The important thing is to get moving a little more each day while you're pregnant to get the best benefits.

▶ Healthy Decisions

If you have had a previous *cesarean delivery*, you will need to think about how you will have your baby this time around and should discuss your options with your health care provider. Another important decision to consider is genetic screening for birth defects.

Vaginal Birth After Cesarean Delivery

If you have had a baby by cesarean delivery in the past, it is important to talk about your delivery plans with your doctor early in your prenatal care. An attempted vaginal delivery after a cesarean delivery is called vaginal birth after cesarean (VBAC) delivery. The success rate for women attempting a VBAC overall is 60–80%. The success rate depends on a variety of factors:

- *Why you previously gave birth by cesarean delivery*—If the reason for your previous cesarean was for arrest of labor, your chance of a successful VBAC is decreased.

- *Whether you have had a prior vaginal delivery*—Women who have had a prior vaginal delivery are more likely than those who have not to have a successful VBAC.

- *Other factors*—Factors that decrease the likelihood of a successful VBAC are increased age of the mother, a higher body mass index (see p. 440), higher predicted birth weight of the baby, and a **gestational age** greater than 40 weeks.

VBAC provides many benefits for women. Women who have a VBAC avoid major surgery and all of the risks that go along with it. Recovery is shorter after a vaginal delivery compared with a cesarean delivery. If you want more children, having a VBAC can help you avoid some of the potential future complications of multiple cesarean deliveries, such as infection, bowel or bladder injury, or hysterectomy.

However, there are some risks involved with a VBAC that may not make it the right choice for every woman. With a VBAC, there is a very small, but serious, risk of rupture of the uterus. Sometimes, even if you choose a VBAC, your health care provider may have to switch to a cesarean delivery during the course of labor, which can happen if problems arise or worsen during childbirth. The highest rate of complications occurs in women who unsuccessfully attempt giving birth by vaginal delivery and who end up giving birth by cesarean delivery.

The type of incision that you had in your uterus—not the one made in your skin—for your previous cesarean delivery is a key factor in deciding whether you should attempt to have a VBAC. This information should be in your medical records. A low transverse (sideways) incision is less likely to rupture than a vertical incision that was made on the upper part of the uterus (high vertical or "classical" incision). Women with high vertical incisions should not have a VBAC because their risk of a uterine rupture in

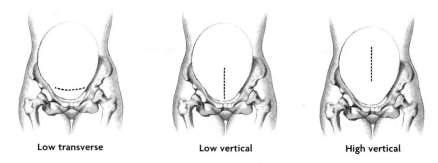

Low transverse   Low vertical   High vertical

Types of uterine incisions for a cesarean birth. The type of incision made in the skin may not be the same type of incision made in the uterus.

labor is increased. If a vertical incision was made in the lower part of the uterus, a VBAC still can be considered.

The following additional factors are considered in the decision to have a VBAC:

- *Previous deliveries*—A VBAC is more likely to be successful if a woman has had at least one vaginal delivery in addition to a previous cesarean delivery. A VBAC can be considered in women who have had two previous cesarean deliveries.

- *Future deliveries*—Multiple cesarean deliveries are associated with additional potential risks. If you know that you want more children, you should keep these risks in mind when making your decision.

- *Existence of a medical problem or pregnancy complication*—Problems with the placenta, problems with the baby, or certain medical conditions during pregnancy may affect whether a VBAC is an option.

- *Need for labor induction*—You can still try to have a VBAC if you are past your due date. However, the success rate for VBAC is decreased if there is a need to induce labor (use drugs or other means to bring on labor). Certain drugs that induce labor (misoprostol and prostaglandins followed by oxytocin) should not be used. Other means of induction can be considered.

- *Type of hospital*—VBAC is not performed in some hospitals. The hospital or other facility where the baby is delivered should be equipped to handle an emergency cesarean delivery if it becomes necessary.

- *Your health care provider*—Some obstetricians do not perform VBACs. You may need to be referred to one who does.

Month 3

The decision whether to try a vaginal delivery or to have a repeat cesarean delivery can be complex. Let your health care provider know if you're interested in trying to have a VBAC with this pregnancy. Together, you and your health care provider can consider the risks and benefits that apply to your individual situation.

Genetic Counseling and Carrier Testing

Early in pregnancy (and sometimes before pregnancy), your health care provider may offer **carrier** testing if your family health history indicates an increased risk for having a child with an inherited birth defect. These inherited diseases are called genetic disorders. They can be passed from parent to child through **genes**. Genes are found on the structures called **chromosomes** in **cells**.

If you are at high risk for having a baby with a genetic disease, genetic counseling and carrier screening can help you and your partner assess your risk of having a baby with the disorder. You may be at high risk of having a child with a genetic disorder if you (or the baby's father) have a family history of that disease. You also are at high risk if you have had a previous child with certain disorders. However, a baby can be born with a birth defect even if the parents do not have these risk factors.

A genetic counselor has special training in genetics. He or she will ask you and your baby's father for a detailed family history. If a family member has a problem, the counselor may ask to see that person's medical records. You also may be referred for physical exams or tests. Using all the information gathered, the counselor will assess the baby's risk of having a problem. The counselor then will explain and discuss the options.

Carrier testing is a way to find out whether a person is a carrier of a particular disorder. A carrier is a person who shows no signs of a disorder but could pass the gene on to his or her children. Carrier testing is available for many, but not all, genetic disorders, including cystic fibrosis, sickle cell disease and other blood disorders, Tay–Sachs disease, and Canavan disease.

It's up to you to decide whether you want carrier testing, but there are some guidelines that you can follow. Cystic fibrosis carrier testing, for example, is available to all pregnant women and should be offered when both partners are of Caucasian, European, or Ashkenazi Jewish ethnicity. Other carrier tests are recommended for people who have certain ethnic backgrounds or who have a strong family history of a genetic disease.

If the test shows you are a carrier, the next step usually is to test the baby's father. If the test shows that both parents are carriers, a genetic counselor can give you more information about the risk of having a baby with the disorder. Further testing may be available to show if the baby has the disorder or is a carrier. Once you know your carrier status, you do not need to be tested in subsequent pregnancies.

❯ Other Considerations

This month, you may notice other changes that may concern you. Your mood may be up one minute, and down the next. These sudden mood shifts can be disconcerting if you were not expecting them. You also may be noticing changes in your skin, such as dark pigmentation on your face or abdomen. Another common concern is what to do if you become sick with the flu, a cold, or a diarrheal illness. There are steps you can take to come through these illnesses safely during pregnancy.

Emotional Changes

Your body is going through big changes now, and so are your emotions. Don't blame yourself if you are sad or moody. The emotions you are feeling—good and bad—are normal. Ask loved ones to support you and be patient. If your emotions are affecting your work or personal relationships and you're concerned about these issues, see your health care provider.

Getting Sick

Pregnant women can get a cold or come down with the flu just like anyone else. Here are some tips to follow if you become sick:

- *Colds*—Catching a cold can make you feel miserable whenever it happens, but getting sick while you're pregnant may make you more miserable than ever. Ask your health care provider about the safety of taking any over-the-counter medication while you are pregnant. Also, get plenty of rest and drink plenty of fluids.

- *Flu*—Flu symptoms are more severe than those of colds. Preg-

❯ Common Symptoms of the Flu

- Fever over 101° F
- Muscle aches and pains
- Extreme fatigue and weakness
- Headache
- Dry cough
- Sore throat
- Loss of appetite

Month 3

nancy can increase the risk for complications from flu, such as pneumonia. Because of the increased risk of flu complications for pregnant women, some of which can be life threatening, your health care provider may prescribe an antiviral drug if the benefits of this treatment outweigh its risks in your specific situation. For antiviral medication to be effective, it must be taken within 48 hours of the onset of symptoms. If you think you are getting the flu, call your health care provider right away. Don't wait for your symptoms to get worse.

All pregnant women should get the flu vaccine. Protection from the vaccine usually begins 1–2 weeks after getting the shot. The protection lasts 6 months or longer. A flu shot is considered safe at any stage of pregnancy. However, the nasal flu mist is not approved for use in pregnant women.

- *Diarrhea*—If you come down with a bout of diarrhea, drink plenty of liquids to avoid getting dehydrated. Call your doctor, too, to report your symptoms and find out whether there are any over-the-counter antidiarrhea medications that you should take.

Skin Changes

During pregnancy your body produces more melanin—the pigment that gives color to skin. These changes are temporary and harmless. This increase in melanin is the reason your nipples become darker, for example. It also causes *chloasma*. This "mask of pregnancy" gives some women brownish marks around their eyes and on their noses and cheeks. Spending time in the sun can make chloasma worse, so protect yourself by wearing sun block and a hat and limiting your exposure to direct sunlight. These marks may fade after the baby's born, when hormone levels return to normal. In many women, the extra pigment produced in pregnancy causes the faint line running from the belly button to the pubic hair to get darker. This line, called the *linea nigra*, has always been there, but before pregnancy it was the same color as the skin around it. It, too, usually fades after delivery.

Stretch marks may appear later in pregnancy. The skin on your belly and breasts may become streaked with reddish brown, purple, or dark brown marks, depending on your skin color. Some women also get them on their buttocks, thighs, and hips. Stretch marks are caused by changes in the elastic supportive tissue that lies just beneath the skin. There are no proven remedies that keep them from appearing or to make them go away. Keeping your belly well moisturized as it grows may reduce itching, though. Once your baby is born, some of these streaks will slowly fade in color.

❱ Prenatal Care Visits

Prenatal care involves tests, physical exams, and imaging exams (such as *ultrasound*) that are performed to monitor the health and well-being of you and your baby. Screening tests are done to see if you or your baby is at risk of certain problems. They are given to people who are not known to be at increased risk for a disorder. Results of screening tests are usually reported as the degree of increased or decreased risk. Other tests, called diagnostic tests, are done to find problems that may occur during your pregnancy. They are given to people who are known to be at an increased risk for a problem, such as people from certain ethnic groups or those who have a medical or family history of certain disorders or problems. A diagnostic test may also be offered if the result of a screening test indicates that you are at increased risk.

Some of the tests that are performed during pregnancy may be mandated by state law. Most commonly, state-regulated tests are those that screen for *sexually transmitted diseases (STDs)*, such as *syphilis* and *human immunodeficiency virus (HIV)*.

No test is perfect. Results can be incorrect. A false-positive result indicates that a disorder is present in a person who does not have the disorder. A false-negative result indicates that a disorder is absent in a person who does in fact have the disorder. In addition, a disorder may be present for which no diagnostic test exists. If you have concerns or questions about any test, talk to your health care provider.

Ultrasound

An ultrasound exam makes an image of your baby from sound waves. These sound waves are produced by a device called a *transducer*. The transducer is either moved across your abdomen, which is called a *transabdominal ultrasound* scan, or is placed in your vagina, which is called a *transvaginal ultrasound* scan. The method chosen depends on what needs to be seen and the gestational age.

A first trimester ultrasound exam is performed for the following reasons:

- Confirm the pregnancy by locating the amniotic sac in which the baby is developing. (More information about when the amniotic sac can be seen is in Chapter 1, "Months 1 and 2 [Weeks 1–8]," p. 39.)
- Estimate the gestational age.
- Determine whether the baby's heart is beating.
- Check whether there is more than one baby.
- Screen for birth defects.
- Examine the uterus and ovaries.

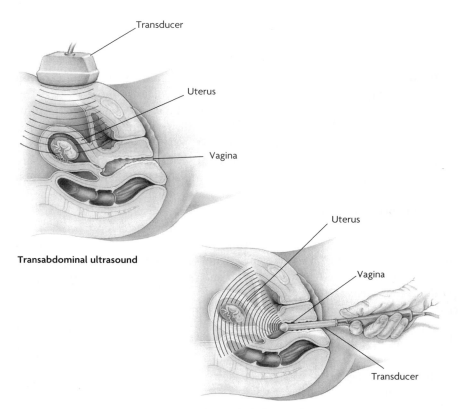

Transducer

Uterus

Vagina

Transabdominal ultrasound

Uterus

Vagina

Transducer

Transvaginal ultrasound

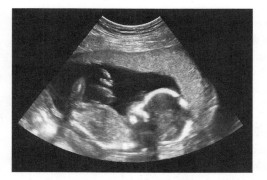

Ultrasound image of a fetus at 17 weeks of gestation

Ultrasound exam. During an ultrasound exam, sound waves are produced by a transducer. These sound waves are reflected off the fetus. The reflected sound waves are changed into pictures that you and your health care provider can view on a screen.

Screening Tests for Birth Defects

Screening tests are available for certain types of common birth defects. Some of the most common birth defects found through screening tests include *neural tube defects*, abdominal wall defects, heart defects, *Down syndrome*, and *trisomy 18.*

Certain screening tests are offered to all pregnant women to assess their risk of having a baby with a birth defect or genetic disorder. If a screening test shows an increased risk of having an affected baby, diagnostic tests may be offered to diagnose the problem. Diagnostic tests include *chorionic villus sampling* and *amniocentesis*. In the past, women at increased risk of having a baby with a birth defect—for instance, women older than 35 years— were offered diagnostic testing first rather than having screening tests. Now, these tests are offered as a first choice to all pregnant women before 20 weeks of pregnancy. It's important, however, to understand the risks of these diagnostic tests, which may include an increased risk of pregnancy loss, before choosing this option. Diagnostic tests are discussed in further detail in Chapter 22, "Birth Defects."

Screening tests can be performed in the first or second trimesters. First-trimester screening is done between 11 weeks and 14 weeks of pregnancy to detect the risk of Down syndrome and trisomy 18. It involves a blood test and an ultrasound exam.

First-trimester screening can be done as a single combined test or as part of a step-by-step process. Second-trimester screening involves a blood test that is done between 15 weeks and 20 weeks of pregnancy. There also is combined screening, in which the results from first-trimester and second-trimester tests can also be used together to increase their ability to detect Down syndrome. These tests also are discussed in further detail in Chapter 22.

The types of screening tests that will be offered to you depend on which tests are available in your area, how far along you are (you cannot have first-trimester screening if you are in your second trimester), and an assessment by your health care provider of which screening tests best meet your needs. Before you have any screening tests, you should be aware of the possibility for false-positive results and false-negative results. Your health care provider should have information about the rates of incorrect results for each test that is offered. You also should understand the advantages, disadvantages, and limitations of each test so that you can make informed decisions.

Pelvic Exam and Pap Test

Your doctor may do a *pelvic exam* and *Pap test*. A pelvic exam is done to assess the size of the pelvis and uterus. During the pelvic exam, you also will be tested for some causes of pelvic infection, such as *gonorrhea* or *chlamydia*. A Pap test may be done to check for changes in the cervix that could lead to cancer, depending on when you had your last Pap test.

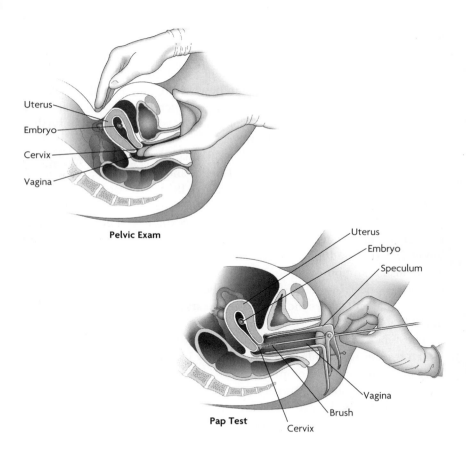

Pelvic exam and Pap test. During a pelvic exam, your health care provider checks your internal organs by inserting one or two fingers into the vagina while pressing on your abdomen with the other hand. For a Pap test, a speculum is inserted into the vagina. A sample of cells is collected from the cervix with a small brush or spatula. The cells are sent to a lab where they are examined for signs of cervical disease.

Lab Tests

The following tests are performed early in pregnancy and may not be done at the same prenatal care visit:

- *Blood type and **antibody** screen*—Your blood type can be A, B, AB, or O. It can also be Rh positive or Rh negative. If your blood cells lack a protein called the Rh **antigen**, your blood is Rh negative. If your blood cells carry the Rh antigen, your blood is Rh positive. Problems can arise when the baby's blood has the Rh antigen and yours does not, a condition called Rh incompatibility. Your body may make antibodies that attack the baby's blood, which can cause the baby to have ***anemia***. This condition requires special care during pregnancy and is also discussed briefly in Chapter 6, "Month 7 (Weeks 25–28)."

- *Hematocrit and hemoglobin*—These tests check for anemia. If your hematocrit and hemoglobin levels are low, you may be advised to increase your intake of iron.

- *Rubella*—Your blood will be checked for immunity to rubella (German measles). If you had this viral infection before or have been immunized against it, you are not at risk for rubella infection.

- *Glucose*—The level of ***glucose*** in your blood is measured to test for ***diabetes mellitus***. For this test, you drink a sugar mixture. An hour later, a blood sample is taken from your arm and sent to a lab. If you have risk factors for diabetes mellitus, this test is done early in pregnancy.

- *Sexually transmitted diseases*—You will be tested for certain STDs, including syphilis, chlamydia, HIV infection, and ***hepatitis B virus***.

- *Urine*—A urine test will be done to determine whether you have bacteria in your urine. If your test result is positive, you will need treatment.

- *Risk screening*—Some screening tests are given to pregnant women who have health conditions, such as hypertension, lung disorders, ***lupus***, and ***obesity***, to make sure these problems do not pose any risk to the baby.

▶ Special Concerns

It's important to be alert to things that may be harmful during pregnancy, including sexually transmitted diseases and domestic violence. Recognizing these risks early will allow you to get the treatment or help you need sooner and prevent harm to yourself and your unborn baby.

Sexually Transmitted Diseases

Sexually transmitted diseases are infections passed from one person to another during sex. Some STDs can be harmful during pregnancy. For instance, if you have an STD, you are more likely to have preterm labor. You are tested for certain STDs early in your pregnancy. Some tests are repeated later in pregnancy, depending on your risk factors. Be honest with your health care provider about your risks. If you do have an STD, you will need treatment. Your partner also should be treated and both of you should not have sex until you finish treatment. There are many different STDs and the treatment for each varies. See Chapter 26, "Infections."

Domestic Violence

An unfortunate reality is that the relationship between you and your partner may not always be a healthy and supportive one. An abusive relationship is one in which one partner subjects the other to emotional or physical abuse. Emotional abuse can take the form of constant name-calling, criticism, and extreme jealousy. In physical abuse, a partner may push, slap, or kick you. But whether the abuse is emotional or physical, it is all considered domestic violence.

Domestic violence (also called intimate partner violence) is a common and tragic problem in the United States. Domestic violence is the leading cause of injury to women in the United States between the ages of 15 years and 44 years and is estimated to be responsible for 20–25% of hospital emergency room visits by women.

Domestic abuse can happen to women of any race, age, sexual orientation, religion, or gender. It can happen to couples who are married, are living together, are of the same sex, or are dating. It happens to people of all socioeconomic and educational backgrounds. Abuse doesn't have to happen every day or every week for it to be classified as domestic violence.

Pregnancy often offers no break from the abuse. In fact, one out of six abused women is first abused during her pregnancy. More than 320,000 women each year are abused by their partners while they are pregnant. Abuse puts both the mother and her baby at risk. An abuser is likely to aim his blows at a pregnant woman's breasts and belly. The dangers of this abuse include miscarriage, vaginal bleeding, low birth weight, and fetal injury.

It isn't easy to admit or realize that the person whom you love, or once loved, or who is the parent of your child, is an abuser. But if you are in a violent relationship, it's vital to take steps to protect yourself and your baby. Abusers often blame others for their own actions. No matter what your partner says, it is not your fault. You do not make it happen. The abuser is the one to blame for the abusive actions.

The first step to breaking the pattern of violence is to tell someone about it. Tell someone you trust—a close friend, a family member, your health care provider, a nurse, a counselor, or a clergy member. Talking about a problem can be a huge relief. The person you confide in may be able to put you in touch with crisis hotlines, domestic violence programs, legal aid services, and shelters for abused women.

Getting ready to leave an abusive relationship can be difficult, but knowing these tips can help:

- Keep any evidence of physical abuse, such as pictures, and write down dates of when the abuse happens.

- Find out where you can go to get help.

- If you are injured, go to the emergency room and report what happened to you.

- Contact your local battered women's shelter and find out about laws and other resources available to you before you have to use them during a crisis.

- Try to set money aside or ask friends or family members to hold money for you.

Once you decide to leave, be prepared for a safe, quick escape:

- You may request a police stand-by or escort while you leave.

- Make a plan for how you will escape and where you will go.

- Hide an extra set of car keys.

- Pack an extra set of clothes for yourself and your children and store them at a trusted friend or neighbor's house. Don't forget toys for the children.

- Take with you important phone numbers of friends, relatives, doctors, and schools, as well as other important items, including the following items:
  —Your driver's license
  —Regularly needed medication
  —Credit cards or a list of credit cards you hold yourself or jointly
  —Pay stubs
  —Checkbooks and information about bank accounts and other assets
  —Birth certificates for you and your children

It's hard to break the cycle of violence. If you do nothing, though, chances are the abuse will happen more often and will become more severe. Leaving your partner or having him or her arrested during your pregnancy takes great courage. But you owe your baby a safe and loving home, and you owe yourself an end to the violence.

For more information or to get help, check the section of your phone book for domestic violence services or hotlines. You also can call the National Domestic Violence Hotline 24 hours a day (see Resources).

YOUR QUESTIONS ANSWERED

Are saunas and hot tubs safe?

Some studies have suggested that sauna and hot tub use may cause an increase in a woman's core body temperature and may lead to birth defects in a developing baby. The American College of Obstetricians and Gynecologists advises pregnant women to remain in saunas for no more than 15 minutes and hot tubs for no more than 10 minutes. It's also suggested that a pregnant woman avoid submerging her head, arms, and shoulders in the hot tub to decrease the areas exposed to heat.

Do I have to get rid of my cat?

No. You may have heard that cat feces are a major source of the infection *toxoplasmosis*, but there's no need to give away your pet. The infection is only present in cats that have access to the outdoors and hunt prey. If your cat never goes outside, only eats cat food, and does not hunt any indoor prey (for example, mice and other rodents), your risk of toxoplasmosis is extremely low. The infection can be very serious for pregnant women. If you have a cat that goes outdoors or may eat prey, have someone else take over cleaning the litter box. (Note that clean cat litter is not dangerous; the feces and the litter that has come in contact with it are what should be avoided.) The litter should be changed daily. If you do it yourself, wear disposable gloves and wash your hands well afterwards. Keep in mind that toxoplasmosis can also be acquired when working with soil or eating raw or undercooked meat. It's essential to wear gloves when gardening and to avoid raw or rare meat.

Is it safe to use my microwave?

You may have heard rumors about radiation being emitted from microwave ovens. However, the levels of emissions are strictly enforced by the FDA and are well below the risk to public health. It's quite safe to continue using your oven unless the microwave door, hinges, or seals are damaged. If you suspect a problem, don't use the oven until it has been repaired or you have purchased a replacement.

Month 3

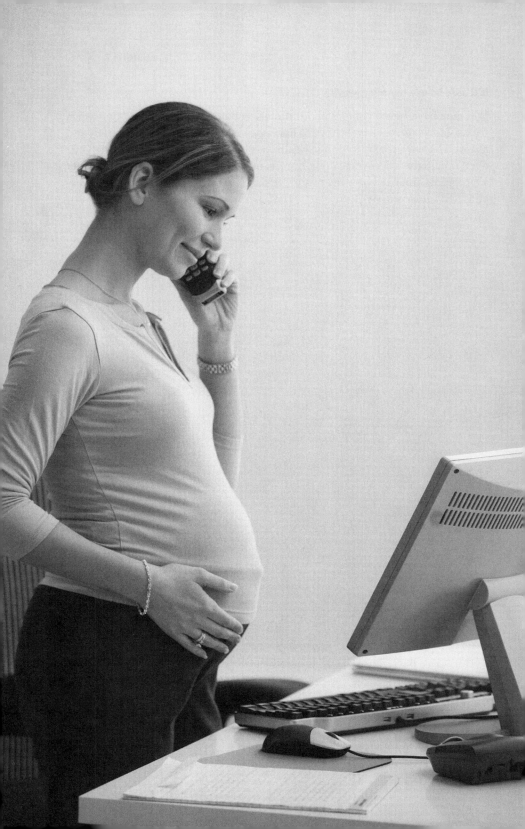

Chapter 3

Month 4
(Weeks 13–16)

YOUR GROWING BABY

Week 13

Your baby is beginning to grow at a quicker pace. The organs are fully formed and will grow even more this trimester. For instance, the spleen is working to produce red blood cells. Your baby's sex **hormones** (**testosterone** and **estrogen**) also are being made. On an **ultrasound**, you may see your baby making breathing-like movements and swallowing amniotic fluid.

Week 14

The eyes are beginning to move, and the arms and legs can now flex. Her hands will soon open and close into fists, and movements such as putting her hands to her mouth are happening more frequently. The organs of taste and smell are developing. Also, the baby's skin is starting to become thicker, and hair follicles are appearing just below the skin surface.

Week 15

The baby is becoming more active now in the **amniotic sac**, rolling around and doing flips. The heart is pumping about 100 pints of blood each day, and the **kidneys** are now producing **urine**.

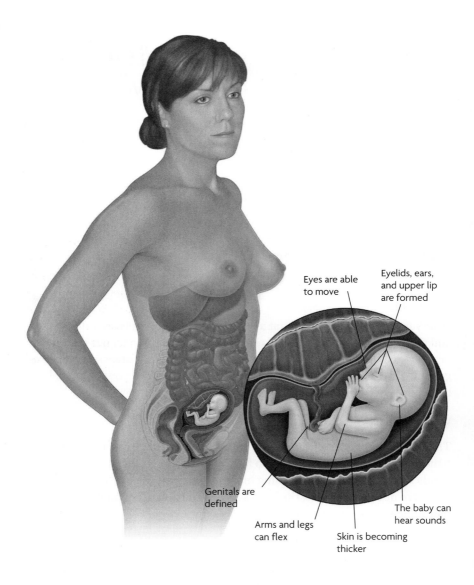

Eyes are able
to move

Eyelids, ears,
and upper lip
are formed

Genitals are
defined

Arms and legs
can flex

Skin is becoming
thicker

The baby can
hear sounds

Mother and baby: Weeks 13–16. Your baby weighs about 5 ounces and is about
6–7 inches long now.

Week 16

Your baby weighs about 5 ounces and is about 6–7 inches long now. Her face has features, such as eyelids, ears, and an upper lip. She can hear sounds now. The digestive system is working, even the stomach. The baby's external genitals also are defined, and you may be able to see them if you have an ultrasound exam.

YOUR PREGNANCY

▶ Your Changing Body

Welcome to the second trimester! Most women feel their best during these next couple of months—so much so that the second trimester is called the "honeymoon period" of pregnancy. Your morning sickness has probably subsided, your energy level may be back to normal, and your pregnancy may be starting to show. The second trimester also marks the time when you can worry a little less because the risk of miscarriage is now lower. And beginning this month, your *uterus* is large enough that it is no longer completely in the pelvis.

▶ Discomforts and How to Manage Them

This month's discomforts may include spider veins and changes in your gums, teeth, and mouth—even strange dreams. You may also experience aches and pains in your abdomen, which can be worrying. It helps to know what pain is normal and what isn't—and when you should call your health care provider.

Lower Abdominal Pain

As the uterus grows, the round ligaments (bands of tissue that support the uterus on both sides) are pulled and stretched. You may feel this stretching as either a dull ache or sharp pain on one side of your belly. The pain may be most noticeable when you cough or sneeze. Not moving for a short time or changing position may help relieve the pain.

If abdominal pain doesn't go away or gets worse, call your health care provider. It could be a sign of a problem.

Month 4

Mouth and Dental Changes

Pregnancy hormones can make your gums swell and bleed, but don't let this keep you from brushing and flossing. Switching to a softer brush may help lessen irritation.

Also, don't cancel your regular dental visit just because you are pregnant. A dental checkup early in pregnancy helps make sure that your mouth stays healthy. Pregnant women are at an increased risk for cavities and gum disease. It's safe to have dental work during pregnancy; just be sure to let your dentist know you're pregnant.

Strange Dreams

It's normal to have unusual dreams—especially in the last trimester—that may be vivid and scary. Experts believe these types of dreams may provide a way for your subconscious to cope with any fears and doubts you have about pregnancy and becoming a mother.

Excessive Salivation

Some women notice that they have excessive salivation during pregnancy, especially when they're nauseated. This condition is more common among women who have severe morning sickness.

The exact cause of excessive salivation is not known, but hormonal changes may be a reason. Also, nausea might make some women try to swallow less, causing saliva to build up in the mouth. If this is a problem for you, tell your health care provider.

Spider Veins

You may have tiny red veins that show up under the skin of your face or legs. Spider veins are a normal part of the changes in your circulation and usually fade once you give birth.

▶ Nutrition

This month may bring food cravings that you didn't expect, which can be a challenge when you are trying to eat a healthy diet. One thing you can do to eat more healthfully is to learn about high and low glycemic foods.

Focus on High and Low Glycemic Foods

As you learn to eat a healthier diet, it may be a good idea to be familiar with which foods have a high and low glycemic index. Foods with a low glycemic index are part of an overall healthier eating plan.

The glycemic index is a ranking of how quickly foods that contain carbohydrates increase your blood *glucose* (sugar) level. A food with a high glycemic index increases blood glucose levels more rapidly than a food with a medium or low glycemic index. Foods with a high glycemic index provide a quick burst of energy, whereas foods with a low glycemic index provide a slower, more even burning of energy. You may feel less hungry when you eat foods with a low glycemic index, and you may be able to sustain higher energy levels for a longer period of time.

Foods with a high glycemic index tend to be white: white breads, potatoes, white rice, and popcorn; however, not all foods with a high glycemic index are white—pretzels also fall into this category. The following foods have a low glycemic index:

- 100% whole-wheat, multigrain, or pumpernickel bread
- Oatmeal (rolled or steel cut), oat bran, and muesli
- Whole-wheat pasta, brown rice, and barley
- Sweet potato, corn, yam, lima or butter beans, peas, and legumes and lentils
- Apples, oranges, and peaches
- Nonstarchy vegetables and carrots

Weight Gain

Eating a healthy diet and gaining a healthy amount of weight during pregnancy is important for your well-being and that of your growing baby. Different stages of pregnancy can present certain challenges to healthy eating. In the first trimester, morning sickness can affect your eating habits. You may crave certain foods or not feel like eating. Usually, though, your appetite increases in the second trimester. Some women again lose their appetites in the third trimester because nausea sometimes returns. Throughout the entire 9 months, however, it is important to stick to a healthy diet to ensure that you and your baby are getting all of the nutrients you need. It's a balancing act that may often prove challenging. See Chapter 13, "Nutrition During Pregnancy," for more detailed information about how to keep eating a healthy diet throughout your pregnancy.

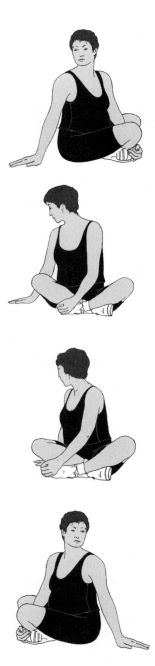

Food Cravings

Pregnant women often have food cravings. Occasionally giving in to these cravings is okay. Cravings can cause problems, however, if you eat only a few types of food for long periods. They also can be less than healthy if you indulge your cravings for one type of food and neglect the rest of your diet.

Some women may feel a strong urge to eat nonfood items such as laundry starch, clay, or chalk. This condition is called *pica*. If you feel these urges, don't indulge in them. Eating nonfood items can be harmful and can prevent you from getting the nutrients you need. Call your health care provider if you think you have pica.

▶ Exercise

You may be feeling much more energized this month, so now is a good time to rev up your exercise routine. Walking is a great way to exercise that doesn't require a gym membership or specialized equipment, and it's already something you've done all your life. This month's exercise will help tone your back muscles, which may be getting a workout in the coming months as your uterus grows larger.

Exercise of the Month: Trunk Twist

This exercise stretches your back, spine, and upper torso.

1. Sit on the floor with your legs crossed.
2. Hold your left foot with your left hand, using your right hand on the floor for support.
3. Slowly twist your upper torso to the right.
4. Switch hands and repeat on the left. Repeat on both sides 5–10 times.

Trunk twist. This exercise is great for stretching your back, spine, and upper torso.

Walking

With your energy rebounding, you may have more motivation to exercise. If you are starting an exercise program, you may be wondering which forms of exercise are easy for the beginner and don't require special equipment.

Walking is a great form of exercise—and one of the easiest. All you need is a good pair of shoes and comfortable clothing. Wear walking shoes or tennis shoes that fit well and give good support, flexibility, and cushioning. If you are not used to exercising, start out slow and easy. Try walking for just 10 minutes at first. If that's easy, add 5 minutes. Keep adding 5 minutes until you can do a brisk walk for 30 minutes every day.

If you need motivation, ask a friend to join you on your walks. If you have other small children, try walking them in their stroller. Make it a family activity.

▌ Healthy Decisions

Some women with medical conditions may have to take time off before the baby is born. If you work outside the home, it's not too early to start thinking about how much time you or your partner will take off after the baby is born. You also may want to give some thought about where you would like to have your baby.

Pregnancy-Related Work Disability

Having a work disability means that health problems keep you from doing your normal work duties. Most pregnancies are not disabling. But for some women with certain health problems, pregnancy may become a disability. A work disability may be partly or totally disabling, which your health care provider will decide. There are two types of pregnancy-related work disabilities:

1. *Disability caused by the pregnancy itself*—Some symptoms of pregnancy may cause short-term or partial disability, such as severe nausea and vomiting. Giving birth also causes short-term disability.

2. *Disability caused by pregnancy complications*—Examples of these complications include **preeclampsia**, **premature rupture of membranes**, and **preterm birth**.

If your health care provider decides that you have a pregnancy-related disability, the appropriate forms must be completed. If your employer wants you to stop working but your health care provider says you can continue, get a letter from the health care provider to give to your employer.

The federal Pregnancy Discrimination Act requires employers that have at least 15 workers to treat workers disabled by pregnancy or childbirth the same as workers disabled by illness or accident. If you are partly disabled by pregnancy and your company gives lighter duty to other partly disabled workers, it must do the same for you. However, because many employers don't offer their workers any disability benefits, they don't have to provide paid leave. If you are not covered by a disability plan at work, you may be able to get state unemployment or disability benefits. For details, contact your local unemployment office.

Maternity Leave

Policies about maternity leave and disability leave vary from company to company and state to state. Only about 4 in 10 working women in the United States get paid leave after giving birth. Others must use sick leave and vacation time or take time off without pay.

The Family and Medical Leave Act protects your right to leave, with certain limits, for pregnancy-related problems or after giving birth. This federal law says you may be on leave up to 12 weeks without pay during any 12-month period and have your job back afterwards.

To qualify for this family leave protection, you must meet the following conditions:

• Work for a company where there are at least 50 employees of the same employer within a 75-mile area (at a branch office, for instance)
• Have worked there for at least 12 months
• Have worked at least 1,250 hours during the past 12 months

You may have to use vacation time or personal or sick leave for some or all of your time off. If your employer provides health care benefits, this coverage must be kept at the same level during the leave period. When you return to work, you must be given the same or an equal job and the same benefits you had when you left. If you use some of the 12 weeks for a difficult pregnancy, it may be counted as part of the 12-week, family-leave entitlement.

Paternity Leave

Paternity leave is the time a father takes off work after the birth of his child. This kind of leave is rarely paid, but most fathers take vacation time or sick

Your Workplace Rights

Three major federal laws protect the health, safety, and employment rights of pregnant working women. If you are denied your rights, contact the agencies listed.

1. *Pregnancy Discrimination Act*—The Pregnancy Discrimination Act requires employers to treat pregnancy as they would treat any other medical condition. That means they must offer the same disability leave and pay as they would to workers disabled by illness or injury. This federal act also makes it illegal to hire, fire, or refuse to promote a woman because she's pregnant. If you think you are the victim of pregnancy discrimination, contact the Equal Employment Opportunity Commission (see Resources). The commission's web site also gives details on how to file a claim.

2. *Occupational Safety and Health Act*—The Occupational Safety and Health Administration (OSHA) requires employers to provide a workplace free from known hazards that cause or are likely to cause death or serious physical harm. It also requires employers to give workers facts about harmful agents. If you think your employer may be breaking these rules, call OSHA, or go to the OSHA web site and click on "Contact Us" (see Resources).

   The National Institute for Occupational Safety and Health (NIOSH) finds workplace hazards, figures out how to control them, and suggests ways to limit the dangers. If you, your union, or your doctor asks it to, this group will inspect your workplace for hazards. Call NIOSH or visit the web site where you can ask an occupational safety and health question (see Resources).

   Certain state and city laws also give workers and unions the right to ask for the names of chemicals and other substances used in the workplace. If you have questions or concerns, ask your employer or call the numbers for OSHA or NIOSH.

3. *Family and Medical Leave Act*—The Family and Medical Leave Act requires employers with 50 or more employees to allow up to 12 weeks of unpaid leave during any 12-month period for the following reasons:

   - The birth, adoption, or foster care of a child
   - To care for a spouse, a child, or a parent with a serious health condition
   - When a worker isn't able to do her job because of her own serious health condition, including a pregnancy-related disability or birth-related disability

To find out more about family and medical leave, contact the U.S. Department of Labor (see Resources). A few states have better leave laws than the federal Family and Medical Leave Act. For details, contact your state's Department of Labor.

Month
4

days when their children are born. Also, many fathers-to-be are taking unpaid leave as part of the Family and Medical Leave Act, which can be used by men too.

Birth Places

The setting in which you give birth can have a major effect on your experience. Many hospitals offer a range of settings; in others, the choice may be limited. There also are freestanding birthing centers that are not in a hospital. The safest places to give birth are thought to be a hospital, a birthing center within the hospital complex that meets the standards jointly outlined by the American Academy of Pediatrics and the American College of Obstetricians and Gynecologists, or an accredited freestanding birth center that meets the standards of the Accreditation Association for Ambulatory Health Care, the Joint Commission, or the American Association of Birth Centers.

Depending on where you live, the following options may be available at the hospital:

• *Labor and delivery*—You go through labor in one room and give birth in another room. You will be transferred to a recovery room and then to a hospital room for the rest of your stay.

• *Labor–delivery–recovery*—You will be in the same room throughout labor and delivery and recovery and then transferred to a hospital room for the rest of your stay.

• *Labor–delivery–recovery–postpartum*—You are in the same room throughout your stay at the hospital.

Your choice will depend on what your area offers, where your health care provider performs deliveries, and what your health insurance will cover. Your health care provider will let you know about the choices available. You can tour the hospitals in your area to see which settings appeal to you.

What about giving birth at home? Although some women choose this option, you should be aware that even the healthiest pregnancies could have complications that arise with little or no warning during labor and delivery. If problems occur, a hospital setting offers the expert staff and equipment to give you and the baby the best care in a hurry. For this reason, the American College of Obstetricians and Gynecologists believes that a hospital, hospital-based birthing center, or accredited freestanding birthing center is the safest place for you and your baby during labor, delivery, and the day or two afterwards.

▶ Other Considerations

Many parents have lots of questions about how their new arrival will affect their finances. This month is a good time to think about financial issues, including health insurance. If you do not currently have health insurance, there are options (see "Health Insurance" on page 74).

Financial Issues

It's no secret that a new baby can drastically alter your family's finances. If you stay home on an extended maternity leave, you and your family will have to adjust to a lower income, and you will have more expenses related to the baby's care:

- *Child care expenses*—Child care can be very expensive. Do some research and compare the costs of different types of care, such as day care centers, home providers, and nannies.

- *Income taxes*—You can claim your baby as a new dependent on your income tax form, so it is a good idea to apply for his or her Social Security number soon after birth. The federal government offers a Child Tax Credit for each child under age 17 years if you meet certain criteria. You also may be able to get a tax credit for the money you spend on child care. If you have

How Much Does Raising a Child Cost?

Many parents-to-be wonder how much it costs to raise a child. The U.S. Department of Agriculture offers a handy online calculator that allows you to estimate these annual costs. The calculator is based on a report called *Expenditures on Children by Families*, a comprehensive study of families across the country. It takes into account how many children you already have, their ages, your marital status, where you live, and your annual income.

After you enter this information and click on "calculate," you will receive a report that breaks down your expenses into several categories: housing, food, transportation, clothing, health care, child care and education, and other expenses. You also can enter specific amounts in each category, if you want.

Note that the calculator applies only to children younger than 18 years—it does not, for example, include the costs of a college education. If you are interested in trying this calculator, go to www.cnpp.usda.gov/calculatorintro.htm.

questions, talk to a tax preparer or check the Internal Revenue Service's web site (see Resources).

• *Being a stay-at-home mom (or dad)*—Can you or your partner afford to stop working and stay home with the baby full-time? Although there are other things to consider when making the decision to stay at home, finances are a major issue. Take a good look at your family's income and expenses and weigh them against the average cost of child care in your area. Also factor in the money you'll save by staying at home, such as decreased spending on work clothes, carryout lunches, commuting costs, or dry cleaning.

Health Insurance

If you have insurance, check to see if your health plan covers complete pregnancy care or only the most routine medical tests and procedures. That could become an issue if problems arise during pregnancy or birth or if the baby has health problems. Check your plan to see how much of the cost it will pay for the following items:

• Obstetric care
• Prenatal tests
• Hospital charges
• Well-baby care
• Postpartum birth control

Also make sure your health care provider and the hospital where you want to give birth are part of your health plan. In many cases, seeing a health care provider or going to a hospital that is "out of network"—meaning not part of the insurance health plan—means that you'll have to pay for some or all expenses yourself.

The Health Insurance Portability and Accountability Act protects most women who switch health insurance plans during pregnancy or who enroll in a plan after they become pregnant. If you change jobs and insurance plans during your pregnancy, you cannot be denied insurance coverage for care related to your pregnancy. It does not matter how long you were with your insurance plan before you switched. Also, your newborn cannot be denied coverage as long as you sign her up for health insurance within 30 days of birth.

If, however, your job does not provide health coverage or you are unemployed, there are still ways you can get health insurance during your pregnancy and after childbirth as follows:

- *Medicaid*—Medicaid is a state-run program that is funded by the federal government. Medicaid provides medical assistance for low-income families and individuals. You can check with your local department of health to see if you qualify and to get more information.

- *State Children's Health Insurance Program*—The State Children's Health Insurance Program provides health coverage to children, up to age 19 years, whose families cannot afford or are not offered health insurance. Families who earn too much to qualify for Medicaid may be able to qualify for the State Children's Health Insurance Program. In most states, families who earn up to about $36,200 a year (for a family of four) are eligible. For little or no cost, this insurance pays for doctor visits, immunizations, hospitalizations, and emergency room visits.

- *Buy your own*—Individuals and families can purchase their own health coverage from major health plans that can be matched to your needs and budget. Check out www.ehealthinsurance.com, where you can compare plan benefits and prices in your part of the country.

- *Discount plans*—Discount health programs, such as Maternity Advantage, can save pregnant women up to 60% on doctor visits, lab work, ultrasound exams, hospital stays, and much more. Maternity Advantage is not insurance but it works with a National Preferred Provider Maternity Network. For a low monthly fee, Maternity Advantage can provide you with a comprehensive maternity plan. You can receive these benefits even after you have found out that you are pregnant.

▶ Prenatal Care Visits

Your prenatal care visit in your fourth month will be much shorter than your first visit. Still, you will have to have some tests and procedures to check your health and your baby's health.

Tests

Your health care provider will do a routine check of your weight and blood pressure and may do a urine test to check for glucose and protein. You may have additional screening tests for birth defects. For example, if you are having second trimester screening for birth defects, it will be performed this month.

Exams

Your health care provider also will monitor how the baby is developing. You may be able to listen to your baby's heartbeat too. Your health care provider may perform an ultrasound exam to check the baby's growth.

▶ Special Concerns

Because infections of the urinary tract and vagina are more common during pregnancy, it is important to know the signs and symptoms of each. Left untreated, some of these infections can result in pregnancy complications. The earlier you receive treatment, the better. Another special concern for pregnant women is stress. Being aware of your stress and taking steps to alleviate it are essential to your health and well-being.

Urinary Tract Infections

Urinary tract infections are infections of the *bladder*, kidney, or *urethra* and are common in pregnancy. If untreated, they can become severe and lead to a more serious kidney infection or preterm labor. These infections can be diagnosed with a simple urine test. It is important, however, to be alert to the signs and symptoms of a urinary tract infection and to call your health care provider if you have any of them:

- Pain when you urinate
- Urge to urinate right away
- Blood in your urine
- Fever
- Back pain

If a urinary tract infection is diagnosed, *antibiotics* will be prescribed for treatment. These medications are safe to take during pregnancy.

Vaginal Discharge

Vaginal discharge often increases during pregnancy. A sticky, clear, or white discharge is normal, and it's usually nothing to worry about. The increased discharge is caused by the normal pregnancy-related changes in the *vagina* and *cervix*.

A discharge, however, that has changed from its normal color; that has a bad odor; or that is accompanied by pain, soreness, or itching in the vaginal area can be a sign of a vaginal infection:

- *Bacterial vaginosis* is an infection caused by an imbalance of the bacteria growing in the vagina. It is the most common cause of vaginal discharge and has a fishy odor. The infection is not a sexually transmitted disease but can be serious enough to cause some women to have a higher risk of having complications, such as preterm birth or premature rupture of membranes.

- Yeast infections usually cause symptoms such as a vaginal discharge that is thick, white, and curd-like; itching around the vagina; and painful urination.

It's important to alert your health care provider to any of these symptoms while you are pregnant. Don't try to treat the infection yourself with over-the-counter medications and never douche while you're pregnant. Your health care provider will treat bacterial vaginosis with antibiotics. Yeast infections are treated during pregnancy with the oral medication fluconazole (Diflucan) or with a vaginal cream or a suppository containing an antifungal cream.

Pregnancy-Related Stress

It is perfectly normal to worry about your pregnancy and whether you are doing all the right things for the baby—what you eat, drink, and feel. The changes happening in your life and thoughts about how your life will change once the baby comes can be stressful. However, it's important to make sure this type of normal stress doesn't become too much, to the point that it makes you anxious or upset every day.

If you think your stress is becoming too much to handle, talk to your family, friends, and especially your health care provider. You will need help to ease your feelings. One good way to start is by realizing that you can't do everything and may need to ask for help sometimes—from your partner, family, and friends. Here are a few more tips that can help reduce your stress:

- Let the household chores go undone sometimes, and use that time to do something relaxing.

- Take advantage of sick days or vacation whenever possible. Spending a day, or even an afternoon, resting at home will help you get through a tough week.

- Get regular exercise. Yoga especially helps to reduce stress.

- Go to bed early. Your body is working overtime to nourish your growing baby, and you need all the sleep you can get.

Month 4

YOUR QUESTIONS ANSWERED

What if I need surgery while I'm pregnant?

Whether having surgery during pregnancy is okay depends on what type of procedure is needed and what types of medications will be necessary. Talk to your health care provider about your particular situation. The decision is based on whether the risks of having the surgery outweigh the benefits of waiting until after you have the baby.

Can I have my regularly scheduled dental X-ray during my pregnancy?

Yes. The amount of radiation in a dental X-ray is extremely low. A dental X-ray doesn't pose any risk as long as it is done with your baby's safety in mind. Be sure to let your dentist know that you are pregnant. Your abdomen, pelvis, and neck area (where the thyroid gland is located) will be covered by a lead apron that will protect you and the baby.

I have terrible allergies. Can I take a prescription medication? What about over-the-counter remedies?

Many people with allergies depend on drugs called antihistamines for relief. Some are available over the counter, and others are available only by prescription. Two antihistamines that have been extensively studied and found to be safe during pregnancy are chlorpheniramine and tripelennamine. However, both of these drugs can cause drowsiness, and they may not be as effective as some of the newer antihistamines. Two newer antihistamines—loratadine and cetirizine—may be considered for pregnant women who can't take chlorpheniramine or tripelennamine. Preferably, these two newer drugs should not be taken during the first trimester of pregnancy.

Oral decongestants help decrease nasal congestion and can be useful in treating allergies. Use of one of the most common decongestants, pseudoephedrine, during pregnancy has been linked to a slightly increased risk of abdominal wall birth defects. For this reason, it has been suggested that women avoid taking this decongestant during the first 3 months of pregnancy. There have been few studies on the safety of two other decongestants, phenylephrine and phenylpropanolamine, during pregnancy, so it is difficult to say whether they can cause harm to an unborn baby.

Another allergy medication available by prescription is corticosteroid nasal spray, such as fluticasone propionate (Flonase) and beclomethasone dipropionate (Beconase). Only one has been tested in humans (Beconase), and it was shown not to cause birth defects. The others, however, have not been tested in humans. Most experts agree that these medications are probably safe to use during pregnancy, especially if the benefits of their use outweigh any potential risk. However, the bottom line on allergy (and all other) medications is to check with your health care provider before taking any over-the-counter drug.

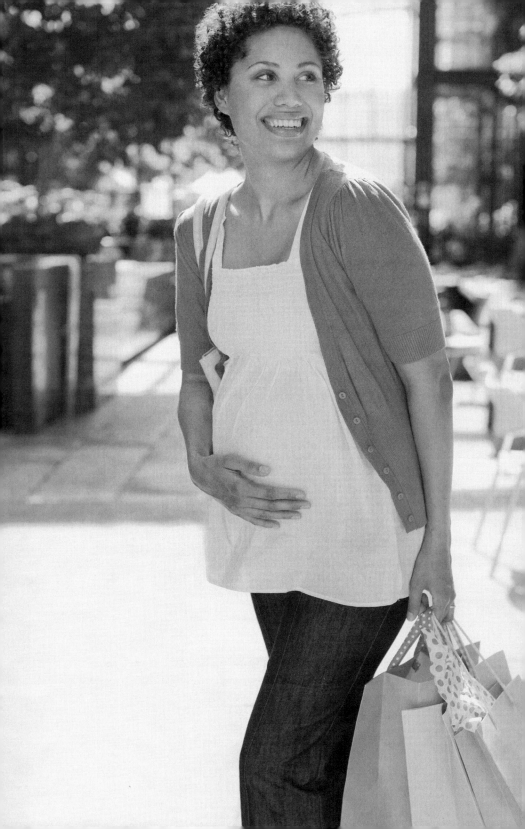

Chapter 4

Month 5

YOUR GROWING BABY

Week 17

The baby is about 9 inches long and weighs about 8 ounces, but in the next few weeks the baby will double his weight. Glands in the skin begin to produce a greasy material called *vernix*. This material acts as a waterproof barrier that protects the baby's skin. The skin will be completely covered with this material by the time the baby is born.

Week 18

Your baby sleeps and wakes regularly and now can be awakened from sleep by noises and your movements. Soft, downy hair, called *lanugo*, is starting to form and will cover your baby's body. This hair helps keep your baby warm inside the womb. In girls, *ovaries* containing eggs have formed, and in boys, the *testes* have begun to descend.

Week 19

Your baby's kicks and turns are stronger now. If you have already felt your baby move, the movements are more noticeable now. The sucking reflex is developing. If your baby's hand floats to his mouth, he may suck his thumb.

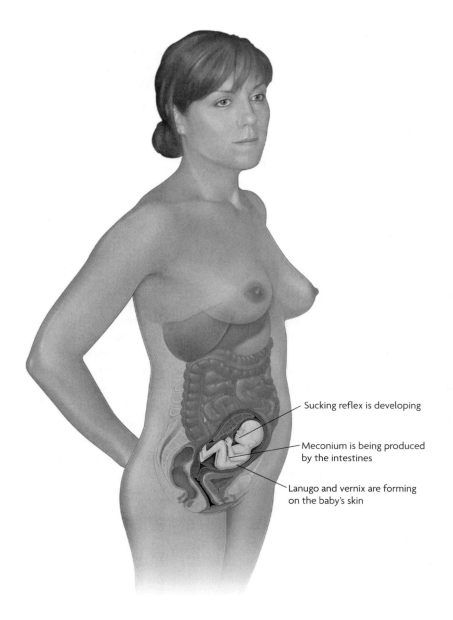

Sucking reflex is developing

Meconium is being produced by the intestines

Lanugo and vernix are forming on the baby's skin

Mother and baby: Weeks 17–20. The baby may weigh as much as 1 pound and is about 10 inches long. You may be able to feel your baby move this month.

Week 20

Your baby may weigh as much as 1 pound now, and he is about 10 inches long. He is swallowing more often. He also is producing *meconium*, a greenish black, sticky by-product of digestion. This substance will accumulate in his bowels, and you'll see it in his first soiled diaper (some babies pass meconium in the womb or during delivery). Your baby's nails grow to the ends of the fingers and may get so long that they will need to be trimmed once he is born.

YOUR PREGNANCY

▶ Your Changing Body

Soon you will feel your baby move for the first time. This is known as *quickening*. Some women, especially those who have had another child, experience quickening as early as 16 weeks. If this is your first baby, however, you may not be aware of your baby's movements until about the 18th week, and sometimes even later.

Another thing you may be noticing now is that your feet are getting bigger. They may continue to increase in size until late in pregnancy. The growth in your feet is partly caused by your weight gain and the swelling from the extra fluid your body retains while you're pregnant, called *edema*. Another reason for this is a *hormone* called relaxin, which loosens the joints around your pelvis so your baby can make his way down the birth canal, and which also loosens the ligaments in your feet, causing the foot bones to spread.

To help with the swelling, soak your feet in cool water and prop them on a pillow as much as you can. You may have to buy new shoes in a bigger size too.

▶ Discomforts and How to Manage Them

If you were not expecting it, nasal congestion may seem like a strange pregnancy symptom. But there is actually a reasonable explanation for that stuffy feeling. You may also feel dizzy at times, and you may find yourself forgetting the simplest things. Another uncomfortable symptom—one that may stay with you throughout the rest of your pregnancy—is low back pain.

Month
5

Congestion and Nosebleeds

During pregnancy, your hormone levels increase, and your body makes extra blood. Both of these changes cause the mucous membranes inside your nose to swell up, dry out, and bleed easily. This may cause you to have a stuffy or runny nose. You also may get nosebleeds from time to time. Here are some remedies:

- Try saline drops or a saline rinse to relieve congestion. (Never use other types of nose drops, nasal sprays, or decongestants without your doctor's approval.)

- Drink plenty of liquids.

- Use a humidifier to moisten the air in your home.

- Dab petroleum jelly around the edges of your nostrils to keep the skin moist.

Lower Back Pain

Backache is one of a pregnant woman's most common problems, especially in the later months. You can probably blame your growing uterus and hormonal changes for your aching back. Your expanding uterus shifts your center of gravity and stretches out and weakens your abdominal muscles, changing your posture and putting a strain on your back. The extra weight you're carrying means more work for your muscles and increased stress on your joints, which is why your back may feel worse at the end of the day. Here are some tips to help lessen back pain:

- Wear low-heeled (but not flat) shoes with good arch support, such as walking shoes or athletic shoes. High heels tilt your body forward and strain your lower-back muscles.

- Do exercises to stretch and strengthen your back muscles.

- Don't bend at the waist to pick something up. If you must lift something, squat down, bend your knees, and keep your back straight.

- Get off your feet. If you have to stand for a long time, rest one foot on a stool or a box to take the strain off your back.

- Sit in chairs with good back support, or tuck a small pillow behind your lower back.

- Use an abdominal support garment (for sale in maternity stores and catalogs). It looks like a girdle and helps take the weight of your belly off your back muscles. Also, some maternity pants come with a wide elastic band that fits under the curve of your belly to help support its weight.

• Apply a heating pad using the lowest temperature setting, warm-water bottle, or cold compress to ease the pain. Be sure to use a towel for wrapping to avoid burns.

Dizziness

Early in your second trimester, it's normal if you feel dizzy or light-headed at times. Your body is going through a lot of changes in circulation, such as less blood flow to your head and upper body. To prevent feelings of dizziness, move slowly when you stand up or change positions. Drinking lots of fluids may help. Also, avoid standing for long periods of time or getting too hot. If you feel dizzy, lie down on your side.

Forgetfulness

You may find it harder to concentrate at work these days or may forget ordinary things that you never did before, such as appointments or tasks. Don't be too alarmed because forgetfulness is common during pregnancy. In the meantime, if it helps, start keeping lists of things to do at work or home to help jog your memory.

Month 5

▶ Nutrition

You may have heard that fish is a good source of omega-3 fatty acids. But you also may have heard that eating some types of fish is not recommended for pregnant women. This month's nutrition focus is aimed at sorting out the latest information on fish. As your appetite increases in the second trimester, you may also be wondering about healthy snacking—which snack foods pack the most nutritional punch and which snack foods you should avoid.

Focus on Omega-3 Fatty Acids

Although you should limit your intake of many high-fat foods in your diet, omega-3 fatty acids are "good" fats that should be part of a healthy diet. Research has shown that omega-3 fatty acids, especially docosahexaenoic acid and eicosapentaenoic acid, may help reduce the risk of heart disease and can slightly lower blood pressure. Results of some research suggest additional benefits, including boosting the immune system and decreasing the symptoms of depression.

A good source for omega-3 fatty acids is fatty fish, such as salmon, tuna, lake trout, and sardines. Pregnant women can eat a variety of fatty fish at least two times a week. About 1 ½ ounces of fish contains 1 gram of omega-3 fatty acids.

Even if you don't like fish, you can still get what you need from other foods. Flaxseed (either as whole seeds or oil) is a good source, and so are canola oil, broccoli, cantaloupe, kidney beans, spinach, cauliflower, and walnuts. One handful of walnuts, for instance, has about 2 ½ grams of omega-3s. Supplements also can be taken, but tell your health care provider before taking any over-the-counter supplement. High doses may have harmful effects.

Fish Precautions

Fish and shellfish can be important parts of a healthy and balanced diet. They are both good sources of protein, omega-3 fatty acids, and other nutrients. However, certain kinds of fish should not be eaten at all during your pregnancy because they contain high levels of a form of mercury that can be harmful to the baby. These are the types of fish you should avoid eating while you are pregnant (or breastfeeding):

• Shark
• Swordfish
• King mackerel
• Tilefish

Common types of fish that are low in mercury are shrimp, canned light tuna (not albacore, which has a higher mercury content), salmon, pollock, and catfish. You can safely eat up to 12 ounces (about two meals) of these fish per week while you're pregnant. If you want to include albacore tuna as part of your two fish meals one week, limit your intake of albacore tuna to no more than 6 ounces for that week. Check local advisories about any mercury or other pollution warnings if you eat fish caught locally. If no information is available, limit your intake to no more than 6 ounces, and don't eat any other fish that week. If you follow these guidelines, you'll get all of the health benefits of fish while reducing your and your baby's exposure to mercury. For more information about fish advisories, go to www.fda.gov. For information about fish advisories in your area, go to www.epa.gov/fishadvisories/advisories.

Healthy Snacking

Usually in the second trimester your appetite increases and you may want to snack more during the day. Snacking is a good way to get the extra calories you need during pregnancy, as long as you choose some healthy snacks that are low in fat and good for you:

- Whole-grain crackers, pretzels, and crispbreads
- Fruits and vegetables
- Nuts and seeds
- Low-fat cheese and yogurt
- Fruit shakes (for example, whip together frozen yogurt, a banana, a splash of fruit juice, and a handful of berries in a blender)

Weight Gain

Steady weight gain is more important in the second and third trimesters, especially if you start out at a healthy weight or you're underweight. In general, you should gain about one third of your total pregnancy weight by your 20th week of pregnancy. If you are gaining weight too quickly, you may have to adjust how much food you're eating and get more exercise.

▶ Exercise

If traditional exercise, such as walking or swimming, does not appeal to you, you may want to try alternative exercise, such as yoga or Pilates. No matter which type of exercise you choose, it's very important to learn a few safety tips. This month's exercise of the month is a safe exercise that stretches and strengthens your back muscles.

Exercise of the Month: Forward Bend

This exercise stretches and strengthens your back.

1. Sit in a chair in a comfortable position. Keep your arms relaxed.

2. Bend forward slowly, with your arms in front and hanging down. Stop if you feel any discomfort on your abdomen.

3. Hold this position for 5 seconds, and then sit up slowly without arching your back. Repeat five times.

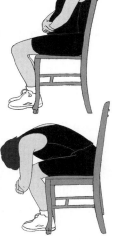

Forward bend. This exercise will help stretch and strengthen your back muscles.

Month 5

Alternative Exercises

Exercise is beneficial for both you and your baby. Walking and swimming are generally safe, but what if neither appeals to you? There are other options that can get you moving, build muscle strength, and help lower your stress:

- *Yoga*—Yoga exercises or postures can stretch and strengthen muscles and help develop good breathing techniques. This age-old practice keeps you limber, tones your muscles, and improves your balance and circulation, with little, if any, impact on your joints. Yoga also is beneficial because it helps you learn to breathe deeply and relax, which may be helpful during labor and birth. Yoga is safe for pregnant women, with the exception of Bikram and other forms of yoga that are performed in a hot environment. Also, some poses aren't recommended for pregnant women, such as those in which you lie flat on your back (after the first trimester) and those that require a lot of abdominal stretching. Tell your yoga instructor that you are pregnant. You may want to consider joining a yoga class that is designed especially for pregnancy.

- *Pilates*—With its focus on healthy breathing and improving flexibility, a Pilates exercise program is a good way to improve posture and build muscle strength. As with yoga, some Pilates moves shouldn't be done during pregnancy. Make sure that your instructor knows that you are pregnant, or join a special class for pregnant women.

- *Tai Chi*—Tai chi involves performing a series of postures or movements in a slow, graceful manner. Each posture flows into the next without pausing. Anyone can do tai chi, and it's known to reduce stress, increase flexibility and energy, and improve muscle strength and balance.

Safe Exercise

Although getting regular exercise is important, it's just as important to be sure you protect yourself from injury. For starters, make sure you have all the equipment you need for a safe workout. Wear shoes that have plenty of padding and that give your feet good support. Wear a sports bra that fits well and gives plenty of support. Here are few more tips on keeping exercise safe:

- Drink enough fluids. Take a bottle of water with you for a drink before, during, and after your workout. If you're getting hot or feeling thirsty, take a break and drink more water or sports drink.

- Begin your workout with stretching and warming up for 5 minutes to prevent muscle strain. Slow walking or riding a stationary bike are good warm-ups.

- Work out on a wooden floor or a tightly carpeted surface. This gives you better footing.

- Don't do jerky, bouncy, or high-impact motions. Jumping, jarring motions, or quick direction changes can strain your joints and cause pain.

- Get up slowly after lying or sitting on the floor. This will help keep you from feeling dizzy or faint. Once you're standing, walk in place briefly.

- Don't do deep knee bends, full sit-ups, double leg lifts (raising and lowering both legs at once), or straight-leg toe touches. After the first trimester, you also should avoid exercises in which you lie flat on your back. This can cut down the blood flow to your baby.

- Follow intense exercise with cooling down for 5–10 minutes. Slow your pace little by little and end your workout by gently stretching. Don't stretch too far, though. Intense stretching can injure the tissue that connects your joints.

Month 5

▶ Healthy Decisions

Do you want to know the baby's sex? You may be able to find out during this month's ultrasound exam. You also may need to decide whether you would like to have some types of genetic screening tests.

Knowing the Baby's Sex

If you'd like to find out whether your baby is a boy or a girl, you usually can do so at the *ultrasound* exam often done around 16–20 weeks. In some cases, it's important for your practitioner to know your baby's sex—for example, if the baby is believed to be at risk for certain congenital conditions. Sometimes it's not possible to determine the sex because the baby is not facing the right way.

The American College of Obstetricians and Gynecologists recommends that ultrasound exams be performed only for medical reasons. Although ultrasonography is generally considered safe, it's not possible to rule out all potential risks. Having an ultrasound exam only to determine the baby's sex is not recommended.

Deciding Whether to Have Genetic Screening

Genetic screening may be recommended or requested during this time in the pregnancy. Most often the results of genetic tests will reveal that the baby is normal. If test results show that the baby may have a birth defect, learn the facts and talk about your feelings with your partner, your doctor, and others with whom you can share your thoughts.

There is no "right" choice in these cases. The decision is based on the values unique to each person. The choice that's right for one woman may not be right for another. Counseling with a genetic expert or other specialist, counselor, social worker, clergy member, or support group may help sort out the issues.

If you find out that your baby has a disorder, you may have to make some difficult choices in a short time. Some women choose to end a pregnancy. Others may choose to continue the pregnancy even if the baby will have a problem. The months before the birth can be used to prepare for and plan for the future, such as learning more about the problem and talking to others who have been through the same situation.

▶ Other Considerations

The second trimester is a good time to travel. If you're planning a trip, you may want to learn about how to take care of yourself away from home. Paying attention to the way you feel is the best guide for your activities—whether you are on the road or at home. The second trimester is also the time when women may begin having problems finding a good position to sleep in.

Travel During Pregnancy

In most cases travel is okay during pregnancy. If you are planning a trip, it's a good idea to check with your doctor about safety measures to take during travel. Most women can travel safely until close to their due dates. Travel may not be recommended for women who have pregnancy complications, however.

The best time to travel is mid-pregnancy (14–28 weeks of pregnancy). After 28 weeks, it's often harder to move around or sit for a long time. During mid-pregnancy, your energy has returned, morning sickness is over, and you are still mobile.

When choosing your mode of travel, think about how long it will take to get where you are going. The fastest way is often the best. Whether you go by train, plane, car, or boat, take steps to ensure your comfort and safety. Here are some tips for healthy travel:

- Have a prenatal checkup before you leave.

- If you'll be far from home, take a copy of your health record with you.

- Know how to locate a health care provider in case you need one. If you need a doctor while traveling in the United States, visit the American Medical Association's web site (see Resources) and search for "Doctor Finder." The American College of Obstetricians and Gynecologists' web

International Travel

If you are planning a trip out of the country, your health care provider can help you decide if foreign travel is safe for you and figure out what steps to take before your trip.

While you are pregnant, you shouldn't travel to areas where there is risk of malaria, including Africa, Central and South America, and Asia. Malaria is a major risk to your pregnancy. If travel to these areas can't be avoided, have your health care provider prescribe an antimalarial drug (a drug to prevent malaria), such as chloroquine or mefloquine. Pregnant women should not take the antimalarial drugs atovaquone and proguanil, doxycycline, or primaquine.

When you are planning your trip, call the International Travelers Hotline at the Centers for Disease Control and Prevention (see Resources). This service has safety tips and up-to-date vaccination facts for many countries. The Centers for Disease Control and Prevention web site also has world travel health facts and special information for traveling while pregnant.

Even if you are in perfect health before going on a trip, you never know when an emergency will come up. Be sure to get a copy of your health record to take with you.

Also, before leaving home, locate the nearest hospital or medical clinic in the place you are visiting. The International Association for Medical Assistance to Travelers has a worldwide directory of doctors who provide quality health care for travelers. Call this agency to obtain a free directory of doctors or visit their web site (see Resources). You must become a member to view their directory of doctors, but membership is free.

If you need to see a doctor who doesn't speak English, it's a good idea to have a dictionary with you of the language spoken. After you arrive, register with an American embassy or consulate. This will help if you need to leave the country because of an emergency.

Deep Vein Thrombosis and Travel

Deep vein thrombosis (DVT) is a condition in which a blood clot forms in the veins in the leg or other areas of the body. It can lead to a dangerous condition called pulmonary embolism, in which a blood clot travels to the lungs. Research has shown that any type of travel lasting 4 or more hours—whether by car, train, bus, or plane—doubles the risk of DVT. This finding suggests that it is not the mode of travel that increases the DVT risk, but the length of time a person remains seated and not moving. Being pregnant is an additional risk factor for DVT.

If you are planning a long trip, you should take the following steps to reduce your risk of DVT:

• Drink lots of fluids.

• Wear loose-fitting clothing.

• Walk and stretch at regular intervals (for example, when traveling by car, make frequent stops to allow you to get out and stretch your legs).

Special stockings that compress the legs below the knee also can be worn to help prevent blood clots from forming. However, talk to your health care provider first before you try these stockings because some people should not wear them (for example, those with diabetes and other circulation problems).

site (www.acog.org) can help you locate an obstetrician; click on "Find an Ob-Gyn." (For international travel, see the box on page 91.)

• Keep your travel plans flexible. Pregnancy problems can come up at any time and prevent you from leaving. Buy travel insurance to cover tickets and deposits that can't be refunded.

• Wear comfortable shoes, support stockings, and clothing that doesn't bind. Wear a few layers of light clothing.

• Take time to eat regular meals to boost your energy. Be sure to get plenty of fiber to ease constipation, a common travel problem.

• Drink extra fluids. Take some juice or a bottle of water with you. In an airplane, the cabin is very dry. Choose water instead of a soft drink.

By Car

During a car trip, make each day's drive brief. Spending hours on the road is tiring, even when you're not pregnant. Try to limit driving to no more than 5 or 6 hours each day. Stop every few hours to stretch, get a drink, and empty

Buckling Up During Pregnancy

For the best protection in a vehicle, wear a lap–shoulder belt every time you travel. The safety belt will not hurt your baby. You and your baby are far more likely to survive a car crash if you are buckled in. Follow these rules when wearing a safety belt:

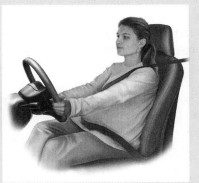

- Always wear both the lap and shoulder belt.
- Buckle the lap belt low on your hip bones, below your belly.
- Never put the lap belt across your belly.
- Place the shoulder belt across the center of the chest (between your breasts)—never under your arm.
- Make sure the belts fit snugly.

The upper part of the belt should cross your shoulder without chafing your neck. Never slip the upper part of the belt off your shoulder. Safety belts worn too loosely or too high on the belly can cause broken ribs or injuries to your belly if you are in an accident.

your bladder. Be sure to wear your seat belt every time you ride in a car or truck, even if your car has an air bag (see box "Buckling Up During Pregnancy"). If you get in a crash—even a minor one—notify your pregnancy health care provider. You may be given tests to check the health of the baby.

By Plane
For healthy pregnant women, air travel is almost always safe during pregnancy. Most airlines allow pregnant women to fly until about 36 weeks of pregnancy, but check with your airline to be sure about their rules. (If you are planning an international flight, however, the cutoff point for traveling on international airlines is often earlier.)

If you have a medical or pregnancy condition that may be made worse by flying or could require emergency medical care, you should avoid flying during your pregnancy. Keep in mind that most common pregnancy emergencies usually happen in the first and third trimesters.

If you're worried about air pressure and cosmic radiation at high altitudes, these issues don't normally cause any problems for the occasional traveler.

Although decreased air pressure during flight may slightly reduce the amount of oxygen in your blood, your body will naturally adjust. Radiation exposure also increases at higher altitudes, but the level of exposure for the occasional traveler usually isn't a concern.

There are concerns, however, for pregnant women whose jobs require them to fly often (such as pilots, flight attendants, or air marshals). Frequent fliers may exceed the cosmic radiation exposure limits set by the federal government. Most airlines, in fact, restrict their flight attendants from flying after 20 weeks of pregnancy. Some even prohibit pilots from flying once pregnancy is diagnosed. If you are a frequent flyer, be sure to check with your doctor about how long it is safe to fly during your pregnancy.

When traveling by air is a must, you can follow these tips to help make your trip as comfortable as possible:

- If you can, book an aisle seat so that it's easy to get up and stretch your legs during a long flight.

- Avoid gas-producing foods and carbonated drinks before your flight. Gas expands at high altitude and can cause discomfort.

- Wear your seat belt at all times. Turbulence can occur without warning during air travel.

- Move your feet, toes, and legs often. If you can, get up and walk around a few times during your flight.

By Ship

Taking a cruise can be fun, but a few commonsense rules apply if you're pregnant. Before you book your trip, make sure a doctor or nurse is on board the ship. Also, check that your scheduled stops are places with modern medical facilities in case there is an emergency.

If you have never taken a cruise, planning your first one while you are pregnant may not be a good idea. Many travelers on cruise ships have the unpleasant symptoms of seasickness, also called motion sickness. Seasickness occurs when conflicting signals about your position from the body, eyes, and inner ear (which controls your sense of balance) are sent to the brain. Seasickness causes nausea and dizziness, and sometimes weakness, headache, and vomiting.

If seasickness usually is not a problem for you, traveling by sea during pregnancy may not upset your stomach. To be on the safe side, ask your health care provider about which medications are safe for you to carry along to calm seasickness. Seasickness bands are useful for some people, although there is little scientific evidence that they work. The bands use acupressure to help ward off an upset stomach. For many people, seasickness goes away on its own after a few days as the body adjusts to the boat's motion.

Another concern for cruise ship passengers is norovirus infection, which can cause severe nausea and vomiting for 1 or 2 days. This infection is very contagious and can spread rapidly throughout cruise ships. People can become infected by eating food, drinking liquids, or touching surfaces that are contaminated with the virus.

There is no vaccine or drug that prevents this infection, but you can help protect yourself from it by frequently washing your hands and by washing any fruits and vegetables before you eat them. If you are pregnant and get this infection (or any other illness that causes diarrhea and vomiting), see a health care provider. Dehydration can lead to certain pregnancy problems. You may need to receive intravenous (IV) fluids.

Sleeping Positions

You may be finding it difficult to get into a comfortable position for sleep. Your belly has grown, and sleeping face down is uncomfortable. Sleeping on your back may not be good for you either because it puts the weight of your uterus on your spine and back muscles. In the second and third trimesters, lying on your back may compress a major blood vessel, making you feel dizzy.

The best position for you is to sleep on your side. Keep one or both knees bent. It may also help to place one pillow between your knees and another under your abdomen, or use a full-length body pillow.

Don't worry if you wake up and find yourself on your back. You won't harm the baby. Also, trust your body. Some pregnant women find that their bodies automatically find the best positions for sleep.

▶ Prenatal Care Visits

The timing of your prenatal care visits during your second trimester depends on your health and any special needs you may have during your pregnancy. Healthy moms-to-be with no known risk factors often need fewer visits than women with medical or obstetric problems.

As long as you and the baby are well, from your first prenatal care visit until 28 weeks of pregnancy, you most likely will have a checkup every 4–6

Month 5

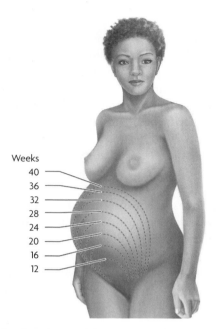

Weeks
40
36
32
28
24
20
16
12

Changes in uterine size. The size of the uterus can help show how long you have been pregnant.

Measuring fundal height. Starting at around the fifth month of pregnancy, your health care provider will measure the height of your uterus to check your baby's growth during each prenatal care visit.

weeks. During your second-trimester visits, you may have the following procedures:

- *Ultrasound examination*—This ultrasound scan is done after approximately 18 weeks of gestation and provides information about your baby's basic anatomy. Also, your health care provider may be able to tell the baby's sex if the baby is in a good position for the genitals to be seen. The amount of amniotic fluid is checked, and the baby's heart activity is assessed. Despite all of the benefits, a normal ultrasound exam does not preclude the possibility of some fetal abnormalities.

- *Fundal height*—As your baby grows, the top of the uterus (the fundus) grows up and out of the pelvic cavity. At about 12 weeks of pregnancy, it can be felt just above the pubic bone. At 20 weeks, it reaches the navel. Starting at this prenatal care visit, your health care provider will start to measure the fundal height—the distance from your pubic bone to the top of your uterus. This measurement allows your health care provider to assess your baby's size and growth rate. As a rule of thumb, the fundal height (in centimeters) should roughly equal the number of weeks you're pregnant. For example, at 20 weeks, the fundal height should be about 18–22 centimeters.

- *Amniocentesis*—If you have decided to have **amniocentesis** but didn't have the test last month, you will have it this month (see Chapter 22, "Birth Defects").

▶ Special Concerns

Asthma is a common respiratory illness that has the potential to become severe in some people. If you have mild or moderate asthma, the risks to your baby are minimal. Severe asthma, however, increases the risk of complications for both you and your baby. If you have asthma, you should learn all you can about your condition and should follow your health care provider's treatment plan exactly.

Insect-transmitted diseases are not as common as asthma, but in some areas of the country, the number of cases of these diseases is increasing. Know which ones occur in your area and take precautionary steps.

Asthma

If you have asthma but keep it well managed, you should be able to have a healthy pregnancy and healthy baby. It is when a woman's asthma is uncontrolled that problems can happen, such as less oxygen getting to the baby.

Month 5

Some women with asthma may find that their symptoms get worse during pregnancy, so seeing your doctor regularly is important. Tell your obstetrician at your first prenatal care visit about your asthma so that the baby's health can be monitored. Although many pregnant women feel uneasy taking medications during pregnancy, if you have asthma, you must continue your medications once your doctor approves them. It's safe to continue using your asthma inhaler during pregnancy.

It's also important to see your allergist or immunologist to learn the best way to manage your asthma while you're pregnant and what, if any, other medications you may need to take.

Insect-Transmitted Diseases

You may live in an area where insect-transmitted diseases, such as Lyme disease and West Nile virus, are prevalent. If so, you should know the signs and symptoms of these diseases. You should also take steps to prevent becoming infected.

Lyme Disease

Lyme disease is caused by a bite from an infected deer tick, which often is hard to see. The first sign of Lyme disease is a sore that may look like a bull's-eye. This sore may go away, but the infection remains. Lyme disease also can cause flu-like symptoms, including swollen or painful joints and muscle aches. A few weeks later, some people get a rash, meningitis (an infection of the coverings of the brain and spinal cord), paralysis of the facial muscles, or heart problems. Antibiotics often will cure the infection.

It is wise to avoid densely wooded areas while you are pregnant. In areas where ticks can be found, wear long-sleeved shirts and long pants tucked into your socks. If you find a tick that has been on you for more than 24 hours, call your doctor.

West Nile Virus

The first case of human infection with West Nile virus occurred in the United States in 1999. Since then, cases have occurred throughout the United States. Although uncommon, infection with the West Nile virus most often is caused by the bite of an infected mosquito. People infected with the West Nile virus may not have any symptoms. In some cases, the infection can lead to West Nile fever or severe West Nile disease. West Nile fever can cause flu-like symptoms, including a fever, body aches, and headache. There is no treatment for West Nile virus infection. It is not yet known whether infection with the West Nile virus during pregnancy can affect the baby.

To protect yourself from mosquito bites, wear long pants and long-sleeved shirts and use insect repellant containing DEET when outdoors. Also, cut down on the time you spend outside at dawn and dusk when mosquitoes are most active.

YOUR QUESTIONS ANSWERED

Can I eat sushi?

It's a good idea to eat only cooked sushi or vegetable sushi during your pregnancy. Although many fish, when fully cooked, are safe to eat, you should avoid all raw or seared fish when you're pregnant. Raw fish, including sushi and sashimi, is more likely to contain parasites or bacteria than cooked fish.

Can I get a massage?

Sure. Massage is a good way to help relax your muscles, improve circulation, and get some well-deserved pampering. The best position for a massage while you're pregnant is lying on your side, rather than facedown. However, some massage tables have a cutout for the abdomen, allowing a pregnant woman to lie face down comfortably. Be sure to let your massage therapist know that you are pregnant if you're not showing yet. Many health spas now offer special prenatal massages done by therapists who are trained to treat pregnant women.

What vaccines are safe during pregnancy?

During your early prenatal care visits, your health care provider will go over your health history and determine whether you need to have any vaccinations while you are pregnant. Some are not safe to get during pregnancy, so unless you are at serious risk of infection, your doctor may decide to wait until after the baby is born. The vaccines that are not safe to get while you are pregnant include those for measles, mumps, and rubella; human papillomavirus; varicella (chicken pox); and tuberculosis. Some vaccines, however, are safe for pregnant women, including the influenza (flu) shot (although the nasal spray is not recommended for pregnant women).

Month
5

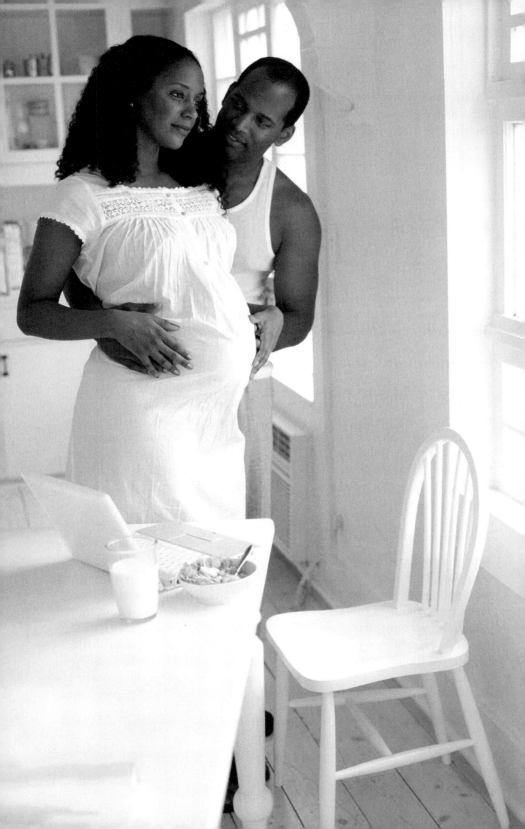

Month 6

(Weeks 21–24)

YOUR GROWING BABY

Week 21

Your baby's fingers and toes are completely formed now, even down to finger prints and toe prints. You may notice jerking movements—it's the baby hiccupping.

Week 22

Although the eyelids are still shut, your baby's eyes are moving behind the lids. Tear ducts also are developing. You may notice the baby responds to sounds now. Loud sounds may make your baby respond with a startled movement and contract her arms and legs.

Week 23

Your baby can respond with movement to familiar sounds, such as the sound of your voice. Now the baby spends about 80% of her sleep time in REM (rapid eye movement) sleep. During this stage of sleep, the eyes move and the brain is very active.

Week 24

The baby has added more weight by this last week of month 6. She now weighs between 1 pound and 1 ½ pound and is about 12 inches long. There also is much more muscle tone than in earlier weeks. The lungs are now fully formed but are not yet ready to function outside the womb.

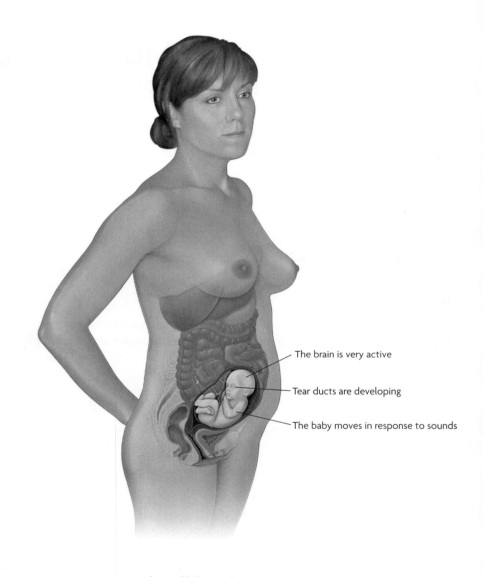

The brain is very active

Tear ducts are developing

The baby moves in response to sounds

Mother and baby: Weeks 21–24. This month, your baby has fingerprints, and you may feel her hiccuping.

YOUR PREGNANCY

▶ Your Changing Body

Week 21 marks the start of the second half of your pregnancy. You'll begin to feel the baby's kicks and to feel stronger movements a lot more now.

▶ Discomforts and How to Manage Them

You may have already experienced acid reflux—otherwise known as heartburn—earlier in your pregnancy. But now, as your uterus grows larger and pushes up against your stomach, heartburn may become more frequent. Other discomforts include hot flashes (caused by pregnancy hormones) and aches and pains (caused by the increased weight of your uterus).

Heartburn

Heartburn is a burning feeling or pain in the throat and chest and is common among pregnant women. Heartburn doesn't mean that something is wrong with your heart. Pregnancy **hormones**, which relax the valve between your stomach and esophagus (the tube leading from the mouth to the stomach), are a main cause of heartburn. When the valve between your esophagus and stomach doesn't close, stomach acids leak into the esophagus. As your **uterus** grows, it adds to the problem by pressing up against your stomach.

If you are bothered by heartburn, try these remedies:

- Eat six small meals per day instead of three big ones (a "grazing" eating pattern).

- Eat slowly and chew your food well.

- Don't drink a lot of liquid with your meals. Drink fluids between meals instead.

- Don't eat or drink within a few hours of bedtime. Don't lie down right after meals, either.

- Try raising the head of your bed. Prop a few extra pillows under your shoulders, or put a couple of books or wood blocks under the legs at the head of the bed.

Month
6

- Avoid foods that are known to make acid reflux worse, such as citrus fruits, chocolate, and spicy or fried foods.

Over-the-counter antacids are safe to use during pregnancy, as long as they do not contain aluminum or a salicylate such as aspirin (avoid Alka Seltzer and Pepto Bismol). Antacids that contain magnesium or calcium are fine, such as Tums, Rolaids, or Mylanta. Read the labels carefully, and if you have any doubts, contact your health care provider.

If you have tried these remedies and your acid reflux persists or gets worse, see your health care provider.

Hot Flashes

If you're feeling hot and sweaty when everyone else says they feel fine, blame your pregnancy hormones and your increased **metabolism**. You are burning more calories and generating more heat. Try to stay cool just as you would on the hottest summer days: wear loose clothing, drink plenty of water, and stay close to a fan or air conditioner for a blast of cool air.

Aches and Pains

It is normal for the extra weight of your growing belly to cause aches and pains as you move around during the day or even when you're trying to rest. Although you may not be able to take the medications you normally would to get rid of the pain, you can find some relief from over-the-counter acetaminophen medications, such as Tylenol, that are safe to use during pregnancy. Don't use aspirin or nonsteroidal antiinflammatory drugs (sometimes referred to as NSAIDs), such as ibuprofen, Motrin, Nuprin, or Advil.

You also might consider alternative ways to relieve the pain. If your muscles are sore and aching, try a warm bath or massage. A heating pad on its lowest setting, or a heat wrap, may help. For mild headaches, try lying down with a cool pack on your head. (Note: If you have a severe headache or if it doesn't go away, call your health care provider.)

❱ Nutrition

Vitamin B and choline are important to your baby's development. Although vitamin B is found in most prenatal vitamin supplements, choline is not. You may want to learn which foods are high in choline and to make sure that your diet includes them. This month, you will also learn about salt and monosodium glutamate, as well as about the different kinds of food poisoning (and how to prevent food-borne illnesses).

Focus on B Vitamins and Choline

B vitamins, including B_1, B_2, and B_6, are key nutrients your growing baby needs. These vitamins supply energy for your baby's development, promote good vision, and help build the *placenta* and other tissues in your body. Your prenatal supplement should provide the right amount of B vitamins that you need each day, but eating foods rich in these nutrients is a good idea too. Foods such as liver, pork, milk, poultry, bananas, whole-grain cereals and breads, and beans are packed with B vitamins.

Choline is another essential nutrient needed during pregnancy. It's important for your baby's brain development and can help prevent some common birth defects. Doctors recommend that pregnant women get 450 milligrams of choline each day. Although the body produces some choline on its own, it doesn't make enough to fulfill all your needs while you are pregnant. It's important to get choline from your diet because the nutrient is not found in most of the prenatal vitamin supplements and multivitamin supplements taken by pregnant women. Make sure your diet contains a healthy amount of foods rich in choline, such as chicken, beef, eggs, milk, and peanuts.

Salt and Monosodium Glutamate

You may be wondering if it is okay to keep eating salty foods while you're pregnant. The answer is yes, but do so in moderation. The recommended daily intake for sodium is 2,400 milligrams, which is the equivalent of 1 teaspoon of table salt. Foods that are extremely high in sodium are frozen processed foods, canned soups and broths, and other processed products. If you have high blood pressure, you may need to restrict your sodium intake to less than 2,400 milligrams.

Another seasoning used in many foods is monosodium glutamate (MSG). It is used a lot to enhance the flavor of many foods, especially Asian food. However, the U.S. Food and Drug Administration (FDA) requires that all foods that contain MSG list this ingredient on the label because some people develop an adverse reaction to it—pregnant or not. However, the FDA hasn't found any evidence that MSG is harmful to a developing baby.

Month
6

Avoiding Food Poisoning

Pregnant women can get food poisoning like anyone else. However, food poisoning in a pregnant woman can have serious consequences for her baby. It's important to know the signs and symptoms of the most common forms of food poisoning so that you can get treatment as soon as possible:

- *Salmonellosis—Salmonella* bacteria are a common cause of food poisoning. These bacteria often are found in raw poultry, fish, eggs, and milk. Salmonellosis (infection with *Salmonella* bacteria) causes vomiting, diarrhea, fever, and abdominal cramps that can last a couple of days. You may become dehydrated earlier than someone who is not pregnant. Dehydration can disrupt the body's chemical balance and has been linked to preterm labor and miscarriage. In addition, one type of *Salmonella* bacteria, called *Salmonella typhi,* can be passed to the baby if you are infected during pregnancy. If you have signs and symptoms of salmonellosis, see your health care provider as soon as possible. You may receive intravenous fluids to prevent dehydration. Drug treatment also may be needed in some cases.

- *Listeriosis—*Listeriosis is a serious infection caused by *Listeria* bacteria found in unpasteurized milk; soft cheeses made with unpasteurized milk, such as feta and brie; hot dogs; luncheon meats; and smoked seafood. Listeriosis can cause fever and other flu-like symptoms, such as chills and aches. Even if the infection doesn't make you seriously ill, it can have very serious effects on your developing baby. If it's not treated right away, listeriosis can cause miscarriage and stillbirth. Pregnant women with listeriosis should be treated with **antibiotics**.

- *Campylobacteriosis—*This infection is caused by bacteria known as *Campylobacter*. Most people who become ill with campylobacteriosis get diarrhea, cramping, abdominal pain, and fever within 2–5 days after being exposed to the bacteria. The illness usually lasts about 1 week. Most cases of the infection are from eating raw or undercooked poultry or from contamination of other foods by raw poultry. Animals also can be infected, and some people have gotten campylobacteriosis from contact with the stool of a sick dog or cat.

- *Escherichia coli—E. coli* are a large and diverse group of bacteria. Although most strains of *E. coli* are harmless, others can make you sick. Some kinds of *E. coli* can cause diarrhea, while others cause urinary tract infections, respiratory illness and pneumonia, and other illnesses. Most often, people are exposed to *E. coli* by eating or drinking contaminated food, unpasteurized (raw) milk, and water that has not been disinfected.

To avoid getting these types of food poisoning, follow these tips:

- Wash your hands and kitchen surfaces with hot, soapy water after you prepare a meal.
- Avoid all raw and undercooked seafood.
- Avoid raw eggs, which can be found in homemade mayonnaise and caesar salad (if you haven't made it yourself, ask whether the dressing has been made with raw egg). Avoid undercooked eggs as well.
- Wash raw fruits and vegetables thoroughly before eating them.
- To prevent listeriosis, don't eat cold cuts, deli meat, or smoked or pickled fish unless they are cooked until they are steaming hot.

Weight Gain

You may have gained between 10 pounds and 15 pounds by this time. If your doctor thinks you are gaining weight too quickly, you may have to adjust how much food you're eating and get more exercise. If you gain too much weight during pregnancy, it often is very difficult to lose after pregnancy, and the extra weight can have negative consequences for your future health.

▶ Exercise

For your aching back and pelvis, try this month's exercise, the backward stretch. Also, if you're thinking about switching things up in your exercise routine, you should know which sports you should avoid while pregnant.

Exercise of the Month: Backward Stretch

This exercise stretches and strengthens the muscles of your back, pelvis, and thighs.

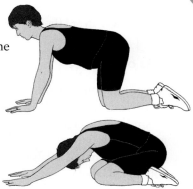

1. Kneel on your hands and knees, with your knees 8–10 inches apart and your arms straight (hands under your shoulders).

2. Curl backward slowly, tucking your head toward your knees and keeping your arms extended.

3. Hold this position for 5 seconds and then return to all fours slowly. Repeat five times.

Backward stretch. This exercise stretches and strengthens the muscles of your back, pelvis, and thighs.

Month 6

Sports to Avoid

Although there are many sports that you can continue doing while you're pregnant, such as walking and swimming, there are some activities that you should avoid because they can be too risky for you and the baby:

- *Downhill snow skiing*—Downhill skiing poses a risk of severe injuries and hard falls. In addition, exercising at heights of more than 6,000 feet carries various risks. If you do engage in physical activities at high altitude, know the signs of altitude sickness (throbbing headache, nausea, vomiting, dizziness, weakness, and difficulty sleeping). Be prepared to descend to a lower altitude and seek medical help if you have any of the signs.

- *In-line skating, gymnastics, horseback riding*—Your balance is affected, and there is a risk of crashes and falls.

- *Water skiing, surfing, diving*—Hitting the water with great force can be harmful. Taking a fall at such fast speeds could harm you or your baby.

- *Contact sports*—Avoid playing fast-paced team sports, such as ice hockey, soccer, basketball, and volleyball. Collisions or falls could result in harm to both you and your baby.

- *Scuba diving*—Scuba diving puts your baby at risk for decompression sickness.

Some sports should be avoided if you haven't done them before. In racquet sports, such as badminton, tennis, and racquetball, your changing body may affect your balance and put you at increased risks for falls. If you're an experienced player, however, you may be more adept at compensating for these changes. If you're not sure about your ability to maintain your balance, you may want to avoid these sports.

Loss of Balance

As you continue to exercise in your second and third trimester, be aware that your growing belly changes how your weight is balanced when you move around. The weight you gain in the front of your body shifts your center of gravity. This puts stress on your joints and muscles—mostly those in the lower back and pelvis. It also can make you less stable and more likely to fall. If you do fall, contact your health care provider if you have bleeding or are experiencing contractions.

▶ Healthy Decisions

With about 3 months to go, now is a good time to give some thought to labor and delivery as well as your baby's care after birth. You have quite a few decisions to make, including how you will feed your baby, whether you want your baby circumcised (if it's a boy), and other important choices. You may also have heard about cesarean delivery on request and are wondering whether it is right for you.

Labor and Delivery: Things to Start Thinking About

It is best to think about your childbirth options and resolve as much as you can well before you give birth. You should also make choices about your baby's birth and care after delivery. Some options you may want to think about ahead of time include the following:

- What kind of childbirth preparation do you want, and what classes are offered nearby?
- Do you want pain relief during labor, or will you try natural childbirth?
- If you have a boy, do you want him circumcised?
- Will you breastfeed your baby? Are there **lactation** classes in your area that you can attend?

Another issue to think about is whom you'd like at your side during labor and delivery. It's a good idea to choose someone who may be best at helping you stay relaxed and calm. A childbirth partner can be a spouse, partner, relative, or close friend. A growing trend is the use of a doula, a layperson who has received special training in labor support and childbirth (doulas are discussed in more detail in Chapter 6, "Month 7 [Weeks 25–28]," p. 124).

If possible, your childbirth partner should come with you to prenatal care visits and tests. Your partner also needs to attend childbirth classes with you because this person has almost as much to learn as you do. Your childbirth partner will help you practice breathing or relaxation exercises. When you're in labor, your partner will coach you through contractions and help you carry out what you learned in class.

Cesarean Delivery on Request

Some pregnant women ask to undergo a **cesarean delivery** even though there is no medical reason it must be done. This type of delivery is known as cesarean delivery on request or elective cesarean delivery. It is estimated that 2.5% of all births in the United States are by cesarean delivery on

Month 6

request. Some women ask for a cesarean delivery because they are anxious about labor and childbirth. Other women are concerned about developing *incontinence* after a vaginal delivery.

Scheduled or not, cesarean delivery is major surgery. If you are considering it, your health care provider will discuss whether it is right for you. Although there are some benefits to elective cesarean delivery, such as a decreased risk of hemorrhage for the mother (compared with a nonelective cesarean delivery, but not compared with a vaginal birth), there also are risks, including a longer hospital stay, an increased risk of respiratory problems for the baby, and greater complications in future pregnancies.

When deciding whether to perform a cesarean delivery on request, your health care provider will consider your specific risk factors, such as your age, body mass index, size of the baby, and plans for future children. Cesarean delivery on request is not recommended for women desiring several children because the risks of several problems, including the possibility of **hysterectomy** (removal of the uterus) and placental problems, increase with each cesarean delivery. Your health care provider should not perform a cesarean delivery on request before your 39th week of pregnancy unless there is a valid medical reason and unless test results show that your baby's lungs are mature. If your baby needs to be born between 34 and 37 weeks (which is called late preterm birth), and if the situation is not an emergency, you may meet with obstetric and pediatric specialists to discuss your options and the potential adverse health consequences that can affect late preterm babies.

If you are considering cesarean delivery on request because you are afraid of the pain of childbirth, talk to your health care provider about the pain relief options that are available and learn all you can about the birth process. Make sure that you will have adequate emotional support during your delivery. Knowing what to expect, including your anesthesia options, may help alleviate your anxiety about vaginal delivery.

Cesarean delivery has not been proved to prevent urinary incontinence. An analysis of the rates of urinary incontinence at 2 years and 5 years after delivery showed no difference by the type of delivery.

▶ Other Considerations

A common concern that many moms-to-be have is whether their baby would survive if they were to give birth prematurely. The answer to this question is complex and depends on many factors.

As your baby grows larger, you may experience a change in how you view your body. How you feel about sex may change too. Also, if you already have children, you may be wondering about the best way to involve them in your pregnancy.

Early Preterm Birth

A baby is considered **preterm** or premature when it is born before 37 weeks of pregnancy. When babies are born before 32 weeks of pregnancy, they are considered to be early preterm. Early preterm babies are at risk for many short-term and long-term problems:

- *Respiratory distress syndrome*
- Bleeding in the brain
- Cerebral palsy and other neurologic problems
- Vision problems
- Developmental delays, such as learning disabilities

Babies born before the 23rd week of pregnancy are not likely to survive. By the 26th week, the chances that your baby will survive are higher—75%—but she will likely face serious lifelong health problems. The chances that a baby born this early will survive depends on several factors, including the type of hospital the baby is born in, the baby's sex and weight, whether medications have been given to the mother to promote the baby's development, and whether there is more than one baby.

Some measures can be taken if you are at risk for preterm labor or have symptoms of preterm labor. Being aware of the symptoms of preterm labor is important; these symptoms are listed in Chapter 6, "Month 7 (Weeks 25–28)."

Body Image

Some women love the way they look during pregnancy. Others don't. Mixed feelings about your pregnant body also are normal. Some days, you'll love your growing body. Other days, however, you'll feel fat and wonder if your body will ever be the same.

Eating a healthy diet and exercising will help you feel better about how you look. If you're in good shape and don't gain more than the suggested weight during pregnancy, you'll have an easier time losing weight after delivery.

Sex

If you're having a normal pregnancy, you and your partner can keep having sex right up until you go into labor. Don't worry; you won't hurt the baby by

Month
6

having intercourse. The **amniotic sac** and the strong muscles of the uterus keep the baby protected.

It is normal to have cramps after sex, as well as spotting. **Orgasm** can cause cramps, and semen contains chemicals called **prostaglandins**, which stimulate uterine contractions. If you have severe, persistent cramping, or if your bleeding is heavy (like normal menstrual bleeding), call your health care provider.

As your belly grows, you'll have to find a position that is most comfortable for you. Let your partner know if anything feels uncomfortable, even if it's something you're used to doing all the time. You may want to try these positions:

- *Side-by-side*—You and your partner can either face each other or your partner can enter you from behind.
- *Woman-on-top*—This position takes the pressure off your belly.
- *Man-behind*—Support yourself on your knees and elbows so your partner can enter from behind.

It's up to you whether you feel up to having sex. Some women do, and some don't. Some women find that their desire for sex changes throughout pregnancy. During the first trimester of your pregnancy, you may have felt too nauseated and tired to have sex. But you may find that your sex drive comes back during the second trimester after morning sickness goes away and you have your energy again. It's also normal for your desire for sex to wane again during the third trimester, particularly in the last month or two. Whatever your mood is, talk with your partner.

If you are having any complications with your pregnancy or you have a history of preterm labor, you may be advised to restrict sexual activity or to monitor yourself for contractions after sex. If you cannot have intercourse, there are other ways to be intimate, such as cuddling, kissing, fondling, oral sex, and mutual masturbation. In some (rare) cases, you may be advised to avoid orgasm. It's important that you ask your health care provider specifically what sexual activity is and is not off-limits.

Involving Your Other Children in Your Pregnancy

If you already have children, they may have many different feelings about your pregnancy and the new baby soon to join the family. Small children may have lots of questions about where babies come from, or they may not want to talk about the baby at all. Some children are eager to be a big brother or sister. Others resent losing center stage to the new baby. A busy teenager with his or her own hobbies and friends may show little interest in your pregnancy and the new baby.

When is the best time to share the news about your pregnancy and talk about the changes soon to come? It really depends on your child. Tell your school-aged children before you tell anyone outside your family. If you don't, they might resent being the last to know. With young children, it's a good idea to wait until they ask about your changing body. The idea of a baby growing inside you may be too hard for small children to grasp before they can see your expanded belly.

▶ Prenatal Care Visits

Your prenatal care visit this month will focus on checking your baby's growth and making sure you are not having any complications. Your weight and blood pressure will be checked. And the doctor will again measure the fundal height. It should now be around 21–24 centimeters.

Be sure to tell your doctor if you are experiencing any symptoms that are causing discomfort. And don't hesitate to ask any questions that may be of concern.

▶ Special Concerns

Preterm birth can occur if labor starts before the end of the 37th week. It's important to recognize the signs and symptoms of preterm labor. If preterm labor is diagnosed early, your doctor may try to postpone birth to give your baby extra time to grow and mature. Even a few more days in the womb may mean a healthier baby.

Have you ever wondered about those keepsake ultrasound facilities you have seen in shopping malls? You may want to think twice about using one. And if you are concerned about a racing heartbeat, rest assured that it is a normal effect of pregnancy (although you should contact your health care provider in certain situations).

Preterm Labor

Call your health care provider right away if you notice any of these signs of preterm labor:

- Change in vaginal discharge (becomes watery, mucus-like, or bloody)
- Increase in amount of vaginal discharge
- Pelvic or lower-abdominal pressure
- Constant, low, dull backache

Month 6

- Mild abdominal cramps, with or without diarrhea
- Regular or frequent contractions or uterine tightening, often painless (four times every 20 minutes or eight times an hour for more than 1 hour)
- Ruptured membranes (your water breaks—either a gush or a trickle)

Diagnosis and treatment of preterm labor are discussed in more detail in Chapter 23, "Preterm Labor, Preterm Birth, and Premature Rupture of Membranes."

Fast or Racing Heartbeat

You may notice throughout your pregnancy that your heart is beating faster. This is normal. It occurs because your heart is pumping more blood faster than normal. You also may be surprised to know that as your pregnancy progresses, your heart pumps up to 30–50% more blood than when you aren't pregnant. These increases in heart rate and blood volume allow the efficient delivery of oxygen and nutrients to the baby through the placenta. Another reason for the faster heartbeat may be caffeine. Pregnant women may be more sensitive to its effects. If you notice that your heart rate stays elevated or if you also have shortness of breath, contact your health care provider right away.

Keepsake Ultrasound Photos

Some centers offer **ultrasonography** to create keepsake photos or videos. However, the American College of Obstetricians and Gynecologists and other experts recommend that, although there is no reliable evidence of physical harm to human *fetuses*, casual use of ultrasonography without a valid medical reason, especially during pregnancy, should be avoided. The use of ultrasonography only to obtain a keepsake picture or find out the sex of the baby without a physician's order may even violate state or local laws or regulations. Ultrasonography is a medical technology that should be used only for medical reasons.

Many parents are excited about the three-dimensional ultrasonography that uses special equipment to show a view of your baby that's almost as detailed as a photograph. However, at the present time, there is no evidence that three-dimensional ultrasonography is any better at diagnosing problems than conventional ultrasonography. Until a clear advantage is established, three-dimensional ultrasonography remains optional, rather than required, at this time.

YOUR QUESTIONS ANSWERED

How do you find a health care provider for your baby?

Pediatricians are doctors who specialize in the care of children. Family physicians also provide health care during childhood. The best time to choose a doctor for your baby is before the baby is born. If you have children who use a doctor you like, check to be sure he or she will take new patients. You may need to choose a new doctor for the baby. Find out if he or she also will care for your older children. If you don't already have a doctor, ask your pregnancy health care provider or friends for recommendations.

If you have health insurance, look for a doctor who is part of your insurance plan. You can choose a pediatrician or a family physician to take care of your baby. Look for a doctor who is board certified.

It's a good idea to have a get-acquainted office visit while you are pregnant. This visit will let you get a feel for how the office is run and what the staff is like. You also can ask the doctor questions you have about the baby.

These are some topics you may want to cover with the doctor:

• *Office visits*—When is the office open? Do you have hours on the weekends or in the evenings? What is the usual length of a visit? Is there a separate waiting room for children who are sick?

• *Personnel*—Will your baby always be seen by the doctor? What other caregivers might be scheduled to see your baby?

• *Phone calls*—Who will answer questions over the phone during office hours? Does the doctor charge for phone calls? How are calls and emergencies handled after regular office hours?

I've been exposed to chickenpox. What should I do now?

If you've been around someone who has chickenpox, you've never had the illness, and you did not get the varicella vaccination before becoming pregnant, tell your health care provider right away. Sometimes steps can be taken to avoid problems and decrease any risk to your baby.

My friend says she had "back labor." What does that mean?

Back labor refers to the intense lower back pain that many women feel during contractions when they're giving birth. Some women even feel it between contractions. It's caused by the pressure your baby's head puts on your lower back. During your prenatal classes, you and your pregnancy partner may learn ways to deal with back labor, such as massage or changes in position.

Month 6

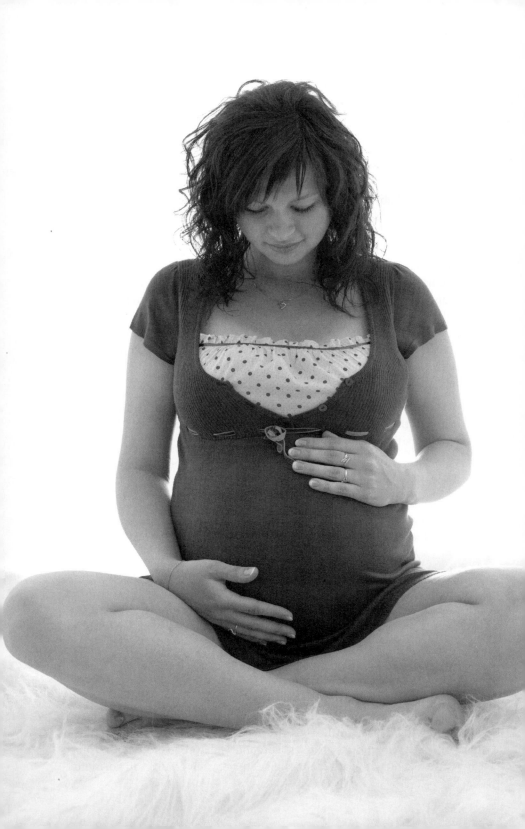

Chapter 6

Month 7

(Weeks 25–28)

YOUR GROWING BABY

Week 25

Your baby is entering a time of rapid growth and further development, particularly of the baby's nervous system. He'll be adding more fat to his body too, which will make the skin look smoother and less wrinkled.

Week 26

Your baby's skin has taken on color because of the melanin that is now being produced. The lungs are starting to produce **surfactant**, a substance that helps inflate the air spaces in the lungs. The highest levels of surfactant production occur during the third trimester.

Week 27

The baby kicks and stretches and can make grasping motions. A smile, especially during REM (rapid eye movement) sleep, may be seen in a baby at this age. At the sound of familiar voices, your baby's heart rate may decrease, which may mean that your baby is calmed by these sounds.

Week 28

The eyes can open and close and sense changes in light. Your baby now weighs about 2 ½ pounds and is about 14 inches long.

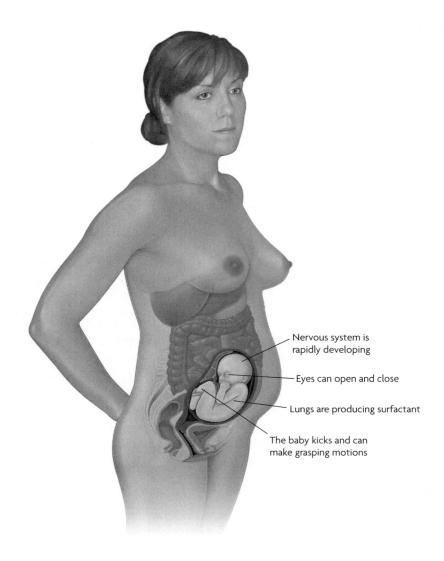

Nervous system is
rapidly developing

Eyes can open and close

Lungs are producing surfactant

The baby kicks and can
make grasping motions

Mother and baby: Weeks 25–28. By the end of this month, your baby will
weigh about 2½ pounds and will be 14 inches long.

YOUR PREGNANCY

▶ Your Changing Body

Welcome to the third—and last—trimester! The end is finally in sight. This can be an active time for many babies, so you will likely feel him kick and roll over a lot more often.

▶ Discomforts and How to Manage Them

The third trimester is a time of rapid fetal growth, and you will probably start seeing—and feeling—the extra weight of your baby. The increasing size and weight of your *uterus* may trigger low back pain and other pains as your body adjusts. Constipation may become a problem. You may also experience "practice contractions" called ***Braxton Hicks contractions***.

Lower Back Pain

Many pregnant women experience low back pain, especially during the later stages of pregnancy. There are several causes that may be responsible for pain in the lower back. One of the most common is the loosening of the ligaments in the sacroiliac joints, the strong, weight-bearing joints in the pelvis, which occurs during pregnancy. To make your baby's passage through your pelvis easier, a hormone called relaxin relaxes the sacroiliac ligaments, making the joint more mobile and flexible. Although this loosening is normal, pain may occur, especially during activities such as getting up from a chair, walking up a flight of stairs, or getting out of a car. If you have these symptoms, see your health care provider. He or she may suggest exercises that strengthen the muscles surrounding the joint. Usually, the problem goes away on its own after the baby is born. However, the more pregnancies a woman has, the greater her risk of sacroiliac joint problems.

Another cause of lower back pain is sciatica, a condition caused by the pressure of the growing uterus on the sciatic nerve. Sciatica causes pain in the lower back and hip that radiates down the back of the leg. Sciatica often resolves on its own after the baby is born. But if you have numbness in your feet or leg weakness with this pain, or if you have severe calf pain or tenderness, you should let your health care provider know.

Month 7

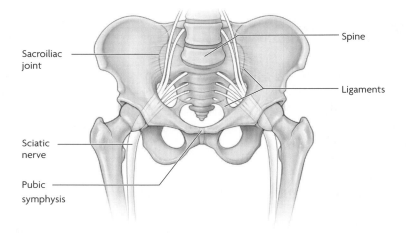

Sacroiliac joint

Spine

Ligaments

Sciatic nerve

Pubic symphysis

Causes of pain during pregnancy. Pregnancy-related changes in the sacroiliac joint, the sciatic nerve, and the pubic symphysis may all cause pain during pregnancy.

Pelvic Bone Pain

The two halves of your pelvis are connected at the front by a joint called the pubic symphysis, which is normally stiff and hardly moves. The hormone that loosens the sacroiliac joints also affects the pubic symphysis, making it more flexible during and just after pregnancy. Sometimes, the increased movement in the joint can cause pain in the pelvic area. To get some relief, try to avoid prolonged standing and heavy lifting. Exercises for the abdomen and pelvic muscles also can help.

Constipation

If you didn't have constipation earlier in your pregnancy, you most likely will have it now, in the later stages. Constipation occurs when you have infrequent bowel movements with stools that are firm or hard to pass. It can occur for many reasons. High levels of **_progesterone_** may slow digestion. Constipation can be aggravated by iron supplements. Toward the end of pregnancy, the weight of the uterus puts pressure on your **_rectum_**, adding to the problem.

Although there is no miracle cure for constipation, the following tips may help:

- Drink plenty of liquids, especially water and prune juice or other fruit juices.

- Eat high-fiber foods, such as fruits, vegetables, beans, whole-grain bread, and bran cereal.

- Walk or do another safe exercise every day to help your *digestive system*.

- Ask your health care provider about taking a bulk-forming agent. These products absorb water and add moisture to the stool to make it easier to pass. If you do take these agents, you need to drink plenty of liquids. Also, remember that you should not take any laxatives without your health care provider's permission.

You also may find that frequent, smaller meals are easier to digest than larger, less frequent meals. Experiment to see what works best for you.

Braxton Hicks Contractions

As early as the second trimester, many women experience Braxton Hicks contractions. Sometimes Braxton Hicks contractions are very mild. They can barely be felt or feel like a slight tightness in your abdomen. Other times, they can be painful. These contractions help your body gear up for birth but do not open the cervix. Braxton Hicks contractions often occur in the afternoon or evening, after physical activity, or after *sexual intercourse*. They are more likely to occur when you are tired or dehydrated, so be sure to drink plenty of fluids to stay hydrated. Braxton Hicks contractions tend to occur more often and become stronger as your due date draws near.

❱ Nutrition

If constipation is a problem for you, you may want to increase your intake of water and fiber. If you are concerned or just curious about whether you are on track for a healthy weight gain, a graph showing the average weight gain by week of pregnancy is included on p. 122, as well as advice for how to handle those well-meaning comments about your weight.

Focus on Water and Fiber

Getting enough water and fiber in your diet are the keys to avoiding or relieving constipation. But water and fiber are useful in other ways. Although most of us don't think water is a nutrient, it is actually an important one that we can't live without. Water performs the following functions:

- Allows nutrients and waste products to circulate within and out of the body
- Aids digestion
- Helps form *amniotic fluid* around the baby

Month
7

While you're pregnant, it's important to drink water throughout the day—not just when you're thirsty. A good goal is to aim for drinking six to eight 8-ounce cups a day.

Fiber also is known as roughage and is found mostly in fruits, vegetables, whole grains, beans, and nuts and seeds. In addition to its well-known benefit of helping with constipation, fiber also can lower your risk of **diabetes mellitus** and heart disease. You should get about 25 grams of fiber in your diet each day. Good sources of fiber are raspberries, apples, bananas, whole-wheat pasta, split peas, and lentils.

A word of caution: if you have not been eating a high-fiber diet and you suddenly introduce lots of high-fiber foods, you may experience gas and bloating as your body adjusts to the increased fiber intake. It's best to introduce high-fiber foods gradually. If you have not been getting your 25 grams a day, increase the amount of grams you take in slightly each day. Remember to drink lots of water as you increase your fiber intake.

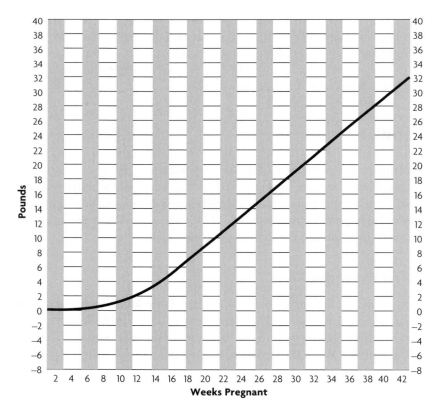

Weight gain during pregnancy. This graph shows how much weight a woman of normal weight should gain throughout pregnancy. Copyright 2009 March of Dimes.

Weight Gain

It is not uncommon for other people to comment on how much weight you have (or haven't) gained. These comments may make you feel that you aren't gaining weight the way you should, and you may become worried or upset. To cope with the comments, first understand that your pregnancy and your weight are your private concerns. A well-timed reply, such as "Thank you for your concern" or "I don't feel comfortable discussing my weight with you," can let your questioner know that his or her comments are off-limits. If you're concerned about your weight, talk to your health care provider. By this stage in your pregnancy, if you have been gaining weight too quickly or too slowly, your health care provider probably has addressed the issue with you already. If not, bring up the issue yourself. The graph on the previous page shows the average weight gain that should take place throughout pregnancy.

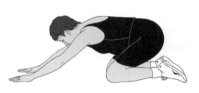

▶ Exercise

This month's exercises focus on helping you ease some of the aches and pains that you may be feeling this month.

Exercise of the Month: Rocking Back Arch

This exercise stretches and strengthens the muscles of your back, hips, and abdomen:

1. Kneel on your hands and knees, with your weight distributed evenly and your back straight.

2. Rock back and forth for a count of five.

3. Return to the original position and curl your back up as far as you can. Repeat 5–10 times.

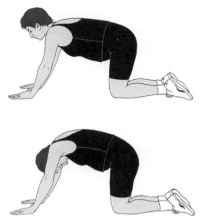

Rocking back arch. This exercise stretches and strengthens the muscles of your back, hips, and abdomen.

Month 7

Swimming

Swimming is good exercise because it uses both your arms and your legs. Although it is a low-impact activity, swimming has good cardiovascular benefits and lets you feel weightless in the water, despite the extra pounds you're carrying. Another good thing about swimming is that it keeps you cool. It also poses a very low risk of injury. Many pregnant women use swimming as a way to exercise right up until their last month.

▶ Healthy Decisions

As your due date nears, you will need to make decisions about many different issues. This month, you may want to concentrate on your birth experience, including whether you would like to use a doula. Another issue to think about this month is whether you will want to save the baby's cord blood. If you decide that you would like to, keep in mind that you need to let your health care provider know at least 8 weeks in advance of your due date.

Doulas

As you and your pregnancy partner discuss the role he or she will have during your labor, you may want to consider hiring a professional labor assistant, or doula. The main role of these trained labor coaches is to help you during childbirth and the postpartum period. They also provide you and your partner with emotional support. Doulas don't have medical training, however, and they don't replace the doctors and nurses caring for you in the hospital.

If you're interested in hiring a doula, ask your health care provider or the instructor of your childbirth class whether they can recommend a few for you to choose from. Ask friends and family members as well. You can also try the association of doulas, DONA International, which has an online locator service (see Resources). Most health insurance plans do not cover doula expenses. Doulas charge different rates for their services, so be sure to ask about their fees.

Birth Plan

Some childbirth education classes will help you draft a birth plan, a written outline of what you would like to happen during labor and delivery. A birth plan might include the setting you want to deliver in, the people you want to have with you, and whether you plan to use pain medications. A birth plan is useful to help your health care provider and labor nurses be aware of your wishes for your labor and delivery.

Keep in mind, though, that having a birth plan does not guarantee that your labor and delivery will go according to that plan. Changes may need to be made based on unexpected events that arise or how your labor is progressing. Remember that you and your health care provider have a common goal: the safest possible delivery for you and your baby. A birth plan is a great starting point, but you should be prepared for alterations as the circumstances dictate.

It's a good idea to go over your plan with your health care provider well before your due date. Your health care provider can advise you about how your plan fits with his or her policies and practice, as well as the hospital's resources and policies. Not every hospital or birthing center can accommodate every request. Nevertheless, a plan can help you make your wishes clear, and discussion about your expectations up front can help reduce surprises and disappointments later.

When writing your birth plan, think about how you would like labor and delivery to proceed. What things do you want during labor and delivery? What would enhance the experience for you? What would make you more comfortable? A sample form that you can use to create your own birth plan is provided on pages 126–127. A separate section is provided for your baby's care that you can give to the baby care staff members. Here are some additional pointers:

- Keep it short.
- Bring two or three copies to the hospital or birth center.
- Don't be surprised if your own wishes change once you are in labor. Give yourself permission to change your plan.

Don't think that you need to have a birth plan before you have your baby. It's not a requirement. If the idea of drawing up a plan doesn't appeal to you, that's perfectly OK.

Cord Blood Banking

Cord blood is blood from the baby that is left in the **umbilical cord** and **placenta** after birth. It contains **cells** called hematopoietic (blood-forming) stem cells. Stem cells can be used to treat some diseases, such as disorders of the blood, **immune system**, and **metabolism**. They also are used to offset the effects that cancer treatments have on the immune system. Other uses are being studied. It's now possible to collect some of this cord blood after birth

Month 7

Birth Plan

Name: _____

Health care provider's name: _____

Your baby's health care provider's name: _____

Type of childbirth education: _____

Labor (Choose as many you wish)
❑   I would like to be able to move around as I wish during labor.
❑   I would like to be able to drink fluids during labor.

I prefer:
❑   An intravenous (IV) line for fluids and medications
❑   A heparin or saline lock (this device provides access to a vein but is not hooked up to a fluid bag)
❑   I don't have a preference

I would like the following people present with me during labor:

_____

It's OK_____ not OK_____ for people in training (medical students, residents, etc) to be present during labor and delivery.

I would like to try the following options if they are available (choose as many as you wish):
❑   A birthing ball
❑   A birthing stool
❑   A birthing chair
❑   A squat bar
❑   A warm shower or bath during labor (not during delivery)

Anesthesia Options (Choose one):
❑   I do not want anesthesia offered to me during labor unless I specifically request it.
❑   I would like anesthesia. Please discuss the options with me.
❑   I do not know whether I want anesthesia. Please discuss the options with me.

Delivery
I would like the following people present with me during delivery:

_____

❑   Unless it needs to be done to ensure the safety of the baby, I would prefer not to have an episiotomy.
❑   I have made prior arrangements for storing umbilical cord blood.

Birth plan. Feel free to make a copy of this plan and to check off your preferences. Remember that it's a good idea to discuss your birth plan with your health care provider well before your due date.

For a vaginal birth, I would like (Choose as many as you wish):

❏ To use a mirror to see the baby's birth
❏ My labor coach to help support me during the pushing stage
❏ For the room to be as quiet as possible
❏ For one of my support persons to cut the umbilical cord
❏ For the lights to be dimmed
❏ To be able to have one of my support persons take a video or pictures of the birth. (Note: some hospitals have policies that prohibit videotaping or taking pictures; also, if it is allowed, the photographer needs to be positioned in a way that does not interfere with performing medical care.)
❏ For my baby to be put directly onto my abdomen immediately after delivery
❏ To begin breastfeeding my baby as soon as possible after birth

In the event of a cesarean delivery, I would like the following person to be present with me: _____

❏ I would like to see my baby before he or she is given eye drops.
❏ I would like one of my support persons to hold the baby after delivery if I am not able to.
❏ I would like one of my support persons to accompany my baby to the nursery.

Baby Care Plan

Feeding the Baby

I would like to (Check one):
❏ Breastfeed exclusively
❏ Bottle-feed
❏ Combine breastfeeding and bottle-feeding

It's OK to offer my baby (Check as many as you wish):
❏ A pacifier
❏ Sugar water
❏ Formula
❏ None of the above

Nursery and Rooming In

I would like my baby to stay (Check one):
❏ In my room with me at all times
❏ In my room with me except when I am asleep
❏ In the nursery but be brought to me for feedings
❏ I don't know yet; I will decide after the birth

Circumcision

❏ If my baby is a boy, I would like my baby circumcised at the hospital or birthing center.

Month 7

and store it in case it's needed by your baby or a family member in the future. Before you make a decision about banking your baby's cord blood, it's important to get all of the facts.

Currently, only a few diseases can be treated with the stem cells from cord blood. The chance that cord blood stem cells will be needed to treat your child or a relative is very low—about 1 in 2,700. However, research is being done to find new uses. Research also may uncover new ways of treating disease that do not involve stem cells.

There also are limitations to how your baby's stem cells can be used. If a baby is born with a genetic disease, the stem cells from the cord blood cannot be used for treatment because they will have the same *genes* that cause the disorder. A child's stem cells cannot be used to treat that child's leukemia, a cancer of the blood. However, stem cells from a healthy child can be used like any other donated organ to treat another child's leukemia. Careful matching of the recipient and donor are done to make sure that the stem cells will work.

Cord blood is kept in one of two types of banks: public or private. Public cord blood banks operate like blood banks. Cord blood is collected for later use by anyone who needs it. The stem cells in the donated cord blood can be used by any person who "matches." There is no fee for storing cord blood in a public bank. Donors must be screened before birth. This screening entails a detailed medical history of the mother and father and their families. Listed are some factors that rule out donating to public banks:

- Travel to certain countries
- Exposure to some vaccines
- Use of illegal drugs
- High-risk sexual behavior
- History of cancer on either side of the family
- Mother or father who were adopted

Many people do not pass the screening required for a public bank. A limited number of hospitals participate in the public cord blood banking option. To find out more about public banks, visit the National Marrow Donor Program web site (see Resources).

The other storage choice is a private bank, which charges a yearly fee. Private banks store cord blood for "directed donation." The blood is stored for use in treating only your baby or relatives.

Whether to donate or store cord blood is up to you. You have three choices:

1. Donate the cord blood to a public bank.
2. Store the cord blood in a private bank.
3. Do not donate or store cord blood.

If you decide to donate or store cord blood, you will need to choose a cord blood bank. Here are some questions to ask yourself when deciding on a bank:

• What will happen to the cord blood if a private bank goes out of business?
• Can you afford the yearly fee for a private bank?
• What are your options if results of the screening tests show you cannot donate to a public bank?

You must let your health care provider know far in advance of your due date (preferably 2 months) if you want to collect and store your baby's cord blood. If you have chosen a private bank, you will need to arrange for the collection equipment to be sent to your health care provider. Also, there usually is a fee charged by your health care provider for collecting cord blood. Often, this fee is not covered by insurance.

Keep in mind that even if you have planned to donate or store cord blood, it may not be possible to collect the blood after delivery. For example, if the baby is born prematurely, there may not be enough cord blood for this purpose. If you have an infection, the cord blood may not be usable.

▶ Other Considerations

Depression and anxiety are serious conditions that can affect a woman's pregnancy. It's important to know the signs and symptoms and to talk to your health care provider if you think you may be experiencing any of them.

Depression, Anxiety, and Stress

For some women, *depression* can occur during a pregnancy or after delivery, even if she has no history of it. However, if you have had depression in the past, you are more likely to have it during pregnancy and after the baby is born.

The signs of depression can seem like the normal ups and downs of pregnancy. A blue mood now and then is normal. However, you may have depression if you are sad most of the time or have any of these symptoms for at least 2 weeks:

• Depressed mood most of the day, nearly every day
• Loss of interest in work or other activities
• Feeling guilty, hopeless, or worthless
• Sleeping more than normal or lying awake at night
• Loss of appetite or losing weight (or eating much more than normal and gaining weight)

Month
7

- Feeling very tired or without energy
- Having trouble paying attention and making decisions

Depression that is untreated during pregnancy may cause problems for you and your baby after delivery. For example, a woman who is depressed may have trouble eating or getting enough rest. She may be more likely to use drugs or alcohol or to smoke. For these reasons, it's important to tell your health care provider if you have any signs or symptoms of depression. Your health care provider also may ask you questions during your prenatal care visits to check whether you are at risk for this condition.

Treatment of depression may include medication and counseling. Support from your partner, family members, and friends also can be helpful. In addition to providing support, they can help you determine if your symptoms are worsening because you may not be the first to notice.

If an *antidepressant* is prescribed, your health care provider and you can determine which drug is best for your individual situation. As with any medication, the benefits of taking an antidepressant drug during pregnancy need to be weighed against the risks. Many studies of the safety of these drugs during pregnancy have been done. It is important for you to know what the evidence is about the particular drug that has been prescribed for you. Keep in mind, though, that not treating depression also can have negative effects on your developing baby.

Another problem that can affect pregnant women is anxiety and stress. Anxiety disorders are the most common psychiatric disorders in the United States—about 18% of all adults have an anxiety disorder. Pregnancy also can trigger a specific anxiety disorder called obsessive–compulsive disorder, or can make existing obsessive–compulsive disorder worse. Anxiety and stress have been associated with some pregnancy problems and a more difficult delivery. If you are experiencing anxiety and stress, tell your health care provider so that you can get the help you need. Treatment may include behavioral therapy to learn coping strategies and relaxation techniques, and sometimes medication.

▶ Prenatal Care Visits

During this month's prenatal care visit, your health care provider likely will track the baby's growth by measuring the fundal height again. It probably will measure between 25 centimeters and 28 centimeters, about equal to the number of weeks of your pregnancy.

Your health care provider will check your weight and blood pressure and may give you a blood test to check for *anemia*—when the blood has too few red blood cells, which can cause fatigue. In addition to checking you for anemia, you are likely to have the following tests:

- *Glucose challenge test*—This test measures your body's response to **glucose** (sugar) and is usually done between 24 weeks and 28 weeks to see whether you have **gestational diabetes**—a type of diabetes mellitus that develops only during pregnancy. The test is done in two steps: 1) you drink a sugary solution, and 2) 1 hour later, a blood sample is taken to measure your sugar level. If the test result is positive, more testing is needed to confirm the diagnosis. Some women who are at high risk for gestational diabetes are given this test earlier in pregnancy. If the earlier test result was negative, you may have a repeat test at 24–28 weeks.

- *Rh antibody screening*—In earlier prenatal care visits, your health care provider tested your blood to see if you are Rh negative or Rh positive. If you tested Rh negative then, you'll probably be tested for Rh **antibodies** this month. These antibodies may be harmful if your baby has Rh-positive blood because it can result in a problem known as Rh incompatibility (see Chapter 24, "Blood Type Incompatibility"). If the test result shows you are not producing antibodies, your health care provider will prescribe an **Rh immunoglobulin** shot to prevent antibodies from forming during your pregnancy.

▶ Special Concerns

Because preterm labor is such a serious issue, each of the remaining month-to-month chapters addresses its signs and symptoms. Other complications that can occur during this time are vaginal bleeding and amniotic fluid problems. Remember, though, that most women do not have any complications during pregnancy. But if you do have unusual signs and symptoms, it's best to see your health care provider right away so that any potential complication can be diagnosed and treated as soon as possible.

Preterm Labor

Preterm birth can happen if labor starts before the 37th week of pregnancy. If you notice any signs and symptoms of preterm labor, call your health care provider right away:

- Change in vaginal discharge (becomes watery, mucus-like, or bloody)

- Increase in amount of vaginal discharge
- Pelvic or lower-abdominal pressure
- Constant, low, dull backache
- Mild abdominal cramps that may feel like menstrual cramps, with or without diarrhea
- Regular or frequent contractions or uterine tightening, (four times every 20 minutes or eight times an hour for more than 1 hour) that are often painless
- Ruptured membranes (your water breaks—whether a gush or a trickle)

Keep in mind, though, that Braxton Hicks contractions may get stronger as your uterus grows. But if they come at regular intervals—four times every 20 minutes or eight times an hour for more than 1 hour—you should contact your health care provider.

Vaginal Bleeding

Vaginal bleeding in pregnancy can have many causes in the third trimester. Sometimes bleeding can become serious and require prompt treatment. You should report any bleeding to your health care provider so that the proper course of action can be taken.

Bleeding may be caused by something minor. Bleeding might occur if the cervix becomes inflamed, for instance. However, some bleeding can be severe and may pose a threat to you or the baby. Heavy vaginal bleeding can suggest a problem with the placenta. The most common problems are *placenta previa* and *placental abruption*. In placenta previa, the placenta lies low in the uterus and covers all or part of the cervix, blocking the baby's exit from the uterus. This condition often causes painless vaginal bleeding. In placental abruption, the placenta starts to separate from the wall of the uterus before the baby is delivered. This condition often causes a constant severe pain in the abdomen; contractions, which may be mild or severe; and heavy bleeding. This condition is very serious and requires prompt attention.

With both placental abruption and placenta previa, the baby may need to be delivered early. If bleeding is severe, you may need a blood transfusion. *Cesarean delivery* may be necessary for either of these conditions. In some cases, the bleeding may stop. If it does, the pregnancy may continue normally, although you will need to be monitored closely.

Amniotic Fluid Problems

The amount of amniotic fluid in your uterus should increase until the beginning of your third trimester. After that, it gradually decreases until you give birth. Sometimes, though, a pregnant women may have too much or too little amniotic fluid, which can cause some discomfort and pain. In addition, abnormal amounts of amniotic fluid could be a sign of potential problems with the baby or the placenta.

During your regular prenatal care visits, your doctor will be monitoring the growth of your uterus. If he or she suspects a problem, you likely will need an additional ultrasound exam to assess the fetal size and amount of amniotic fluid.

YOUR QUESTIONS ANSWERED

What kind of birth control should I use after I have the baby? What if I want my tubes tied?

If you are not ready for another baby right away, talk to your health care provider about which method of birth control is good for you. What you were using before pregnancy might not be a good choice now. For example, birth control pills that contain *estrogen* affect your milk supply if you plan to breastfeed. Other methods that do not contain estrogen may be better if you are breastfeeding.

If you're considering *sterilization*, talk to your health care provider about your wishes ahead of time (see Chapter 12, "The Postpartum Period"). Tubal ligation, in which the fallopian tubes are cut, can be performed after delivery, often while you are still in the hospital. This procedure requires a small abdominal incision. The operation is easy to do after birth because the *fallopian tubes* are easy to access at this time. Another type of sterilization, called hysteroscopic sterilization, can be performed 3 months after childbirth. This method involves inserting an instrument called a hysteroscope into the uterus though the *vagina* and placing a small device into each fallopian tube. The devices cause scar tissue to form, which blocks the fallopian tubes and prevents the *egg* from being fertilized. Because it takes up to 3 months for the scar tissue to completely block the fallopian tubes, you are not immediately sterile after this procedure, and you must use another form of birth control during this time. A procedure called a *hysterosalpingography* usually is performed at the 3-month mark to confirm that the tubes are blocked.

Month
7

You should not have sterilization if you have any doubts about having another child. Sterilization is intended to be permanent. If you are sure, you may want to talk with your partner about **vasectomy**, which is equally effective and not as major a surgery as tubal ligation. If you are not sure, there are many forms of birth control that you can use that provide long-term, but reversible, protection against pregnancy. These forms include the intrauterine device and the injectable contraceptive. Make sure you explore all of the options so that you know what's available and what would best suit your needs.

Is breastfeeding really the best way to feed my baby?

Yes. Although there are a few exceptions (for example, if you are infected with **human immunodeficiency virus [HIV]**), breastfeeding is by far the best way to feed your baby. Breast milk contains all of the nutrients to nourish your baby fully. It contains antibodies that help your baby's immune system fight off illnesses. The protein and fat in breast milk are better used by the baby's body than the protein and fat in formula. Babies who are breastfed have less gas, fewer feeding problems, and often less constipation than those given formulas. They also are at lower risk for **sudden infant death syndrome**. But breastfeeding isn't just good for babies; it's good for mothers too. It's convenient, cheaper than formula, and always available. Breastfeeding burns calories, helping you lose those extra pounds you gained during pregnancy. By releasing the hormone **oxytocin**, breastfeeding helps your uterus contract and return to its normal size more quickly. It also may lower your risk of **osteoporosis**. The American Academy of Pediatrics and the American College of Obstetricians and Gynecologists recommend exclusive breastfeeding for at least the first 6 months of life. Breastfeeding can continue up to 1 year of age or for as long as a mom and her baby want.

What is vitamin D deficiency? How can I prevent it?

Vitamin D deficiency happens when a person does not get enough of the vitamin in her daily diet. It has long been known that vitamin D is crucial for healthy bones. Some research also suggests that vitamin D may play a role in preventing certain types of cancer and **autoimmune disorders**. It is recommended that pregnant women get 200 international units of vitamin D in their diet daily (the same as nonpregnant women). Although vitamin D can be made in the body through exposure to sunlight, most people do not get enough vitamin D through sunlight exposure alone. Food sources of vitamin D include fortified milk; fatty fish, such as salmon and mackerel;

and fish liver oils. If your health care provider suspects that you may be vitamin D deficient, a test can be done to measure the levels in your body. Vitamin D supplements may be recommended if your levels are too low.

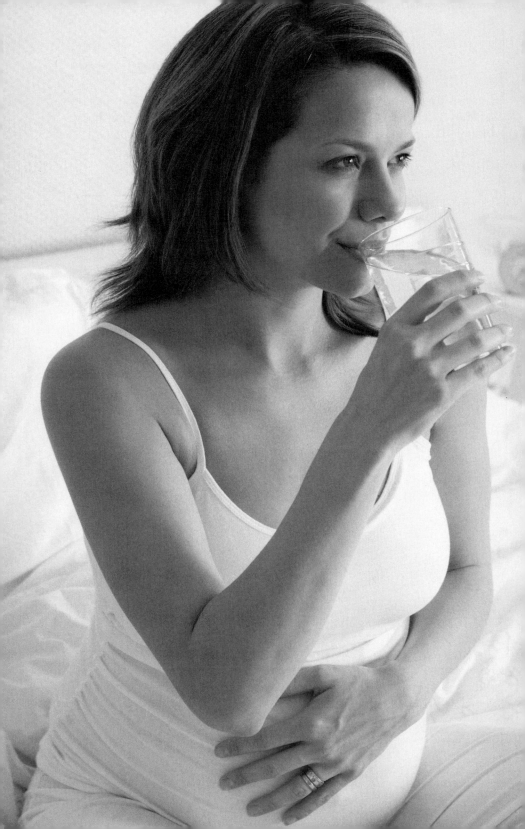

Chapter 7

Month 8
(Weeks 29–32)

YOUR GROWING BABY

Week 29

With her major development finished, the baby gains weight very quickly. During the last 2½ months of pregnancy, one half of the baby's weight at birth will be added. Your baby is going to need plenty of nutrients to complete her growth.

Week 30

This week, the fine hair that covered the baby's body *(lanugo)* begins to disappear. Some babies, however, never fully rid themselves of lanugo and are born with patches of it on their shoulders, back, and ears. Meanwhile, the hair on the baby's head starts to grow and thicken. Some babies are born with a full head of hair, although it normally is lost within the first 6 months of life.

Week 31

The baby's brain is growing and developing rapidly. Parts of the brain can now control the body's temperature too, and she is not just relying on the temperature of the ***amniotic fluid***. The bones harden, but the skull remains soft and flexible.

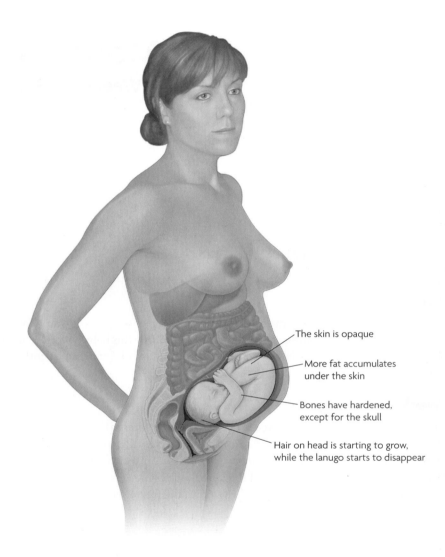

The skin is opaque

More fat accumulates under the skin

Bones have hardened, except for the skull

Hair on head is starting to grow, while the lanugo starts to disappear

Mother and baby: Weeks 29–32. With major development now complete, your baby will put on weight rapidly in the last 2 months.

Week 32

More fat is accumulating under the skin, which changes the skin from being "see-through" to opaque. The baby is about 18 inches long and weighs about 5 pounds.

YOUR PREGNANCY

▶ Your Changing Body

You're reaching the homestretch of your pregnancy now. You are probably excited but anxious as well. In these last weeks, your body is working hard to help your baby fully develop. As a result, you may find that you tire more easily, just as you did during the first trimester.

▶ Discomforts and How to Manage Them

By this month, your *uterus* has expanded to midway between your breasts and navel. The size of your uterus may now be causing some unpleasant side effects.

Shortness of Breath

In these later weeks of pregnancy, you may start to experience shortness of breath from time to time. Your uterus is now starting to take up more room in your abdomen, pressing the stomach and the diaphragm (a flat, strong muscle that aids in breathing) up towards the lungs. Although you may feel short of breath, your baby is still getting enough oxygen. To help breathe easier, move more slowly, and sit or stand up straight to give your lungs more room to expand. If there is a major change in your breathing or if you have a cough or chest pain, call your health care provider right away.

Hemorrhoids

Pregnant women often have hemorrhoids—painful, itchy varicose veins in the rectal area. The main causes of hemorrhoids are the extra blood flow in the pelvic area and the pressure that the growing uterus puts on *veins* in

Month 8

the lower body. Constipation can make hemorrhoids worse because straining during bowel movements traps more blood in the veins.

Hemorrhoids often improve after the baby is born. Talk to your doctor about using over-the-counter creams and suppositories. You also can try these tips for relief (or to avoid the problem in the first place):

- Eat a high-fiber diet and drink plenty of liquids.

- Keep your weight gain within the limits your doctor suggests. Extra pounds can make hemorrhoids worse.

- Sitting for a long time puts pressure on the veins in your pelvic area. Get up and move around to shift the weight of your uterus off these veins.

- If you do get hemorrhoids, apply an ice pack or witch hazel pads to the area to relieve pain and reduce swelling.

- Try soaking in a warm (not hot) tub a few times a day.

Varicose Veins and Leg Swelling

The weight of your uterus pressing down on a major vein called the inferior vena cava can slow blood flow from your lower body. The result may be sore, itchy, blue bulges on your legs called varicose veins. These veins also can appear near your *vagina*, *vulva*, and *rectum* (see "Hemorrhoids"). In most cases, varicose veins do not cause significant problems and are more of a cosmetic issue.

Varicose veins are more likely to occur if this isn't your first pregnancy. They also tend to run in families. Although there is nothing you can do to prevent varicose veins, there are ways to relieve the swelling and soreness and perhaps help stop them from getting worse:

- If you must sit or stand for long periods, be sure to move around often.
- Don't sit with your legs crossed.
- Prop up your legs—on a couch, chair, or footstool—as often as you can.
- Wear support hose that do not constrict at the thigh or knee.
- Don't wear stockings or socks that have a tight band of elastic around the legs.

Leg Cramps

Cramps in the lower legs are another common symptom in the second and third trimesters. During late pregnancy, you may experience sharp, painful cramps in your calf that can awaken you from a sound sleep. It was once thought these cramps were caused by not getting enough calcium or potassium in your diet, but experts no longer think these deficiencies are the reason. No one is sure what actually causes leg cramps. If you're bothered by them, the following tips may help:

* Stretch your legs before going to bed.
* If you experience a cramp, flex your foot, which often brings immediate relief.
* Massage the calf in long downward strokes.

Fatigue

Most women find that they are more tired during the third trimester than they were during the second trimester. Feeling tired is normal at this time. Your body is working hard to support a developing new life, and your increasing size may make it difficult for you to find a comfortable sleeping position. Try to get as much rest as you can, even if it's a short 15-minute nap during the day. Continue to exercise and eat healthily because both will help boost your energy.

Itchy Skin

Some women find that their skin is very itchy during pregnancy, especially the skin over the expanding abdomen and breasts. If you're bothered by itchy skin, drink plenty of water to keep your skin hydrated. Applying a moisturizer to your skin in the morning and at night also can help. Adding cornstarch to your bath water may help as well. If, however, your itching is severe or you have a rash, let your health care provider know. Some skin conditions that can occur during pregnancy should be treated.

▶ Nutrition

It's important to stick to a healthy diet in these last weeks of pregnancy. Eating well will give you more energy and will ensure that your baby is getting the nutrients she needs.

Focus on Calcium

Calcium is a mineral that is used to build your baby's bones and teeth. You should get 1,000 milligrams of calcium each day (teenagers younger than 19 years need 1,300 milligrams a day). During pregnancy, if not enough calcium is present in the diet, the calcium that is needed for the baby's development is taken from the mother's bones. Dairy products are great sources of calcium,

Month 8

as are dark, leafy greens; fortified cereals, breads, and juices; almonds; and sesame seeds. Your health care provider also may recommend calcium supplements if your diet does not contain enough calcium.

◗ Exercise

Even if you are feeling more tired, you should still try to keep up with your exercise routine. Monitor how you feel, and stop if you are out of breath or feeling winded. You may find that learning some relaxation techniques will be helpful as you count down these final weeks.

Exercise of the Month: Leg Lift Crawl

This exercise strengthens the muscles of your back and abdomen:

1. Kneel on your hands and knees, with your weight evenly distributed and your arms straight (hands under your shoulders).

2. Lift your left knee and bring it toward your elbow.

3. Straighten your leg back. Do not swing your leg or arch your back. Repeat on both sides 5–10 times.

Relaxation Techniques

Relaxation techniques are a great way to help reduce the stress of pregnancy and any anxiety you have about your upcoming childbirth. It's important to do your best to stay calm and stress-free so that you can conserve energy in these coming weeks. Learning some basic relaxation techniques can improve your health in many ways:

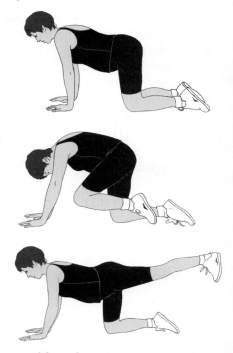

- Slows your heart rate
- Lowers your blood pressure
- Slows your breathing rate
- Reduces your need for oxygen

Leg lift crawl. This exercise strengthens the muscles of your back and abdomen.

- Increases blood flow to major muscles
- Reduces muscle tension

Listening to music or getting a massage are two easy ways to relax. Try burning a scented candle that has a calming aroma, such as lavender, and just closing your eyes and resting. You may want to find a class in your neighborhood or buy or rent a DVD that teaches the relaxation techniques of yoga, tai chi, or meditation. Whatever you do, just make sure it calms you for some part of your day, whenever you're feeling most stressed.

▶ Healthy Decisions

Planning and making decisions may seem like all you and your partner are doing these days, but rest assured, planning can help make your life less stressful. If you have a boy, you and your partner will have to decide whether to circumcise him. You also need to decide what kind of child care you will use if you are going to work outside the home after the baby is born. Just as you're thinking about your child's day care arrangements, it's important to start getting ready for your labor and delivery too.

Circumcision for Boys

Circumcision means cutting away the *foreskin*—a layer of skin that covers the tip of the penis. An anesthetic will be used to lessen the pain. Circumcision usually is done soon after birth and before the baby leaves the hospital.

For some parents, circumcision is a religious ritual. It also can be a matter of family tradition or personal hygiene. Studies show that there are some medical benefits of circumcision, including a slightly decreased risk of urinary tract infections during the first year of life; a lower risk of getting cancer of the penis (although this cancer is very rare to begin with); a slightly lower risk of getting a sexually transmitted disease, including infection with *human immunodeficiency virus (HIV)*, the virus that causes *acquired immunodeficiency syndrome (AIDS)*; and a lower risk of infection of the foreskin. However, these medical reasons are not sufficient to recommend circumcision for all infant boys, and the American Academy of Pediatrics believes the decision is up to the parents. If you want your son circumcised, tell your health care provider ahead of time. Also, check with your insurance provider because the procedure may not be covered.

Month 8

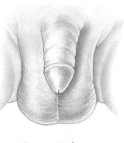
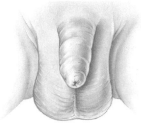

Circumcised penis
Uncircumcised penis

Circumcision. In this procedure, the baby's foreskin is removed.

Child Care

If you are planning to return to work after having the baby, finding good child care will be a top priority for you and your partner. Give yourself some time to figure out which option is best for your family. You may want to arrange child care during these final weeks before the baby arrives. Ask around for recommendations for child care; your friends, neighbors, and co-workers are all good sources of information.

There are three basic child care options: 1) care in your home, 2) care in a caregiver's home, or 3) care in a child care center. If you want to hire someone to care for your baby in your home (such as a nanny or au pair), contact agencies that focus on child care placements. Keep in mind that this type of care can be very costly. To cut costs, some parents share a caregiver with another family. The caregiver in these "share-care" setups is paid to watch two babies in one family's home.

A less costly option is having a relative or a licensed provider care for your baby in their home. In most cases, these caregivers watch more than one child.

Child care centers are yet another option. This type of setting may take care of many groups of children of all different ages. Some accept babies as young as 6 weeks, and some do not take infants until they are out of diapers, so be sure to ask questions while you're doing your research.

As you and your partner begin your search, be prepared to ask prospective child care providers some very detailed questions (see the box).

Getting Ready for Delivery

There is a lot you can do to help delivery go as smoothly as possible. You can start by practicing with your partner all the exercises you learned in childbirth classes, such as breathing, relaxation, stretching, or meditation. You

Finding Good Child Care

Getting answers to the following questions can help you find a child care provider who is right for you and your baby:

1. **Gather the facts.** Make a list of child care providers, family child care homes, and child care centers in your area. Then find out the following:

   Where is it located? _____

   Does the provider care for infants? _____

   What hours are available? _____

   Is it open year-round (do they work during holidays)? _____

   What's the cost for care? _____

2. **Check it out.** If you are thinking about family home or center care, visit more than once. Make an appointment the first time. If you like what you see during this visit, drop in the next time. (If drop-in visits aren't allowed, keep looking.) Find out:

   Is the facility clean, safe, and well-equipped? _____

   Are there enough care providers (one adult per three to four infants, four to five toddlers, or six to nine preschoolers)? _____

   Are the caregivers attentive and loving? _____

   Do the children seem happy and well cared for? _____

   What's a normal day like? _____

   What's served at meal and snack times? _____

3. **Set up an interview.** Schedule a chat with a family child care provider, nanny, or center director. Have your baby with you and note how the caregiver responds to him or her. Ask the following:

   What experience and training do the care providers have? _____

   _____

   Have they cared for infants before? _____

   For an individual caregiver, why did she leave her last job? _____

   _____

   For a center, what's the staff turnover rate? _____

   Do the care providers have training in first aid and CPR? _____

   Are they willing to give your child prescribed medications? _____

   What plans are in place in case of a medical emergency? _____

   Is the home or center licensed, or is the caregiver certified? _____

   Can you visit during the day to breastfeed? _____

Finding Good Child Care, *contined*

4. **Check credentials.** Never leave your baby with someone until you have checked out his or her background. Ask for the following:
   - The document showing that the home or center is licensed or registered or that the caregiver is certified; call the licensing agency to ask about any complaints.
   - Written policies on philosophy, procedures, or discipline
   - References from other parents who have used the caregiver, home, or center; call at least three other parents

5. **Try it out.** Once you have chosen a caregiver, do a few "practice" runs before you go back to work. This way, if anything strikes you as being "off," you still have time to keep looking. It also will help you and your baby get used to the setup before your maternity leave ends.

also can have the answers to the following questions well before your delivery day:

- What number do I call when I go into labor?
- Should I go straight to the hospital or call the doctor's office first?
- At what point in my labor should I leave for the hospital?
- Have I filled out all the paperwork needed to begin my maternity leave and collect disability pay?
- Do I need to register at the hospital before I check in for delivery? If so, have I done this?
- When can family and guests visit me after I have the baby?
- What friends and family do we need to spread the news to once the baby arrives?
- Do we have their phone numbers or e-mail addresses?
- Have I purchased an infant car seat, and do I know how to install it?
- Have I made arrangements for care of my other children and pets while I'm in the hospital?

▶ Other Considerations

Women now have many choices about childbirth preparation methods. There is something out there for everyone. This month also is a good time to familiarize yourself with your anesthesia options, and a hospital tour may make you feel more secure as your due date approaches.

Childbirth Preparation Methods

Childbirth preparation is a means of coping with pain and reducing the discomfort associated with labor and delivery. Childbirth preparation classes are available that teach these various techniques. The most common methods of preparation—Lamaze, Bradley, and Read—are based on the theory that much of the pain of childbirth is caused by fear and tension. Although specific techniques vary, childbirth methods seek to relieve discomfort through the general principles of education, support, relaxation, paced breathing, and touch. Here is a brief description of some of these methods:

- *Lamaze*—The Lamaze method of childbirth was invented in the 1950s by French obstetrician Dr. Fernand Lamaze. This method is based on the idea that a woman's inner wisdom guides her through childbirth. Lamaze childbirth education helps women gain confidence in their bodies and learn to make informed decisions about pregnancy, birth, breastfeeding, and parenting. To learn more about this method, go to the Lamaze International web site (see Resources).

- *Bradley*—The Bradley method views childbirth as a natural process and is based on the belief that a healthy pregnancy and birth can be achieved through education, preparation, and support from a childbirth coach. This method involves the active participation of the mother and her coach during the labor process and teaches a variety of relaxation techniques. Information about the Bradley method is available online (see Resources).

- *Read*—One of the first methods to introduce the concept of prepared childbirth, the Read method seeks to eliminate fear and anxiety by educating mothers and coaches about labor and delivery. The Read method is explained in the book *Childbirth Without Fear,* written by its founder, Dr. Grantly Dick-Read.

- *Hypnobirthing*—This method teaches relaxation and self-hypnosis techniques. Information regarding this method is available online (see Resources). The instructors have gone through extensive training. The goal is to teach women how to harness the body's natural painkilling chemicals —endorphins—to achieve a natural and fear-free childbirth.

With all of the choices available, you're likely to find something that appeals to you and your individual beliefs. As you consider your options, keep the following tips in mind:

Month 8

- Contact the instructor, if possible. The instructor's approach and knowledge are important factors in determining whether the class is right for you. Call or e-mail the instructor to ask questions and get a sense of how the class is taught.

- Find out the location and schedule. Is the class offered nearby? What is the schedule? How many weeks does it meet? You want to find a class that fits your lifestyle and schedule.

- Figure in the cost. Find out how much the class costs and what's included in the fee. Also, check whether your insurance policy covers all or part of the cost.

- How many people are in the class? Some classes are small and offer individual attention. Others are larger. Talk with your childbirth partner about whether a small or large class is more suitable for you and your needs.

Don't think, though, that you have to select a particular childbirth method. It's not a requirement for giving birth. Your nurses and health care provider will give you the instructions and information you need while you're at the hospital or birthing center.

Hospital Tour

Most hospitals offer tours of where you'll give birth, and it's a good idea to take advantage of this opportunity if it's available. In fact, if you're taking childbirth education classes at the hospital where you'll be giving birth, you'll probably get a tour at some point during the course. If it will be your first time at the hospital, going for a tour also will give you a chance to learn the quickest route there and where to park the car when it's time for the birth. During the tour is a good time to ask about the hospital's policies on whether your partner can be in the room during labor and delivery (even *cesarean deliveries*), whether your partner can stay overnight in the room with you and the baby, and whether your partner can take pictures or videos of the birth.

Pain Relief During Labor

You may want to start thinking about whether you would like pain relief during labor and delivery. You don't have to decide now, but it's a good idea to know your options. Even if you do make a decision now, you may change your mind once you're in labor.

Each woman's labor is unique. The amount of pain a woman feels during labor may differ from that felt by another woman. Pain depends on many factors, such as the size and position of the baby, the strength of contractions, and how you handle pain.

Some women take classes to learn breathing and relaxation techniques to help cope with pain during childbirth. Others may find it helpful to use these techniques along with pain medications.

There are two types of pain-relieving drugs—*analgesics* and *anesthetics*. Analgesics lessen the pain, while anesthetics block all pain and sensation. Some forms of anesthesia, such as general anesthesia, cause you to lose consciousness. Other forms, such as regional anesthesia, remove all feeling of pain from parts of the body while you stay conscious. General anesthesia usually is not used for vaginal births.

Not all hospitals are able to offer all types of pain relief medications. However, at most hospitals, an *anesthesiologist* will work with your health care team to help you choose the best method. See Chapter 10, "Labor and Delivery," for more discussion about pain relief during labor.

Bed Rest

Your health care provider may recommend bed rest during the late stages of your pregnancy. Bed rest often is recommended if you show signs of *preterm* labor, if you are having a multiple pregnancy, or if you have high blood pressure. However, there is no scientific evidence that bed rest helps alter the course of pregnancy.

If bed rest is recommended, talk to your health care provider about whether you need to stay in bed or whether you can do some forms of activity. If you get bored, use the time to write letters and make "to-do" lists for your partner or family to help with tasks that need to be done. Surround yourself with books, magazines, puzzles, your MP3 player, and a stack of DVDs—whatever it takes to help make the time in bed as pleasant as possible.

▶ Prenatal Care Visits

During the third trimester, your health care provider will ask you to come in for more frequent checkups, usually every other week beginning at week 32 and every week beginning at week 36.

Like your earlier visits, your health care provider will check your weight and blood pressure and ask about any symptoms you may be experiencing.

Month
8

Your health care provider also will check your baby's size and heart rate. A vaginal exam may be done to check whether your *cervix* has started preparing for birth.

▶ Special Concerns

As in previous months, you should know the signs and symptoms of preterm labor. You should also be alert to the signs and symptoms of *premature rupture of membranes,* a condition that occurs in 1 out of 10 pregnancies.

Preterm Labor

Preterm labor is still a problem to watch out for during this month of pregnancy, but babies born now have a better outcome than those who are born earlier. If you notice any of the signs and symptoms of preterm labor (see Chapter 6), call your health care provider right away. Remember that *Braxton Hicks contractions* may start to intensify as you approach your due date. It's normal to have these contractions during the later stages of pregnancy. If they become regular or persist, that's a sign to contact your health care provider.

Premature Rupture of Membranes

In most cases, when your water breaks, it's followed by other signs of labor. When doctors refer to your water breaking, they are referring to the rupture of the *amniotic sac* that holds the amniotic fluid. When the membranes rupture when the pregnancy is at term but before labor begins, it is called premature rupture of membranes (PROM). When the membranes rupture before 37 weeks of pregnancy, it's called preterm PROM.

Call your health care provider if you have any leakage of fluid from your vagina. The health care provider will want to see you to evaluate if your membranes have ruptured. Other reasons for fluid leakage are *urine* leakage, cervical mucus, vaginal bleeding, or a vaginal infection. PROM is diagnosed on the basis of your medical history, physical exam results, and lab test results. It is confirmed when there is amniotic fluid in the vagina. Labor frequently starts after the membranes rupture. If it does not and the pregnancy is at term, labor is often induced. If the pregnancy is not at term, a decision needs to be made about whether to deliver the baby. More information about PROM can be found in Chapter 23, "Preterm Labor, Preterm Birth, and Premature Rupture of Membranes."

YOUR QUESTIONS ANSWERED

I had some leakage of amniotic fluid. My health care provider diagnosed premature rupture of membranes, but it seems to have stopped on its own. Is it OK for me to have sex?

No. Sex is not recommended if you have been diagnosed with premature rupture of membranes. It can increase the risk of infection and bring on labor.

Are there any particular signs or symptoms that should alert me to call my doctor?

In your eight month of pregnancy, you should be aware of the signs of pre-term labor and premature rupture of membranes and call your health care provider if you experience any of them. Also call if you have any vaginal bleeding, a fever, severe abdominal pain, or a severe headache. But again, it's always a good idea to be safe and cautious, so if you have any symptoms that cause you concern, don't hesitate to call your health care provider.

I am *lactose intolerant*. How can I get all the calcium I need if I can't eat dairy products?

Lactose intolerance is also known as lactase deficiency and means you cannot fully digest the milk sugar (lactose) in dairy products. Pregnant women with this condition still need to get the daily amount of calcium in their diet to nourish their baby's growing muscles and organs. These tips can help lessen the symptoms of lactose intolerance without limiting your calcium intake:

- Try different kinds of dairy products. Not all dairy products have the same amount of lactose. For example, hard cheeses such as Swiss or cheddar have small amounts of lactose and generally cause no symptoms.

- Buy lactose-free products, such as Lactaid. They contain all of the nutrients found in regular milk and dairy products.

- Get calcium from other foods. Good sources are pink canned salmon; almonds; calcium-fortified breads and juices; dark leafy greens like spinach, kale, and collard greens; and molasses.

Month
8

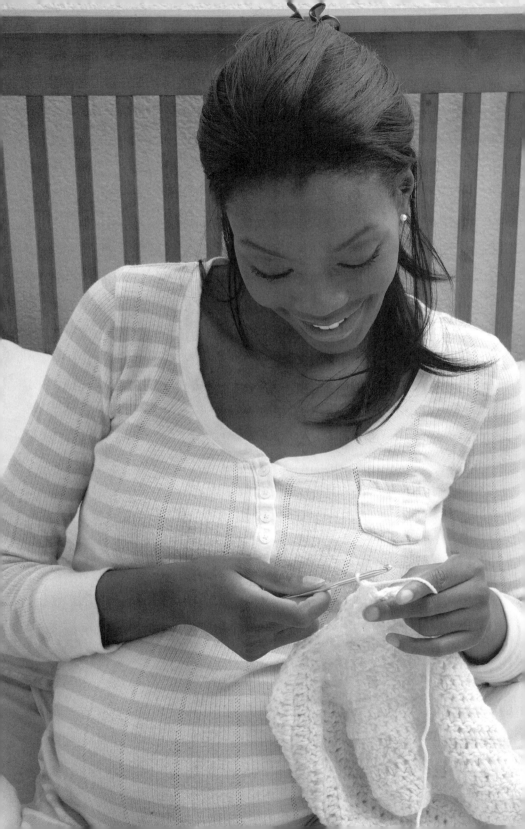

Chapter 8
Month 9
(Weeks 33–36)

YOUR GROWING BABY

Week 33

The baby is gaining weight more quickly—about ½ pound a week—as he gets ready for birth in a few weeks. He weighs about 5½ pounds and is about 20 inches long. Babies at this stage won't get too much longer than 20 inches but will add on weight.

Week 34

Your baby is developing definite sleeping patterns. His skin is less wrinkled because of the fat that's been added underneath.

Week 35

The lungs are now more mature and getting ready for the baby to breathe on his own at birth. The circulatory system is complete, and so is the musculoskeletal system.

Week 36

How big is the baby now? He's probably around 6 pounds and filling up all the space in the *amniotic sac*. There's not much room for rolling around and turning somersaults. You will continue to feel kicks and fetal movement.

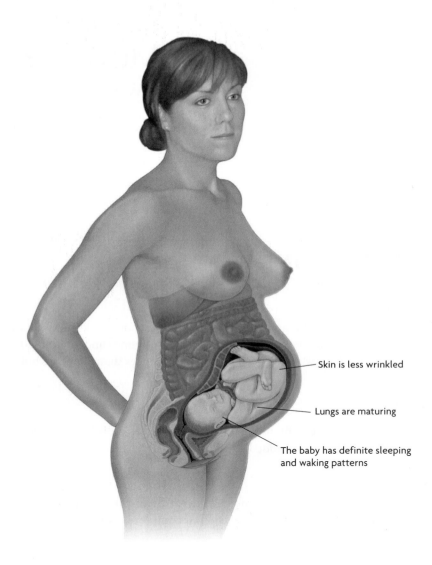

Skin is less wrinkled

Lungs are maturing

The baby has definite sleeping
and waking patterns

Mother and baby: Weeks 33–36. This month, your baby will most likely
gain about 2 pounds of weight but won't get much longer than 20 inches.

YOUR PREGNANCY

❱ Your Changing Body

Today starts the ninth month of pregnancy. It's probably a busy time for you as you prepare your life, your home, and your family to welcome the new baby.

❱ Discomforts and How to Manage Them

This month, the discomforts of pregnancy are probably at their peak. Remember to take good care of yourself and get plenty of rest during these last weeks.

Frequent Urination

In the final weeks of your pregnancy, you'll feel more pressure on your bladder as the baby moves deeper into your pelvis. You will urinate much more often during the day and may have to go several times during the night.

Some women also leak *urine* during these later weeks, especially when laughing, coughing, or sneezing. This, too, is caused by the baby pressing on your bladder. These problems will likely go away once you give birth.

Prelabor (Braxton Hicks Contractions)

As you near your due date, **Braxton Hicks contractions** may get stronger. You may even mistake them for labor. It's easy to be fooled by these prelabor contractions. If you have contractions, time them. Note how long it is from the start of one contraction to the start of the next. Keep a record for an hour and also jot down how your contractions feel. The time between contractions will help tell you if you are truly in labor. When it's true labor, your contractions will come at regular intervals, get closer together, and can last 30–90 seconds. The intensity of the contractions is also important. It's more likely to be true labor if you have trouble walking and talking during a contraction.

Even a doctor, midwife, or nurse can have a hard time telling prelabor from the real thing. He or she may need to observe you for a few hours to decide. A vaginal exam also will be done to see if your **cervix** is opening.

No matter what your watch says about the timing of contractions, it's better to be safe than sorry. If you think you may be in labor, call your health care provider.

Trouble Sleeping

It's normal for insomnia to return in these last few weeks of pregnancy. It's also normal for it to be almost impossible to find a comfortable position to sleep. Try not to worry about losing sleep. Make your bedroom as comfortable as possible, use as many pillows as you need to prop yourself up and get support, and get a few hours of rest whenever you can.

Leg Swelling and Pain

Most pregnant women have some swelling in their legs and feet. To relieve the swelling, stay off of your feet as much as you can. Prop your legs up on a pillow or use a footrest during the day. Comfortable, supportive shoes may help relieve some of the discomfort.

Pelvic Pressure

The baby will soon settle into position to get ready for birth, and you may feel him settling deeper into your pelvis. This sensation often is called "dropping," and it will cause some increased pressure in the pelvis, bladder, and hips. There is not much you can do about the pressure other than try to stay off your feet when you are most uncomfortable. Soaking in a warm bath may give some relief.

Numbness

If you have numbness or tingling in your hands, fingers, or toes, it is a normal reaction caused by your body's swelling tissues pressing on the nerves. In severe cases, you may develop carpal tunnel syndrome. Carpal tunnel syndrome is caused by the compression of a nerve within the carpal tunnel, a passageway of bones and ligaments in the wrist. These symptoms usually go away after you give birth and the tissues return to normal. However, if you have these symptoms, don't hesitate to mention them to your health care provider at the next prenatal care visit. Splints and resting the affected hand are typically used to treat these symptoms during pregnancy.

❯ Nutrition

Continue your healthy eating, and make sure you are drinking plenty of water. Your baby needs all the nutrients he can get in these last few weeks to fully mature and be ready for birth. You'll need the energy a healthy diet provides too.

Focus on Vitamin C

Getting the right daily amount of vitamin C is important for a healthy immune system as well as for building strong bones and muscles. During your pregnancy, you should get at least 85 milligrams of vitamin C each day (80 milligrams if you are younger than age 19 years). You can get the right amount in your daily prenatal vitamin supplement, but you can also find vitamin C in foods such as citrus fruits and juices, strawberries, broccoli, and tomatoes.

❯ Exercise

Keep up with your exercise this month. Go for walks and continue the strengthening and stretching exercises you learned early in your pregnancy. Don't forget, you can still do your yoga poses too. Yoga will help with your breathing exercises once labor begins. You can review with a yoga instructor about which poses are appropriate for late pregnancy.

Exercise of the Month: Upper Body Bends

This exercise strengthens the muscles of your back and torso:

1. Stand with your legs apart, knees bent slightly, with your hands on your hips.

2. Bend forward slowly, keeping your upper back straight until you feel the muscle stretch along your upper thigh. Repeat 10 times.

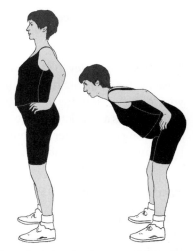

Upper body bends. This exercise strengthens the muscles of your back and torso.

❱ Healthy Decisions

There are many important decisions for you and your partner to make this month—from how you want to give birth to how to feed your baby.

Positions for Childbirth

By now you and your health care provider probably have discussed how you want to give birth—in a standard bed or whether you'd like to use some other positioning options that may be available at your hospital or birthing center:

- *Birthing bed*—A bed that can be adjusted to numerous positions for you, such as squatting, sitting on the end of the bed with your feet supported, or lying on your side.

- *Birthing chair*—A chair that has been especially designed to allow giving birth in a seated position.

- *Birthing stool*—A frame that stabilizes and supports you while you squat.

- *Birthing ball*—A large rubber ball that you can sit on during labor and allows you to rock back and forth on a soft surface.

- *Birthing pool or tub*—During labor, you get in a tub of water that is large enough for both you and your childbirth partner, if desired. It is not recommended to give birth in water. Many hospitals do not have a tub or pool, so be sure to check first if you are interested in this option.

There are pros and cons of each type of birthing position. Birthing stools and chairs allow you to take advantage of gravity as the baby descends through the birth canal. A disadvantage is that it may be difficult for the health care provider to assist with the birth. Giving birth in a bed may make it easier for your health care provider to provide assistance, but lying on your back or side doesn't allow gravity to do its work. Think about all of your options and ask lots of questions. Find out which options your hospital or birthing center offers. Often, women do not know how they want to give birth until they're in labor.

Your Baby's Hospital Stay

Your baby may stay in the nursery at the hospital, or you may have the option of having the baby with you at all times in your room (called "rooming in"). Rooming in is a good way to get to know your new baby. It's also the best way to get started breastfeeding. However, having the baby stay in the hospital

nursery may be a good choice as well, especially if you are exhaust
had a difficult labor. The baby will be brought to your room from the n
for feedings.

Packing for the Hospital

The last thing you want to be doing once labor starts is tossing items into a suitcase in a panic. To avoid this, pack your bag a few weeks before your due date. Leave it in a handy place, such as a hall closet or the trunk of your car.

You can't pack everything ahead of time—you will need some things in the meantime, such as your glasses and slippers (see the box). Make a list of these last-minute items that need to be packed before you leave for the hospital, and put the list in a place that will trigger your memory, such as on the refrigerator door.

Don't worry if you forget something. A friend or family member can bring you whatever you need. The hospital also may have some items, but you may be charged for them.

Feeding Your Baby

Deciding whether to breastfeed or bottle-feed your new baby is a personal decision that each new mother should make on her own. There are a few important facts that you need to know when making this decision. Most experts agree that breastfeeding is the best way to feed your baby. The American Academy of Pediatrics as well as the American College of Obstetricians and Gynecologists recommend exclusive breastfeeding for at least the first 6 months of life. Breastfeeding can continue up to 1 year of age (and beyond, if that's what you and your baby want).

Breastfeeding gives newborns the perfect food, with numerous advantages over baby formula. It also can help you lose weight quicker after giving birth. Breast milk is good for several reasons:

- It is always available.

- It is free.

- It contains active infection-fighting white blood cells and antibodies that give increased protection against infections in the first months of a baby's life, when these infections can be the most serious.

- It contains the perfect proportion of nutrients that your baby needs, including protein, carbohydrates, fats, and calcium.

/ant to Pack

_____ card, photo ID, and hospital registration forms

_____ age

_____ Lip balm

_____ An old nightgown or nightshirt (if you don't want to wear a hospital gown)

_____ A bathrobe, slippers, and socks

_____ Glasses, if you wear them (you may not be allowed to wear contact lenses)

_____ Lollipops or hard candies to keep your mouth moist

_____ An MP3 or CD player and some soothing music

_____ Camera

For your hospital stay:

_____ Two or three nightgowns (be sure the gowns open at the front if you plan to nurse)

_____ Two or three nursing bras and a dozen or so nursing pads

_____ Sanitary pads

_____ A few pairs of socks and panties

_____ Toiletries, such as toothbrush, toothpaste, and deodorant

_____ Contact lenses, if you wear them

_____ A notepad and pen

_____ Change for the vending machines

_____ Phone numbers of people you want to call after the birth

_____ Magazines or other reading material

For discharge from the hospital:

_____ A receiving blanket and clothes for your newborn to wear home

_____ Loose-fitting clothes for you to wear home

_____ Infant car seat

- It is easily digestible.

- It contains important fatty acids that promote brain development.

- It protects the baby against certain conditions, such as asthma, ear infections, and **obesity**, and lowers the risk of **sudden infant death syndrome.**

There are numerous advantages for the mom who breastfeeds as well. Women who breastfeed tend to lose weight more quickly after the birth. It also helps the **uterus** contract and return to its normal size more rapidly, which decreases postpartum bleeding. Breastfeeding reduces the risk of ovarian and breast cancer and also may reduce the risk of type 2 **diabetes mellitis** and **postpartum depression.**

Bottle-feeding is the other option for feeding your baby. Here is what you should know about bottle-feeding:

- Infant formulas have gotten better at matching the ingredients and their proportions to that of human milk. However, some babies need to try several formulas before the right one is found.

- It gives the mom some flexibility, because using the bottle allows more than one person to feed the baby (although this option is also possible with breast milk if you pump it into a bottle).

- It can be expensive. Remember that you will need to buy infant formula, nipples, and bottles.

- It's time-consuming. You will need to keep the bottles clean and sterilized so you always have a bottle ready at feeding time.

Chapter 14, "Feeding Your Baby," provides more detailed information about how to feed your baby. If you need more questions answered to help make a decision between breastfeeding or bottle-feeding, ask your health care provider. You also can go online to the La Leche League International web site. This organization aims to help mothers breastfeed worldwide (see Resources). The American Academy of Pediatrics also has extensive information about breastfeeding (see Resources).

▶ Other Considerations

Now is the time to shop for a car seat if you haven't done so already. Is the baby's room ready? Do you have all the clothes and supplies you'll need once the baby comes home? The last few weeks are always a busy time for new parents as they make sure they are prepared to bring the baby home from the hospital.

Preparing Your Home for the Baby

A trip to any baby supply retailer or a look at the many online baby supply web sites will give you plenty of ideas about what you'll need at home to get ready. Talk to other new moms as well to get an idea of what products they used and liked best.

This also is a great time for you and your partner to start lining up family and friends who will want to pitch in once the baby arrives. Don't be afraid to ask for help. And if anyone offers to help, don't be modest. You'll welcome the extra pair of hands once you're at home and spending some sleepless nights with the new baby. Make a list of some things you can use help with, such as the following tasks, and ask family and friends to take their pick:

• Cook a few meals and place them in the freezer for later.
• Go grocery shopping.
• Help with the laundry.
• Help out with your other children.
• Take care of family pets.

Remember that you may need help for at least a couple of weeks. Make sure that you have help lined up for the weeks ahead and not just the first couple of days after the baby comes home.

Buying a Car Seat

You will not be able to take the baby home from the hospital unless you have a car seat already secured in your car. By law, your baby must ride in a car seat at all times.

All infants should ride rear-facing in the back seat starting with their first ride home from the hospital. They should remain rear-facing until they have reached at least 1 year of age and weigh at least 20–22 pounds. Children should not ride in the front seat of a car until they are age 12 years because of the risk of injury associated with the passenger air bag inflating.

There are two types of rear-facing car safety seats: 1) infant-only seats and 2) convertible seats. An infant-only seat is for babies who weigh up to 20–22 pounds. Most infant-only seats are made to pop out of a base; that way you can carry the seat by its handle or place it in a special stroller. An infant-only seat must be replaced when your baby reaches 20–22 pounds. The other kind of seat, the convertible seat, isn't as portable as an infant-only seat, but it can be used for infants and toddlers who weigh up to 40 pounds.

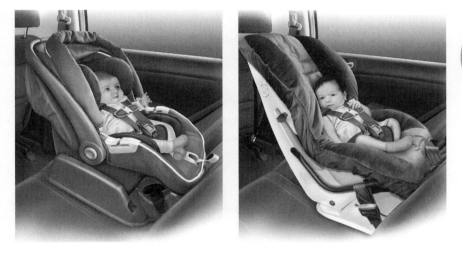

| Infant car seat | Convertible car seat |

Types of car seats. An infant car seat (*left*) is made for infants weighing up to 20–22 pounds. A convertible seat is for babies and toddlers weighing up to 40 pounds.

Many moms pass on baby supplies to new mothers once their own children no longer use them. Be careful, however, with used car seats. If you do borrow or reuse a car seat, you need to make sure that you know its history, such as whether it's been in an accident. Check the seat carefully for missing parts and defects. If you find any problems, do not use the car seat. The label with the car seat's model number should still be attached, and the instructions should be included with the car seat. If you can't afford to buy a seat, some communities and hospitals have programs for new parents to borrow an approved safety seat at no charge.

Once you have the car seat, it's important to install it correctly. Even the best car seat won't protect your baby if it's not installed properly. Some fire departments and other local agencies will check the placement of your car seat. If your infant seat has a base, practice putting it in and out of the base properly to make sure you know how it is done before leaving the hospital.

Preparing for Breastfeeding

Many mothers-to-be wonder if there's anything they should do to get ready to breastfeed. The truth is, there is very little you need to do to prepare your breasts for breastfeeding other than purchasing a good nursing bra.

Tips for Buying and Installing a Car Seat

Some safety seats will fit in your car better than others. A well-designed seat that is easy to use is the best for you and your child. When buying a seat, keep these tips in mind:

- Know whether your car has the LATCH system. LATCH stands for Lower Anchors and Tethers for Children. Special anchors, instead of safety belts, hold the seat in place. Newer cars and trucks will have the LATCH system. If either your car or your safety seat is not fitted with LATCH, you will need to use safety belts to install the car safety seat.

- Try locking and unlocking the buckle while you are in the store. Try changing the lengths of the straps.

- Try the seat in your car to make sure it fits.

- Read the labels to check weight limits.

- Do not decide just based on price. Seats that cost more are not always better.

When installing the seat, follow these tips:

- If you are using the LATCH system, place the seat on one side of the back seat, facing the rear.

- If you are using the safety belts, place the seat in the middle of the back seat, facing the rear.

- Lock the seat into its base, if it has one. The base should not move more than 1 inch when pushed front to back or side to side. If you are using the safety belts, make sure the lap part of the belt is tightly fastened to the car seat frame.

If you have questions about installing a car seat, contact your local fire department or other local agency, which may be able to check your seat's placement and make sure it's properly installed.

There usually is no need to put lotion on your breasts. Your nipples are already producing what they need for their protection. Also, do not use soap on your breasts because soap can dry them out. When you bathe or shower, rinsing with clear water is fine.

If you have any questions about breastfeeding before the baby arrives, contact the lactation specialist at your hospital or your local La Leche

League chapter. Keep in mind, though, that the nurses at the hospital will show you how to breastfeed the baby once you give birth, so you won't be on your own to learn the proper technique. In fact, if you want to breast-feed, your nurses will make sure you're feeding the baby well before you are allowed to leave the hospital.

▶ Prenatal Care Visits

During your last month of pregnancy, you'll have health care appointments every week—right up to the time you give birth. At these visits, your health care provider will check your weight, blood pressure, and **urine** as usual. Fundal height will be measured again and the heartbeat will be monitored. You may have a vaginal exam to check whether your cervix is preparing for labor. Your health care provider also may estimate the baby's weight and determine her position in the uterus. A head-down position is called a **vertex presentation**. If the feet or buttocks are facing down, this position is called a **breech presentation**. If your baby is in a breech position, there is still plenty of time for her to turn so that she's in the vertex position. If the baby still hasn't turned by about week 36, your health care provider may try a technique called external cephalic version.

At one of your prenatal care visits during weeks 35–37, you will be screened for group B streptococci (GBS). You won't be tested if you had a previous baby with GBS infection or if you have had GBS in your urine during this pregnancy. Group B streptococci are common bacteria that are usually harmless in adults, but babies who become infected can sometimes become critically ill. If you test positive for GBS, you will receive **antibiotics** during labor so that it is not passed to the baby. It's important for you to know what your GBS status is after you are tested. If you go into labor far from home or if your health care provider is not available, it will be helpful for your caregivers to know whether you need to receive antibiotics during labor.

Depending on your risk factors and state laws, you may have the following screening tests. Some are repeat screenings of earlier tests:

- Human immunodeficiency virus (HIV)
- Syphilis
- Chlamydial infection
- Gonorrhea

❯ Special Concerns

You should still be aware of the signs and symptoms of **preterm** labor (see Chapter 6, "Month 7 [Weeks 25–28]"). Many of the warning signs can occur in a normal pregnancy, however. If you have any doubts, contact your health care provider.

Preeclampsia

Preeclampsia is a medical condition of pregnancy that can occur after 20 weeks of pregnancy. It is estimated that preeclampsia occurs in 5–8% of all pregnancies, and it occurs primarily in first pregnancies. This condition can affect all organs of the mother's body, including the kidneys, liver, brain, and eyes. It also affects the **placenta**.

Preeclampsia is diagnosed by your health care provider when your blood pressure is elevated above a certain point and when protein is found in your urine. Preeclampsia may cause the following signs and symptoms:

• Headache
• Vision problems
• Pain in the upper abdomen
• Sudden weight gain (more than 2 pounds in a week)

If you notice any of these symptoms, call your health care provider right away. Chapter 18, "Hypertension," gives more details about how preeclampsia is diagnosed and treated.

External Cephalic Version

Most babies move into a head-down position a few weeks before birth. If the baby's buttocks, or buttocks and feet, are positioned to come out first, this is called a breech presentation. Sometimes, the baby can be turned into a head-down position by **external cephalic version**, also known as cephalic version. Cephalic version can be done after 36 completed weeks of pregnancy. Cephalic version involves lifting and turning the baby inside the uterus from the outside. There is some risk of complications with this procedure (see more information in Chapter 11, "Operative Delivery, Cesarean Delivery, and Breech Presentation"). If the baby is still in the breech position by the due date, a **cesarean delivery** may be the best option.

YOUR QUESTIONS ANSWERED

I'd like to get a pedicure, since I can't see, let alone reach, my feet. I've heard you can get infections from pedicures. Is this true?

While it is true that you can get fungal nail infections if the instruments used for your pedicure are not sanitized, this happens very rarely. Pedicures are a great way to pamper yourself during pregnancy, so indulge yourself and enjoy! To reduce the small risk of a fungal infection, bring along your own pedicure tools.

How soon after I have my baby can I start breastfeeding?

As soon as the baby is delivered, you can start breastfeeding, if you feel up to it. A healthy baby is perfectly capable of breastfeeding in the first hour after birth. Keeping your baby directly next to your skin also is the best way to maintain her body temperature. Your labor nurses can help you and your baby get into the right position.

I have inverted nipples. Can I still breastfeed?

Yes, breastfeeding is still possible. You first should determine whether your nipples are truly flat or inverted—there are degrees of inversion, and your nipples may not be completely flat. The way to find out is to pinch your nipple. If it does not become erect, then it is flat. If it does not protrude, it is truly inverted. However, many babies can exert enough suction to draw the nipple out on their own. Before the baby is born, you can wear breast shells, which provide gentle traction on the nipples. You also can wear breast shells for 30 minutes at a time after the baby is born. Keep in mind that a nurse or lactation specialist will be on hand at the hospital to provide assistance.

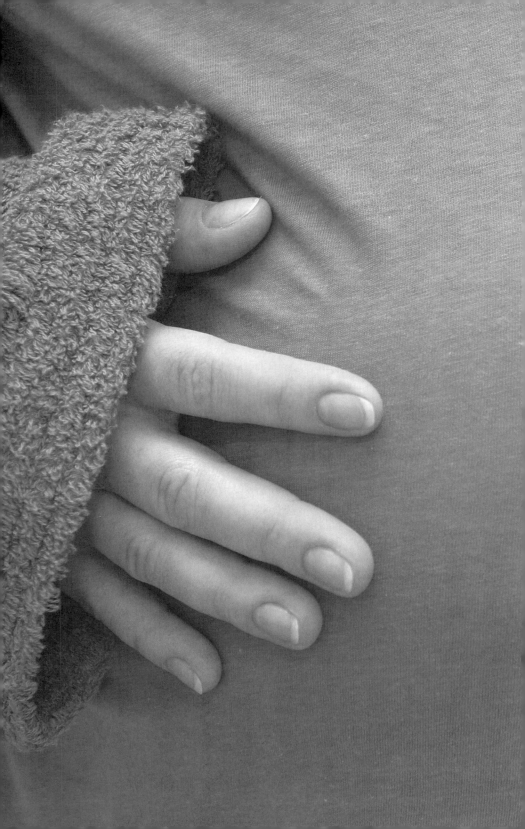

Chapter 9
Term
(Weeks 37–40)

YOUR GROWING BABY

Week 37

The *lanugo* (body hair) that has covered the baby and kept her warm throughout the time in the womb has mostly been shed. She is still adding fat all over—the elbows, knees, and shoulders—and now her body is about 16% body fat.

Week 38

Your baby could be born any day now. Eighty-five percent of babies are born within 2 weeks of their due dates.

Week 39

At birth, the brain will weigh about 14 ounces. After birth, the brain continues to increase in size and weight. By the time your baby is 1 year old, the brain will weigh 20 ounces.

Week 40

The baby is ready to be born. By now, her head may have dropped into position in your lower pelvis. At 40 weeks, she weighs about 6–9 pounds and is probably between 18 inches and 20 inches long.

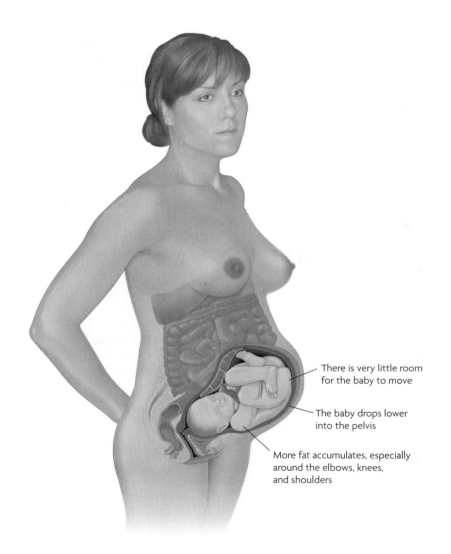

There is very little room for the baby to move

The baby drops lower into the pelvis

More fat accumulates, especially around the elbows, knees, and shoulders

Mother and baby: Term (Weeks 37–40). Your baby is now ready to be born.

YOUR PREGNANCY

▶ Your Changing Body

You've reached the end of your pregnancy! In these final weeks before your due date, you probably can't wait until the pregnancy is over. This month, your **uterus** will finish expanding; it has grown from only about 2 ounces before you were pregnant to about 2 ½ pounds now.

▶ Discomforts and How to Manage Them

You're probably very uncomfortable now. Walking is an effort, and lying down not much better. Many women report sleepless nights during the last few weeks. It may be difficult to get in and out of the car. You may be getting bored with just waiting for the baby to come, or you may be keyed up and anxious.

Try to keep your mind off the waiting. Spend some quality time with your partner, read a good book, or go see a movie (you won't be able to for a while once the baby comes). Staying active will help the days pass more quickly.

Frequent Urination

The uterus is bigger than it has ever been now and it is pressing much more on your bladder, causing many trips to the bathroom throughout the day. But don't cut back on drinking plenty of liquids during this time because your body needs the fluids more than ever now.

Snoring

If your partner says you've been snoring a lot more than usual, blame it on normal changes in breathing during pregnancy. If your snoring is a real problem, try sleeping with nasal strips across the bridge of your nose or using a humidifier in your bedroom.

▶ Nutrition

It's not unusual for symptoms of mild nausea to return in the final weeks of pregnancy. In fact, some women even lose a few pounds. Nausea may be a sign that labor is starting. If nausea is severe or persists, call your health care provider.

In these last weeks, you may feel better eating four or five small meals during the day, instead of three big ones. If mild nausea is a problem for you, try to eat bland foods, such as the BRATT diet (banana, rice, applesauce, tea, and toast). Just remember that you must keep eating regularly throughout the day. You and the baby will need the energy to cope with the strain of labor and birth.

Focus on Docosahexaenoic Acid

Docosahexaenoic acid (DHA) is an omega-3 fatty acid (see Chapter 4, "Month 5: [Weeks 17–20]") found in fish such as salmon and tuna as well as flax seeds and their oil. While research is still being conducted to learn more about its effects, some studies suggest that DHA plays a role in the development of the brain both before and after the baby is born. The U.S. Food and Drug Administration states that DHA also may be useful in helping to protect against heart disease in adults. Keep in mind that although fish are good sources of DHA, pregnant women are advised to avoid certain fish that may contain high levels of mercury (see p. 86). Eating fish that are low in mercury, such as shrimp, salmon, and halibut, however, is safe.

What to Eat if You Think You Are Going Into Labor

If you think you're in the early stages of labor, you may be wondering whether you can eat and if so, what. Here are the latest guidelines from the American College of Obstetricians and Gynecologists about eating and drinking during labor:

- If you are having a planned *cesarean delivery* or a repeat cesarean delivery, you should not eat any solid food for 6–8 hours before your surgery is scheduled. Depending on your hospital's or health care provider's policies, you may have small amounts of clear liquids up to 2 hours before surgery. Clear liquids include water, fruit juices without pulp, carbonated beverages, tea, and sports drinks.

- Women who are having an uncomplicated labor can have small amounts of clear liquids during labor. However, because it's not possible to predict whether you will need a cesarean delivery, you won't be allowed to eat solid foods during labor at the hospital.

- Women with certain conditions that may increase their risk of problems with *anesthesia*, such as *obesity* or *diabetes mellitus*, may be told to further restrict their intake of food and liquids beyond these guidelines.

Your health care provider or the hospital or birth center may have their own policies regarding eating and drinking during labor. You need to know these policies before your labor starts, so be sure to ask at one of your prenatal visits.

▶ Exercise

Exercise this month will be a challenge. Try the back press, which stretches your back muscles and does not involve a lot of movement. Now is a good time for you and your partner to practice the breathing exercises you learned in childbirth class. Practice now while you are relaxed so you both remember exactly what to do once labor starts.

Exercise of the Month: Back Press

This exercise strengthens your back, torso, and upper body:

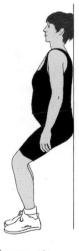

1. Stand with your back against a wall, with your feet 10–12 inches away from it.

2. Press the lower part of your back against the wall.

3. Hold for 10 seconds. Repeat 10 times.

Breathing Exercises

Different childbirth methods teach different breathing techniques. Most, however, are based on the concept that concentrating on your breathing can distract you from the pain of contractions and help you relax. Many also teach you how to use a focal point—imaging a peaceful, tranquil scene that you associate with being calm and relaxed.

Back press. This exercise strengthens your back, torso, and upper body.

If you haven't attended childbirth classes, don't worry. Once you are in labor, the nurses will give you plenty of instructions on how to relax and breathe during the different stages of labor.

▶ Healthy Decisions

When do you go to the hospital? What about children in the delivery room? These are common decisions that you may be faced with during these last weeks.

When to Go to the Hospital

During the final weeks, you and your partner will no doubt spend anxious moments wondering when is the right time to go to the hospital. It will depend mostly on whether your water breaks and the timing and intensity of your contractions. Your health care provider will give you clear instructions as you approach your due date, so follow them exactly.

Children in the Delivery Room

Some families invite their older children into the delivery room to witness their sibling's birth. Only you can know if this is right for your child—or for you. If you would like to make your baby's birth a family affair, talk with your health care provider first. Find out what the hospital policy is about children in the delivery room. Many won't allow young children to be present. If your other children are going to be in the room, each needs to have their own adult support person. Even if your child isn't with you during delivery, he or she can meet the new brother or sister shortly after birth.

▶ Other Considerations

Sometimes it's hard to tell if labor is starting or if it is simply a false alarm. There may be times when you wonder, "Is this it?" Telling real labor from prelabor often is difficult, even for health care providers. While you are waiting for labor to begin, some women wonder whether it is still OK to have sex. Some women also may experience a burst of energy, commonly called the "nesting instinct."

Knowing When You're in Labor

Many women think they are in labor when they are not. Painful contractions don't always signal true labor. Painless ones don't always mean prelabor, either. Each woman feels pain differently, and it can differ from

Things to Do This Month to Get Ready

- Put a waterproof sheet or mattress cover on your bed to protect it in case your water breaks during the night.

- Wash and organize the baby's clothes. Some advise leaving the tags on and only washing them if you're sure your baby is going to need them. You may want to wait if you think you will be returning baby clothes to the store. However, you can always donate any clothes that you don't end up using.

- Line up your helpers. Make sure everyone knows what they're to do and when they're to do it. You may want to make a schedule to see on what days you may be shorthanded and to avoid an overload of people on any one day. Also, keep in mind that you may still need helpers a few weeks after the birth, not just in the first few days.

- Prepare meals that can be frozen and defrosted easily. Soups, stews, and casseroles are great to have on hand and easy to microwave when needed.

- Write in a journal. You may want to write down your thoughts and feelings as you get ready for the birth. Your child may enjoy reading your journal later on, and you'll have a record of how you felt during this special time.

one pregnancy to another. Nevertheless, there are certain changes in your body that signal labor is near. Keep in mind, however, that not all women experience these signs. Once labor really starts, things may move quickly. Your water may break, your contractions will come faster and more often, and your baby may be born within hours. The more you know in advance about what to expect during labor, the better prepared you will be for the actual event (see Chapter 10, "Labor and Delivery").

Having Sex

If you and your partner feel the desire, it is perfectly OK to have sex right up to the time you give birth, unless your health care provider has told you otherwise. Some women find *sexual intercourse* uncomfortable in the final weeks of pregnancy. You and your partner can give each other pleasure in ways that do not involve intercourse, including oral sex and mutual *masturbation*.

Term

Nesting

Many moms-to-be approaching their due dates feel a strong urge to complete work projects and organize the house for the baby. This urge is known as the "nesting instinct." While there is no scientific evidence to prove that there is such a thing, many women attest that it indeed exists.

If the nesting urge strikes, go ahead and do what you need to do in order to satisfy your feelings. However, remember not to overdo it, and don't exhaust yourself. Ask for help. You need to conserve your energy for labor and delivery as well as for caring for the new baby.

▶ Prenatal Care Visits

You usually will see your health care provider once a week this month until you go into labor. Your weight, blood pressure, and uterus size will be measured just as last month. The baby's position will be checked, and you will be asked about the baby's movements. Your **cervix** may be checked to see if it has started preparing for labor.

▶ Special Concerns

Although **preeclampsia** can occur earlier in pregnancy (any time after 20 weeks), it most commonly occurs in the last weeks of pregnancy. For some women, rupture of the membranes signals the start of labor, as well as vaginal spotting. Heavy bleeding, however, may be a sign of a problem that needs to be checked by your health care provider.

Signs of Preeclampsia

Preeclampsia may cause the following signs and symptoms:

* Headache
* Vision problems
* Pain in the upper abdomen
* Sudden weight gain (more than 2 pounds in a week)

If you notice any of these symptoms, call your health care provider right away. Chapter 18, "Hypertension," gives more details about how preeclampsia is diagnosed and treated.

Rupture of Membranes

You may feel a trickle or a gush of fluid at the beginning of labor or during labor. When your membranes rupture, also known as your water breaking, the fluid-filled amniotic sac that surrounds the baby has broken. Call your health care provider if your membranes rupture, and follow his or her instructions. Once your membranes rupture, your health care provider will want to make sure labor begins soon if it hasn't already. Also, if you have tested positive for group B streptococcus infection, you will need to receive *antibiotics* (see Chapter 8, "Month 9 [Weeks 33–36]").

Changes in the Baby's Movement

You may notice that the baby's movement is different now from the movements you felt in previous weeks. It's normal for movements to feel different because there is less room in the uterus. The rate of movement is actually the same; it just doesn't feel the same to you.

Your health care provider may have you monitor the baby's movements by keeping track of how long it takes for you to feel 10 movements. To do this test (which is sometimes called a "kick count"), choose a time when the baby usually is active. Often, a good time is after you've eaten a meal. Each baby has its own level of activity, and most have a sleep cycle of 20–40 minutes. Call your health care provider if it takes longer than 2 hours for the baby to make 10 movements.

Vaginal Spotting

If you have light spotting in weeks 37–40, it could be a sign that labor is beginning. Vaginal discharge that is pink or slightly bloody is known as the "bloody show." If vaginal bleeding is heavy—as heavy as a normal menstrual period—it could be a sign of a problem. In this situation, contact your health care provider right away.

Some women also pass the thick mucus plug that seals off the cervix during pregnancy a few weeks before or at the start of labor. Passage of the mucus plug may be a signal that your cervix is opening.

▶ Postterm Pregnancy (Weeks 40–42)

A *postterm pregnancy* is one that lasts 42 weeks or longer. Women who are having a baby for the first time or who have had postterm pregnancies before may give birth later than expected. A pregnancy often lasts longer than expected because the exact time when you became pregnant is not known. Postterm pregnancy is not all that rare—7% of pregnancies last 42 weeks or longer.

If your due date has come and gone, your health care provider most likely will do some form of fetal evaluation to check your baby's health. If you don't start labor on your own by 41 or 42 weeks, your health care provider will discuss the option of inducing labor with you.

Risks

When a pregnancy goes longer than 40 weeks, it can increase the risks to the baby's and mother's health. After 42 weeks, the *placenta* may not work as well as it did earlier in pregnancy. Also, as the baby grows, the amount of *amniotic fluid* may begin to decrease. Less fluid may cause the **umbilical cord** to become pinched as the baby moves or as the uterus contracts. Postterm pregnancies also double the mother's risk of needing a cesarean delivery.

Despite these risks, most women who give birth after their due dates have healthy newborns. When a baby is not born by the due date, certain tests can help the doctor monitor the baby's health. Some tests, such as a kick count, can be done on your own at home. Others are done in the doctor's office or in the hospital. These are called *electronic fetal monitoring* and include the *nonstress test*, *biophysical profile*, assessment of amniotic fluid levels, and *contraction stress test* (see Chapter 28, "Testing to Monitor Fetal Health," for a detailed description of these tests).

Cervical Ripening

In preparation for labor and delivery, the cervix begins to soften, thin out (a process called effacement), and open (called dilation). Your health care provider will perform a vaginal exam in the last few weeks of pregnancy to see if your cervix has started these processes. If you've gone past your due date and your cervix has not begun these changes, your health care provider may recommend cervical ripening to make your cervix ready for labor.

Several techniques of cervical ripening are available, including devices designed to open the cervix or medications containing *prostaglandins*, chemicals that are made by the body that ripen the cervix and cause uterine contractions. There are different types of dilators that are used. *Laminaria* is a natural or artificial substance inserted into the cervix that expands when it absorbs water. A catheter, or small tube, also can be used to dilate the cervix, as well as special dilators. Medications include misoprostol, which can be given in a tablet that is taken by mouth or placed in the **vagina** or as a vaginal gel, and prostaglandins, which are inserted into the cervix or vagina.

The decision to use cervical ripening is based on several factors, including whether the risks outweigh the benefits. There is an increased risk of infection with the use of dilators. Risks of cervical ripening medication include an increase in the rate and strength of uterine contractions and changes in fetal heart rate. Monitoring of the baby's heart rate and the strength of uterine contractions is done for at least a short period of time after medications for cervical ripening are given.

Labor Induction

In cases in which continuing the pregnancy is more risky than delivering the baby, the health care provider might induce (bring on) labor. More than one method of labor induction may be used. Some of the methods used to induce labor also can speed up a labor that's not progressing as it should. There are several methods for inducing labor:

- *Stripping the membranes*—Your health care provider inserts a gloved finger through your cervix and sweeps a finger over the thin membranes that connect the amniotic sac to the wall of your uterus. You may feel some intense cramping and have spotting when this is done. Stripping the membranes causes your body to release prostaglandins.

- *Rupturing the amniotic sac (breaking your water)*—If your water has not broken already, breaking it can get contractions started or make them stronger. Your doctor may make a small hole in the amniotic sac. This is called an amniotomy. Most women go into labor within hours of their water breaking. If labor does not begin, another method may be used to bring on contractions to decrease the risk of infection.

- *Misoprostol*—This medication stimulates uterine contractions. It can be used to induce labor when the cervix is not ready for labor. It can be given orally or vaginally.

- *Oxytocin*—**Oxytocin** is a natural hormone in your body that causes contractions or makes contractions stronger. Your doctor may give you the synthetic (man-made) form of oxytocin through an intravenous tube in your arm. Contractions usually start about 30 minutes after oxytocin is given.

The risks of labor induction depend on the method chosen and include:

- Change in fetal heart rate
- Increased risk of infection in the woman and baby

- Umbilical cord problems
- Overstimulation of the uterus
- Uterine rupture (rarely)

To help prevent these problems, the fetal heart rate and force of contractions may be monitored with some types of induction. To avoid uterine rupture, misoprostol followed by oxytocin is not used in women who have had a previous cesarean delivery or a scar from other surgery on the uterus.

Old Wives' Tales

You may have heard other mothers talk about ways you can make labor start on your own. Many women believe doing such things as taking long walks, having sex, or eating spicy foods can bring on labor. There is, however, no evidence that any of these methods work.

One nonmedical method of labor induction that is somewhat more effective is nipple stimulation. Research on this method found that it did bring on labor in some women, but only when the cervix was ready for labor. However, you should not attempt to bring on labor with nipple stimulation without your health care provider's supervision.

YOUR QUESTIONS ANSWERED

What is an *episiotomy* and why might I need one?

An episiotomy is a procedure in which a small cut is made to widen the opening of your vagina when you're giving birth. It may be done to assist delivery of the baby or to avoid tearing the skin at the opening of the vagina. Episiotomies used to be performed routinely, but current guidelines from the American College of Obstetricians and Gynecologists suggest restricting their use. It is helpful to discuss this issue with your health care provider be-

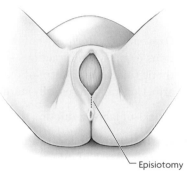

Episiotomy. An episiotomy is a cut made between the vaginal opening and the anal opening in order to widen the passage for the baby. They are no longer considered routine but may be needed in special situations.

Episiotomy

fore labor. Ask about his or her rate of episiotomy and the situations in which it could be performed.

I've heard about operative delivery. What is it and when is it done?

In an operative delivery, the baby is delivered using forceps or vacuum extraction (a special suction cup). Operative delivery is done for a variety of reasons. The baby's heartbeat may have become slow or erratic, or the woman may have become too tired to push. See Chapter 11, "Operative Delivery, Cesarean Delivery, and Breech Presentation" for more details about operative delivery.

What determines whether my planned vaginal birth has to be done by cesarean delivery instead?

Although you and your health care provider may have planned a vaginal delivery, sometimes a cesarean delivery may be needed. There are many circumstances that can make a cesarean delivery necessary, including certain medical conditions, labor not progressing, and the baby being in a **breech presentation**. See Chapter 11 for more discussion of cesarean delivery.

Part II
Labor, Delivery, and the Postpartum Period

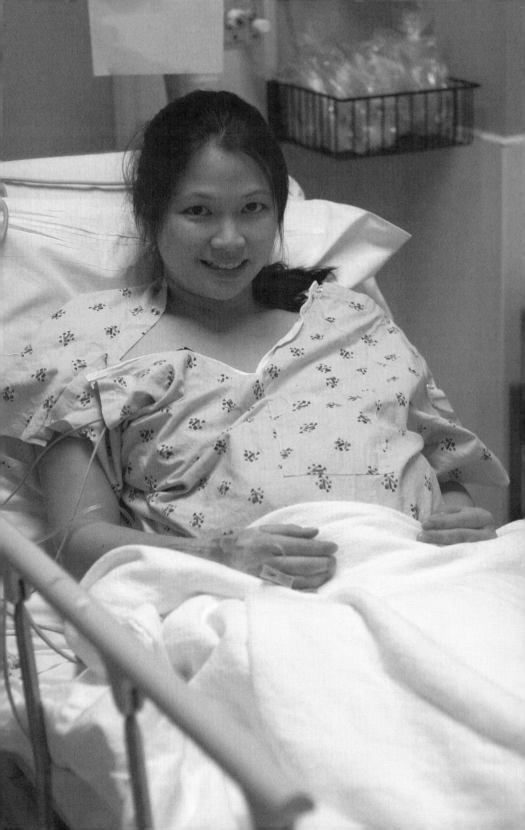

Chapter 10
Labor and Delivery

L abor occurs when a woman has regular contractions that result in a change in her *cervix*. Although for most women, real labor is noticeably different than prelabor, that's not always the case. It's relatively common for a woman to think she is in true labor when she is not. However, if you are having contractions that occur before 37 weeks and that are regular and consistent over a 1- to 2-hour period, it is important to notify your prenatal care provider.

Once labor really starts, it usually is steadily progressive. For a woman having her first baby, labor typically lasts 12–18 hours. For women who have given birth before, it typically lasts 8–10 hours. However, every woman is different. Your labor may not be like your sister's or your friend's. It may even differ with each child. Despite these differences, labor and delivery usually follow a pattern. The more you know about what to expect during labor, the better prepared you will be once it begins.

Stages of Childbirth

Labor and birth are divided into three different stages—Stages 1, 2, and 3. Stage 1 is labor; Stage 2 is the "pushing and delivery phase," in which you actively participate in pushing the baby out; and Stage 3 is delivery of the *placenta*.

When reading the following sections, it is important to remember that every woman's labor is unique to her. The descriptions of the typical labor below may not exactly describe what you ultimately experience.

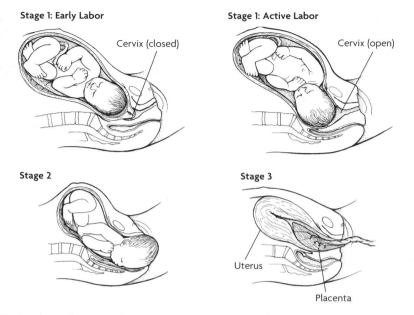

Stage 1: Early Labor

Cervix (closed)

Stage 1: Active Labor

Cervix (open)

Stage 2

Stage 3

Uterus

Placenta

The three stages of childbirth. In Stage 1, the cervix dilates. In Stage 2, the cervix completely dilates, and the mother pushes the baby out of the vagina. In Stage 3, the placenta detaches from the uterus and is delivered.

Common Terms

You may hear your health care provider and nurses use specific terms to describe how your labor is progressing:

- *Effacement*—Thinning of the cervix. Normally, your cervix looks like a tube that connects the top of the **vagina** to the bottom of the **uterus**. It's about an inch long. As your labor progresses, the cervix will start to draw up and thin out until it is right up against the uterine wall. Effacement is estimated in percentages, from 0% to 100% (completely thinned). Effacement makes it possible for your cervix to stretch and for the baby to pass through the opening.

- *Dilation*—The amount that the cervix has opened. It is measured in centimeters, from 0 centimeters to 10 centimeters (fully dilated).

- *Ripening*—The process of softening, thinning, and dilation of the cervix in preparation for birth.

- *Station*—The location of the presenting part—usually the baby's head—in the birth canal. The ischial spines, the bony parts of the pelvis that stick out into the birth canal, are used as a reference point. Station is measured in numbers, describing the position of the presenting part relative to the

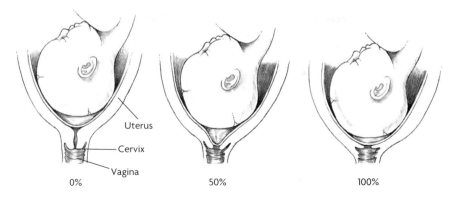

Effacement. During effacement, your cervix draws upward and becomes part of the lower uterus. It is measured in percentages, from 0% (no effacement) to 100% (full effacement).

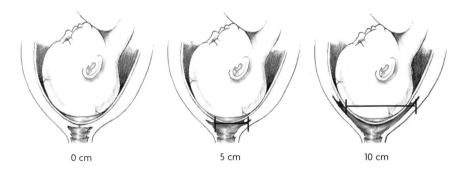

Dilation. During dilation, the opening of the cervix enlarges. It is measured in centimeters, usually from 0 centimeters (no dilation) to 10 centimeters (fully dilated).

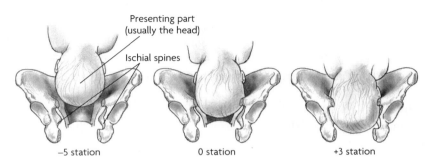

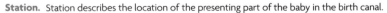

Station. Station describes the location of the presenting part of the baby in the birth canal.

ischial spines. A negative station (from –1 to –5) means that the presenting part is above the spines. At –5, the baby is 5 centimeters above the spines. A positive station (from +1 to +5) describes a presenting part that has progressed down the birth canal. At +5 the *fetus* is ***crowning*** and is visible on a pelvic examination just at the opening of a woman's vagina.

Stage 1: Early Labor

Stage 1 is divided in two separate phases: early labor and active labor. The beginning of early labor can be difficult to define but describes the process of having regular contractions before the cervix dilates to 4 centimeters. You may hear this stage described as "latent labor." Some women will have cervical dilation of 1–4 centimeters without apparent labor occurring because of the quiet prelabor processes that occur in the late part of pregnancy. Dilation of 4 centimeters is a somewhat arbitrary benchmark that is used to define when a woman is in labor rather than in the prelabor phase.

What Happens During Early Labor

During early labor, you will begin to have mild contractions that will be anywhere from 5 to 15 minutes apart and will last about 60–90 seconds. The contractions gradually will get closer together, and toward the end of early labor, they are less than 5 minutes apart. During these contractions, you may feel pain or pressure that starts in your back and moves around to your lower abdomen. When this happens, your belly will tighten and feel hard. Between contractions, the uterus relaxes and your belly softens. These contractions are doing vital work. They help dilate the cervix and help push your baby lower into the pelvis.

The first stage of labor is almost always the longest. How long it lasts is different for every woman. For some, it's a few hours. For others, it's longer. For first-time moms, the average is from 6 hours to 12 hours.

You probably will spend most of early labor at home, waiting for the contractions to get closer together. Your health care provider most likely will have given you instructions on when to leave for the hospital, so follow them exactly. If you are not sure about what to do, call your health care provider.

What You Can Do

During early labor, you should try to stay as relaxed as possible. Staying relaxed will help your cervix thin out and dilate. You may want to alternate active movements with rest. Here are some things you can do during early labor:

- Go for a walk.
- Take a nap.

- Take a shower or bath.
- Play some relaxing music.
- Do relaxation and breathing techniques taught in childbirth class.
- Change positions often.
- Make sure you have everything you need for the hospital.

Slow, relaxing breathing may be helpful during this stage:

- Take a deep, cleansing breath at the beginning of the contraction.
- Breathe slowly, focusing on the in-and-out movement of your breath.
- Try counting during the contraction.
- At the end of the contraction, take a deep, cleansing breath.

How Your Labor Coach Can Help
Your labor partner can be a big help to you during Stage 1 of childbirth, both emotionally and physically. Now is the time to help you with the strategies you both learned in childbirth class about how to relax and cope with the pain. Other ways to help include:

- Keep you distracted by playing cards or other games.
- Massage your back and shoulders.
- Time your contractions.
- Place a heating pad or ice pack on your lower back.
- Make phone calls with you.

Stage 1: Active Labor

When active labor begins, your contractions will have progressed and are coming closer together. Active labor is typically considered to have started when a woman is having regular contractions and her cervix has dilated to 4 centimeters. It's hard to know when that precisely occurs, so when your contractions are stronger, closer together, and regular, it's time to go to the hospital.

What Happens When You Check In
Each hospital has its own procedures. After you are admitted, the next steps may vary. The following sequence is what usually happens:

- *Consent forms*—These forms vary, but most spell out who will be taking care of you, why a procedure is being done, and the risks involved. Read this form and be sure to ask about anything that's not clear. Signing the consent form means that you understand your medical condition and agree to the care described. You may need to sign separate consent forms for **anesthesia** and for **cesarean delivery**.

- *Triage room*—Before you are admitted to the hospital, the hospital staff will determine whether you are in labor. You'll be taken to a special triage room, or this may be done in the hospital's emergency department. If you are found to be in labor, you will be taken to a hospital room. If you're not in labor, you'll be told to return home.

- *Room assignment*—You'll be taken to a hospital room. In some hospitals you will stay in the same room for both labor and delivery. Other hospitals have a separate delivery room.

- *Changing clothes*—You'll be asked to put on a hospital gown. Ask the nurse if you want to wear your own gown, but keep in mind that it may get stained or ruined.

- *Vital signs*—Your pulse, blood pressure, and temperature will be checked.

- *Lab tests*—A **urine** or blood sample may be taken.

- *Physical exam*—You'll eventually be given a vaginal exam to see how much your cervix has dilated.

- *Intravenous line*—An intravenous line may be placed in your arm or wrist so that medications and fluids can be administered if you need them.

- *Fetal monitoring*—Your baby's heart rate and your contractions likely will be monitored with **electronic fetal monitoring**.

Once you're in your hospital room, a labor-and-delivery nurse will be checking on you from the time you check in until after your baby is born. These nurses are trained to help women through the physical and emotional demands of labor. In teaching hospitals, a resident doctor, student nurse, or medical student also may be a part of your birth team.

Your own health care provider may be there from start to finish, or he or she may arrive shortly before you give birth. During this stage, the following things will be closely monitored:

- Your heart rate and blood pressure
- The time and length of your contractions
- How much your cervix has dilated
- The baby's heartbeat, with either an electronic fetal monitor or a special stethoscope

What Happens During Active Labor

Active labor generally is when the cervix dilates from 4 centimeters to 10 centimeters. Contractions get stronger and come as often as 3 minutes apart, and each one lasts about 45 seconds. Active labor can last about 4–8 hours. During this time, you may experience the following:

- Your water may break if it hasn't already.
- You'll have back pain if the baby's head presses down on your backbone during contractions.
- Your legs may cramp.
- You may feel the urge to push.
- You may feel nauseated.

What You Can Do
Your contractions will become more intense, so focus on your breathing and take each contraction one at a time. Let your childbirth partner and nurse help you through all the breathing and relaxation exercises. When each contraction passes, try to relax and don't think about the next one. It may help to move around in the bed to find a position that is most comfortable for you. There are some other things you can do now:

- If you feel like it and your health care provider says it's OK, walk the halls.
- Urinate often because an empty bladder gives your baby's head more room to move down.
- Ask for pain relief if you want it (see "Pain Relief During Labor" later in this chapter).
- If you feel the urge to push, tell your health care provider. Don't give in to the urge just yet—pant or blow to keep yourself from bearing down.

How Your Labor Coach Can Help
You'll depend on your labor partner more and more as the labor pains intensify. Let him or her help you through the pain-management methods you learned in childbirth class. Your partner also can help in the following ways:

- Apply counterpressure to your back: press firmly on the lower back or massage with knuckles or tennis balls.
- Flex your feet to help relieve your leg cramps.
- Act as a focal point during contractions.
- Offer comfort and support.
- Give you ice chips or hard candies if you want.

Helping Labor Along
Sometimes if your labor isn't progressing as quickly as it should, your health care provider may decide to augment your labor by rupturing your membranes (if they haven't already ruptured) or giving you a drug called Pitocin, a synthetic form of **oxytocin,** the **hormone** that causes the uterus to contract.

This drug increases the frequency and duration of your contractions (see p. 179). Labor is augmented if contractions are thought to be infrequent or mild enough that they won't cause the cervix to dilate and the woman is in active labor.

Transition to Stage 2

Towards the end of the active phase of labor, it is common for labor to intensify. For many, this will be the toughest stage and the most painful. If you've been given an epidural or other pain medication, however, the pain may not be as intense. The contractions come closer together and can last 60–90 seconds. With each contraction, you may start to feel an urge to bear down. You'll feel a lot of pressure in your lower back and rectum. This can feel like the urge to move your bowels, but much stronger. Tell your health care provider or nurse as soon as you feel like pushing. He or she will check your cervix to see how much it has dilated. Until your cervix is fully dilated and your health care provider or nurse gives you the go-ahead, you should try not to push. Pushing before your cervix is fully dilated can exhaust you as well as cause some swelling of the cervix, which may prevent it from fully dilating. Controlling your breathing or blowing air out in short puffs can help you resist bearing down. The transition phase does not last too long, maybe 15–60 minutes. You should be ready to start the Stage 2 soon.

Stage 2: Pushing and Delivery

This stage can last anywhere from 20 minutes to 3 hours or more. It's different for every woman and for every pregnancy. The second stage of labor results in the baby's birth but typically is the most work for the mother. Once your cervix is fully dilated, you can begin to push your baby out. During Stage 2, you'll notice a change in the way your contractions feel. They may be slower, come 2–5 minutes apart, and last about 60–90 seconds.

What You Can Do

If you have been in a standard labor room, you'll be moved to a room for delivery. If you are in a labor–delivery–recovery room, your health care provider and nurse will help you get into a good delivery position. Many women give birth to their babies while propped up in bed, with their legs braced against foot rests. There are other birth positions you can try (lying on your side, for instance) as long as your health care provider approves.

Once your health care provider gives you the go-ahead, bear down with each contraction or when you are told to push. As the baby moves down the birth canal, your attendants will tell you how to help your baby along. When the baby's head appears at the opening of your vagina, you'll feel a burning or stinging feeling as the **perineum** stretches and bulges. This is normal.

After the head emerges from the birth canal, the baby's body turns. First one shoulder slips out, and then the other. After the shoulders are delivered, the rest of the baby's body follows quickly. Your health care provider or your labor coach then will cut the **umbilical cord**. The blood in the umbilical cord (called cord blood) routinely is obtained for newborn blood tests, such as blood type.

How Your Labor Coach Can Help
Your labor partner can hold your hands and talk to you through the contractions. Offering words of support can be a big help. Tell your partner where you want him or her to stand. By standing at your shoulder, he or she can offer emotional and physical support as you give birth to the baby. From this spot, your coach will have the same view that you do of the baby's birth.

Stage 3: Delivery of the Placenta

After your baby is delivered, one more part of childbirth remains, delivery of the placenta. This last stage is the shortest of all. It likely will last from just a few minutes to about 20 minutes.

During this stage, you will still have contractions. They will be closer together and less painful. These contractions help the placenta separate from the wall of the uterus. Then the contractions move the placenta down into the birth canal. Once there, a push or two by you will help expel the placenta from the vagina. Some health care providers help deliver the placenta by reaching inside the vagina to the uterus and grasping the placenta. If you had an **episiotomy** or tear, it will be repaired. If you have elected to store cord blood, it's collected either before or after delivery of the placenta.

These contractions also help your uterus return to its smaller size. As the uterus shrinks, the blood vessels that brought nutrients and oxygen to the placenta and removed wastes are sealed, which helps control blood loss.

Pain Relief During Labor

Every woman's labor is different. The amount of pain you feel during labor may be completely different from the pain your mother, sister, or girlfriend had with her labor and may be different even from pain you may have experienced in prior deliveries. Pain depends on many factors, such as the size and position of the baby and the strength of contractions.

Despite the expected pain of labor, however, some women worry that receiving medication to relieve the pain will somehow make the experience less natural. But many women find that pain relief gives them better control over their labor and delivery. Don't be afraid to ask for pain relief if you need it.

There are two types of pain-relieving drugs, *analgesics* and *anesthetics*:

1. Analgesics relieve pain without total loss of feeling or muscle movement. They do not stop pain completely, but they do lessen it. In most cases, analgesics are given through a shot either into a muscle or through an intravenous line.

2. Anesthetics block most feeling, including pain and muscle movement. Some forms of anesthetics, such as general anesthetics, cause you to lose consciousness. Other forms, such as regional anesthetics, remove most pain from selected parts of the body while you stay conscious. You may still feel pressure, however. You'll be given anesthetics if you are having a cesarean delivery, and it is optional for labor.

Talk with your health care provider about your options. In some cases, he or she may arrange for you to meet with an *anesthesiologist* before your labor and delivery. An anesthesiologist will help you pick the best method.

Analgesics

Like other types of drugs, analgesics can have side effects. Most are minor, such as nausea, feeling drowsy, or having trouble concentrating. Sometimes other drugs are given with analgesics to relieve nausea. Systemic analgesics are not given right before delivery because they may slow the baby's breathing at birth.

Local Anesthesia

Local anesthesia provides numbness or loss of sensation in a small area. It does not, however, lessen the pain of contractions. Local anesthesia is helpful when an episiotomy needs to be done and repaired or when any vaginal or perineal tears that happened during birth are repaired. Local anesthesia can be given late in the second stage of childbirth to numb the perineum.

Local anesthetics rarely affect the baby. There usually are no side effects after the local anesthetic has worn off.

Regional Anesthesia

Regional analgesia tends to be the most effective method of pain relief during labor and causes few side effects. Epidural anesthetics, spinal blocks, and combined spinal–epidural blocks are all types of drugs used for regional anesthesia to decrease labor pain. They are termed "regional" because they act on a specific area of the body.

Epidural Block

Epidural blocks cause loss of some feeling in the lower areas of a woman's body, yet she remains awake and alert. An epidural block may be given soon after contractions start or later as labor progresses. An epidural block with more or stronger medications can be used for a cesarean delivery or if a vaginal birth requires the help of forceps or vacuum extraction.

How It Works. An epidural block is given in the lower back. During the procedure, you will be asked to sit or lie on your side, with your back curved outward. After the procedure, you may be allowed to move but not to walk around.

Before the block is performed, the skin will be cleaned and a local anesthetic will be used to numb an area of the lower back. A needle is inserted through the skin into the epidural space in the spine. After the epidural needle is placed, a small tube (catheter) is inserted through it, and the needle is withdrawn. Small doses of the medication can then be given through the tube to reduce the discomfort of labor. The medication also can be given continuously without another injection. In some cases, the catheter may touch a nerve. This may cause a brief tingling sensation down one leg.

Because the medication needs to be absorbed into several nerves, it may take a short while for it to take effect. Pain relief will begin within 10–20 minutes after the medication has been injected.

Although an epidural block will make you more comfortable, you still may be aware of your contractions. You also may feel vaginal exams and some pressure as the baby's head descends. The anesthesiologist will adjust the degree of numbness for your comfort and to assist labor and delivery. This may cause a bit of temporary numbness, heaviness, or weakness in the legs.

Side Effects and Risks. Although most women do not have problems with the use of an epidural block, there may be some drawbacks to using this pain relief method:

• An epidural block can cause your blood pressure to decrease. This, in turn, may slow your baby's heartbeat. To prevent this, you'll be given fluids through an intravenous tube before the drug is injected. You also may need to lie on your side to improve blood flow.

• After delivery, your back may be sore from the injection for a few days. However, an epidural block should not cause long-term back pain.

• Some women (less than 1 out of 100) may get a headache after the procedure. A woman can help decrease the risk of a headache by holding as still as possible while the needle is placed. If a headache does occur, it often subsides within a few days. If the headache does not stop or if it becomes severe, treatment may be needed.

• When an epidural block is given late in labor or a lot of anesthetic is used, it may be hard to bear down and push your baby through the birth canal. If you cannot feel enough when it is time to push, your anesthesiologist can adjust the dosage.

Serious complications are very rare:

• The veins located in the epidural space become swollen during pregnancy. There is a risk that the anesthetic could be injected into one of them. Signs that this has occurred include dizziness, rapid heartbeat, a funny taste, or numbness around the mouth when the epidural is placed. Tell your health care provider right away if you have any of these signs.

• If the level of anesthetic is too high, your chest muscles may be affected, and it could be hard for you to breathe.

As long as your analgesic or anesthetic is given by a trained and experienced anesthesiologist, there's little chance you'll run into trouble. If you think an epidural block may be the choice for you, bring up any concerns or questions you have with your health care provider.

Spinal Block

A spinal block—like an epidural block—is done with an injection in the lower back. For this procedure, you must sit or lie on your side in bed while a small amount of a drug is injected into the spinal fluid to numb the lower half of the body. It brings good relief from pain and starts working fast, but it lasts only an hour or two. It usually is used for cesarean delivery and only rarely in late labor or for a vaginal delivery.

Combined Spinal–Epidural Block

A combined spinal–epidural block has the benefits of both types of pain relief. The spinal part helps provide pain relief right away. Drugs given through the epidural provide pain relief throughout labor. Some (but not all) women may be able to walk around after the block is in place. For this reason, this method sometimes is called the "walking epidural."

General Anesthesia

General anesthetics are medications that cause you to lose consciousness and experience no pain. *General anesthesia* puts you to sleep. It often is used when regional anesthesia is not possible or is not the best choice for medical or other reasons. It can be started quickly and causes a rapid loss of consciousness. Therefore, it often is used when an urgent cesarean delivery is needed.

A major risk during general anesthesia is caused by food or liquids in a woman's stomach. Labor usually causes undigested food to stay in the stomach. During unconsciousness, this food could come back into the mouth and go into the lungs where it can cause damage. To avoid this, eating or drinking may not be allowed or may be restricted once labor has started. A tube will be placed in your throat after you are asleep to help you breathe. This may cause a sore throat after you wake up.

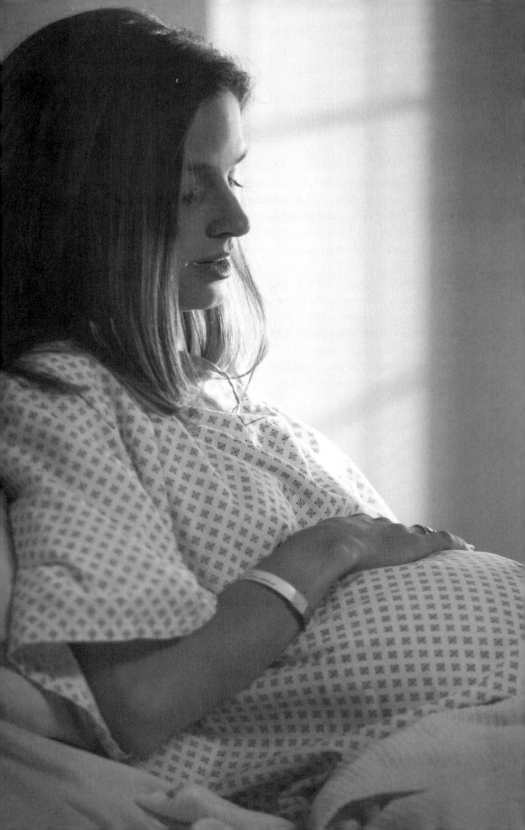

Chapter 11
Operative Delivery, Cesarean Delivery, and Breech Presentation

O nce labor really starts, it usually is steadily progressive. No one can predict just how the birth of a baby will proceed. Sometimes the birth happens fairly quickly and there are no problems. With some births, however, the mother may push for hours and not make much progress. With others, problems may occur during labor. If your doctor thinks that continuing labor or a vaginal delivery would be unsafe for you or your baby, he or she may decide that the best option is to deliver the baby another way—either by operative delivery or *cesarean delivery*.

Operative Delivery

In some cases, your doctor may need to help delivery along by using *forceps* or a vacuum device. This type of delivery is called operative delivery. Operative delivery is done in about 10–15% of vaginal deliveries for several reasons:

- Your baby's heartbeat becomes slow or erratic.
- You become too tired to push.
- The baby's position makes delivery harder.

Types of Operative Delivery

There are two types of operative delivery—forceps delivery and *vacuum extraction*:

- *Forceps delivery*—Forceps look like two large spoons. They are inserted into the *vagina* and placed around the baby's cheekbones and jaw. The

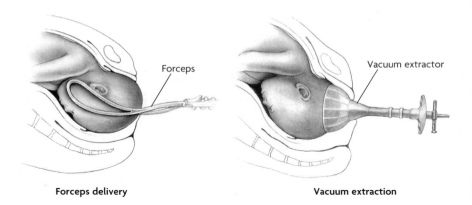

Forceps

Vacuum extractor

Forceps delivery

Vacuum extraction

forceps are then used to gently guide the baby's head out of the birth canal.

- *Vacuum extraction*—A small suction cup is inserted into the vagina and pressed to the baby's head. Suction holds the cup in place. A handle on the cup then allows the doctor to apply gentle, well-controlled traction and help the baby through the birth canal while you continue to push.

Risks

In most cases, using these tools to help delivery causes no major problems, and both have been found to be safe to use. There is, however, some risk that forceps delivery or vacuum extraction can bruise the baby's head. Forceps may tear the vagina or cervix. Uncommonly, more serious injuries to the baby can occur. Your doctor should discuss these risks with you before operative delivery is performed.

Cesarean Delivery

Most babies are born through the mother's birth canal. However, in many pregnancies, a baby is delivered through an incision in the mother's abdomen and **uterus**. This is known as a cesarean delivery. Cesarean deliveries are very common. In fact, 31% of the babies born in 2006 were delivered this way. The rate of cesarean deliveries has increased 50% since 1996.

Why You Might Need One

A cesarean delivery may be needed if circumstances occur during labor that make a cesarean delivery a safer choice than a vaginal delivery. A cesarean delivery also may be planned ahead of time because of certain problems or conditions.

The following reasons may make a cesarean delivery necessary:

- *Labor fails to progress*—One of the most common reasons why doctors perform cesarean deliveries is because labor slows down or stops. About one in three cesarean deliveries is done for this reason. For example, you may be experiencing contractions, but they are too weak or too infrequent to dilate the cervix wide enough for the baby to move through the vagina. Sometimes, even if your cervix dilates enough, the baby may be too big for your pelvis, or the baby's position may not allow passage in a safe and timely manner.

- *Labor is too stressful for the baby*—The baby's heart rate may become abnormal during labor or *fetal monitoring* may detect signs of other problems.

- *Umbilical cord problem*—If the **umbilical cord** becomes pinched or compressed, the baby may not get enough oxygen.

A cesarean delivery also may need to be scheduled even before you go into labor. Reasons for a scheduled cesarean delivery include the following conditions:

- *You had a previous cesarean delivery*—A previous cesarean delivery may mean that you'll need a cesarean delivery this time too.

- *You're having more than one baby*—If you are having two or more babies, you may need to have a cesarean delivery. Many women having twins are able to have a vaginal delivery. However, if the babies are being born too early or are not in good positions in the uterus, a cesarean delivery may be needed. The likelihood of having a cesarean delivery increases with the number of babies you are carrying.

- *You have a large baby or a small pelvis*—Sometimes a baby is too big to pass safely through a woman's pelvis and vagina. This condition is called **cephalopelvic disproportion**.

- *Your baby is in a breech presentation or is lying in a position that makes vaginal delivery dangerous*—If you are in labor and your baby is in a **breech presentation** (with buttocks or feet closest to the vagina), your doctor may feel that a cesarean delivery is the safest way for delivery. If the baby is transverse (lying sideways in the uterus rather than head-down), a cesarean delivery is the only choice for delivery.

• *You request it*—Some pregnant women decide to undergo a cesarean delivery even when there is not a medical reason why it must be done. This is known as "cesarean delivery by request." It is important to discuss this option with your health care provider in advance and explore your reasons carefully before deciding to request a cesarean delivery. As with any major surgery, cesarean delivery carries some risks. These risks increase with the number of cesarean deliveries that you have. See the detailed discussion "Cesarean Delivery By Request" on pages 109–110.

• *You have placenta problems.*—*Placenta previa* is a condition in which the placenta is below the baby and covers part or all of the cervix, blocking the baby's exit from the uterus. Placenta problems also can cause heavy bleeding.

• *You have a medical condition that may make vaginal birth risky*—For example, a cesarean delivery may be done if a woman has an active herpes infection during labor.

What Happens During a Cesarean Delivery

The process of cesarean delivery can vary, depending on the reason why the cesarean delivery is being done. However, in most cases, cesarean deliveries follow a similar procedure.

Anesthesia

To numb pain during your cesarean delivery, an *epidural block*, *spinal block*, or *general anesthesia* will be used. An *anesthesiologist* will talk with you about which type of pain medication you prefer and will take your wishes into account when deciding which method is best for you. Whether you have general, spinal, or epidural anesthesia will depend on your health and that of your baby, as well as why the cesarean delivery is being done.

If you already have an epidural *catheter* in place and then need to have a cesarean delivery, usually your anesthesiologist will be able to inject more medication or a different medication through the same catheter to increase your pain relief. The anesthetic will numb the entire abdomen for the surgery. Although you will not feel any pain, there may be a feeling of pressure.

Preparing You for Surgery

Before the cesarean delivery proceeds, a few steps are done to prepare you for surgery:

• Your blood pressure, heart rate, and breathing will be monitored during the surgery. An oxygen mask will be placed over your nose and mouth or a tube will be placed in your nose to make sure you and your baby get plenty of oxygen during surgery.

• A nurse will wash your abdomen and, if needed, hair between the pubic bone and navel may be trimmed. The abdomen will be swabbed with an antiseptic, and sterile drapes will be placed around the area of the incision.

• A catheter will be inserted into the **bladder**. The catheter keeps the bladder empty so that it's not injured during surgery.

Making the Incision

Once your abdomen is cleaned and you are asleep or numb from the anesthetic, the doctor will make the abdominal incision:

• The incision is made through the skin and the wall of the abdomen and goes from side to side, just above the pubic hairline (transverse), or up and down (vertical).

• The doctor gently spreads apart the abdominal muscles and cuts through the lining of the abdominal cavity. The abdominal muscles usually are not cut.

• When the doctor reaches the uterus, another cut is made in the uterine wall. This incision also can be transverse (side to side) or vertical (up and down). In most cases, a transverse incision is made. This type of cut is done in the lower, thinner part of the uterus. It causes less bleeding and heals with a stronger scar. A vertical incision may need to be done if you have had placenta previa or if the baby is in an unusual position. You should ask your doctor what type of incision was made in your uterus because the type of incision is a factor in deciding whether you can have a vaginal birth in the future.

Removing the Baby

The doctor lifts the baby out through the incisions. The umbilical cord then is cut, and the baby is passed to the nurse.

Afterbirth and Closing the Incisions

After the baby is delivered, the placenta is removed from the uterus. The doctor then closes the incisions made in the uterus and abdominal wall with stitches that will later dissolve on their own in the body. The incision in your skin, however, will be closed with stitches or surgical staples that will have to be removed later by your doctor.

Risks

Like any major surgery, cesarean delivery involves risks. Problems occur in a small number of women. Although they usually can be treated, in very rare cases, complications can be serious or even fatal:

- The uterus, nearby pelvic organs, or skin incision can get infected.

- You can lose blood. A blood transfusion may be needed in a few cases. In very rare cases, a *hysterectomy* (surgical removal of the uterus) may need to be done if bleeding cannot be controlled.

- You can develop blood clots in the legs, pelvic organs, or lungs.

- Your bowel or bladder can be injured.

- You can have a reaction to the medications or types of anesthetics that are used.

Recovery

If you are awake for the surgery, you probably can hold your baby after the surgery is completed. You will be taken to a recovery room or directly to your hospital room. Your blood pressure, pulse rate, breathing rate, and abdomen will be checked regularly.

If you are planning on breastfeeding, be sure to let your doctor know. Having a cesarean delivery does not mean you won't be able to breastfeed your baby. If all is going well for you and your baby, you should be able to begin breastfeeding soon after delivery.

You may need to stay in bed for a while. The first few times you get out of bed, a nurse or other adult should help you.

Soon after surgery, the catheter is removed from the bladder. You will receive fluids intravenously after your delivery, until you are able to eat and drink. The abdominal incision will be sore for the first few days. Your doctor can prescribe pain medication for you to take after the anesthetic wears off. There are many different ways to control pain. Talk to your doctor about your options.

The usual hospital stay after a cesarean delivery is 2–4 days. How many days you will have to stay depends on why you needed the cesarean delivery and how long it takes for your body to recover.

Back at Home

Once you are permitted to go home, you will need to take special care of yourself and limit your activities. Take it easy. You just had major surgery, and it will take a few weeks for your abdomen to heal. During the weeks you recover from the surgery, you may experience:

- Mild cramping, especially if you are breastfeeding
- Bleeding or discharge for about 4–6 weeks
- Bleeding with clots and cramps
- Pain in the incision

Your doctor will tell you not to place anything in your vagina or have sex for a few weeks in order to prevent infection. Give yourself time to heal before doing any strenuous activity. If you have a fever, heavy bleeding, or the pain gets worse, call your doctor right away.

Breech Presentation

By 3 or 4 weeks before the due date, most babies change position in the uterus so their heads are down near the birth canal. This is called a **vertex presentation**. If the baby does not change position, she may be in a breech presentation. It happens in 3–4% of babies who are born full-term. It occurs more frequently in preterm babies.

Although the reasons why a baby is in a breech position are not always known, it is more common if one or more of the following conditions occur:

- You have had more than one pregnancy.
- You are having twins.
- The uterus has too much or too little **amniotic fluid**.
- The uterus is not normal in shape or has abnormal growths (**fibroids**, for example).
- The placenta covers all or part of the opening of the uterus (placenta previa).

Occasionally babies with certain birth defects also will stay in a breech presentation at term, but most babies in a breech presentation at term are otherwise normal.

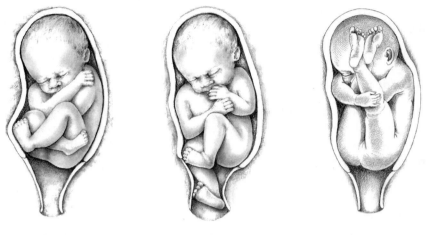

Complete breech   **Footling breech**   **Frank breech**

Breech presentations. In a breech birth, the baby's buttocks, feet, or both may be in place to come out first during birth.

The Baby's Position

To plan for delivery of a baby in a breech presentation, your health care provider will do a physical exam to find out how the baby is positioned. If the baby is in a breech presentation—and depending on your and the baby's condition—the health care provider may try to turn the baby's head down. This procedure is known as *external cephalic version*.

To turn the baby, the health care provider places his or her hands at certain points on your abdomen, then lifts and turns. In some cases, a second person may help turn the baby or watch the baby with *ultrasound*. Most often, external cephalic version is not tried until you are at least 36 weeks' pregnant. If it is done before this time, the baby may go back to a breech presentation.

The baby's heart rate is checked with fetal monitoring before and after external cephalic version. If any problems arise with you or the baby, external cephalic version will be stopped. Sometimes, a drug is given to you first to relax the uterus, which may make it easier to turn the baby. You also may receive pain relief, such as an *epidural block*.

External cephalic version usually is done near a delivery room. If problems occur, the baby then can be delivered quickly, by cesarean delivery if necessary. More than half of attempts at external cephalic version succeed. Some babies, though, move back into a breech presentation. If that happens, the procedure may be tried again. But it tends to be harder to do as the time for birth gets closer. As the baby grows bigger, there is less room for her to move.

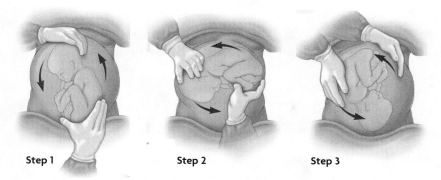

Step 1   Step 2   Step 3

External cephalic version. In this procedure, the health care provider attempts to lift and turn the baby from a breech presentation to a vertex (head-down) presentation. Reprinted from Beckmann CRB, Ling FW, Barzansky BM, Herbert WNP, Laube PW, Smith RP. Obstetrics and gynecology. 6th ed. Baltimore: Lippincott Williams & Wilkins; 2010.

Delivery

If your baby is in a breech presentation, your health care provider will talk with you about the best type of birth for you and your baby. If the baby can be turned with version, vaginal birth may be an option. If the baby is in a breech presentation as the time of delivery nears, cesarean delivery may be best.

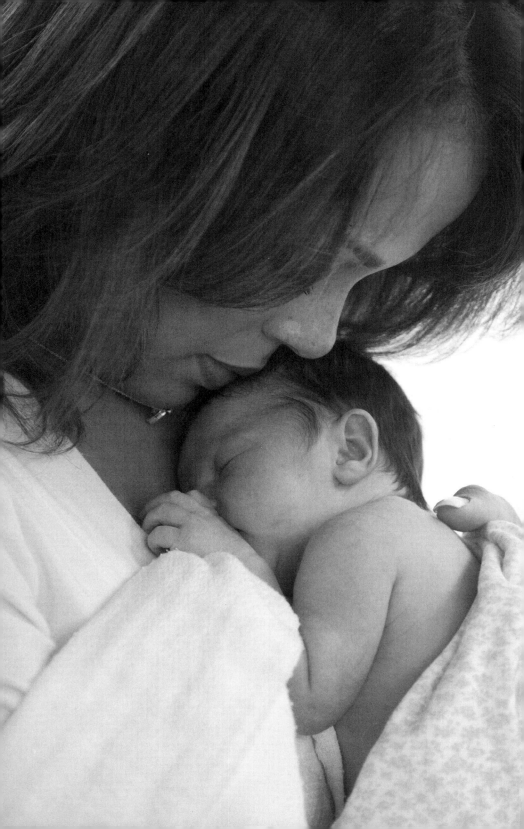

Chapter 12
The Postpartum Period

It may be hard to believe that childbirth is over and that this baby is really yours. The postpartum period can be a time of joy and happiness, as well as fatigue and sometimes sadness. If you know what's happening to your body and emotions, you can better face the ups and downs of the first few months of being a mom.

Right After the Baby Is Born

In the moments after birth, you will most likely be able to hold and cuddle your baby. Your caregivers also will be busy assessing your newborn's health, as well as checking on your condition to make sure all is well.

Your Baby's Apgar Score

Your baby's health will be assessed with the Apgar test 1 minute after birth and then again 5 minutes after birth. The *Apgar score* rates five newborn features: heart rate, breathing, muscle tone, reflexes, and skin color. Each of these features is given a score of 0, 1, or 2. Then all the scores are added, with a maximum possible score of 10. Most babies have an Apgar score of 7 or more at 5 minutes after birth. Few babies score a perfect 10 (see Table 12-1).

The Apgar score is used to check the baby's condition right after delivery. It also is a good way to measure how well the baby adjusts to the outside world in the minutes after birth. The Apgar score does not show how healthy your baby was before birth, nor does it predict how healthy your baby will be in the future.

Table 12-1 The Apgar Score

Component	Score 0	Score 1	Score 2
Heart rate	Absent	Fewer than 100 beats per minute	More than 100 beats per minute
Respiration	Absent	Weak cry or hyperventilation	Good, strong cry
Muscle tone	Limp	Some flexing of arms and legs	Active motion
Reflexes (response to airway being suctioned)	No response	Grimace	Cries or withdraws; coughs; sneezes
Color*	Blue or pale	Body is pink; hands and feet are blue	Pink all over

In babies with dark skin, the mouth, lips, palms, and soles are examined.

Your Baby's First Breath

During pregnancy, your baby got oxygen through the **placenta** and **umbilical cord**. In the moments after birth, your newborn takes his first breath of air. It's not just the lungs that must be working and able to fill with air seconds after delivery. All the related body parts, such as muscles around the lungs and airways leading from the mouth and nose, must also be ready to start working.

After birth, there's more pressure outside the lungs than there is inside them. This pressure causes the lungs to expand and fill with air. As a result, the baby may start crying. Many babies cry on their own at birth. Others don't cry right away. Instead, they simply start breathing.

After birth, your baby's breathing is closely monitored. If the baby isn't breathing well, steps may be taken to help. Often, this simply means rubbing the baby's body to wake him up a bit. Sometimes the baby may be given oxygen.

Maintaining the Baby's Temperature

The temperature inside your **uterus** is fairly stable. Before birth, your baby was kept warm by your body. After birth, your baby enters a place that's much cooler. Your newborn also is wet with **amniotic fluid**. The baby can lose a lot of heat as the moisture on his skin evaporates. If the baby is given to you right after birth, the best way to keep the baby warm is to hold him close to your skin. A towel or blanket will be used to dry off the baby.

Although newborns have built-in controls to keep body temperature even, they do not work as well as an adult's do. A newborn can easily get too hot or too cold. It's important to monitor the baby's environment and make sure that the baby is dressed appropriately.

Getting to Know Your Baby

You'll never forget the first time you see your new baby. As a new mom, you may have lots of questions about the way your newborn looks and acts. Knowing what's normal and what to expect from this time in your baby's life will help you relax and enjoy watching your baby grow.

Your Baby's Weight

One of the first questions people ask after a baby arrives is how much he weighs. In fact, that's one of the first things doctors and nurses at the hospital want to know too. There's no such thing as a right weight for a newborn. There is a range that is thought to be normal for most babies. Most full-term babies weigh between 5 1/2 and 9 1/2 pounds. The average weight is 7 1/2 pounds.

The weight often depends on how close a baby is born to the due date. Babies born early tend to weigh less than those born at term (37–42 weeks after your last menstrual period). Babies born late tend to weigh more. In the first 3 days after birth, it is normal for a baby to lose a very small amount of weight before beginning to gain.

How Your Baby Looks

If you're used to seeing newborns on television, you may be surprised to know that most shows use babies who are a few months old to portray newborns. Real newborns look a lot different the first few days:

- The body may seem scrunched up because a new baby draws his arms and legs up close, into the so-called fetal position. This is the way he fit into the close confines of your uterus. Even though the baby has more room now, it'll take a few weeks for him to stretch out a bit.

- The face may be slightly swollen, and the area around his eyes may be a little puffy for a few days.

- The baby's head may be long and pointy for a few days or weeks. Why? Babies have two soft spots on the top of their heads where the skull bones haven't yet joined. These soft spots make the head flexible enough to fit through the birth canal.

• Right after birth, the baby's genitals may be swollen. The swelling usually is caused by extra fluid that has built up in the baby's body. In girls, the **labia** may be swollen because of the high levels of maternal **hormones** that she was exposed to in the uterus. Boys may have extra fluid around their testicles that may make their **scrotums** appear swollen. This swelling usually resolves within days.

How Your Baby Acts

Most newborns' basic needs and responses to the outside world are the same. Even so, each baby has a unique personality right from the start.

The way one baby behaves and interacts with people can be very different from the way another newborn acts. Some babies are quiet and calm. This is likely to be true of babies who seemed quiet in the uterus. Other babies are bundles of energy from the start. They cry and kick with vigor and demand around-the-clock attention.

After the stress of birth, most newborns are very alert for the first hour or so. This is a good time to nurse, talk to, or just hold your new son or daughter.

When this alertness fades, the baby will get sleepy. Don't worry if your newborn seems very drowsy or sleeps a lot for the next few hours or even days. After all, you are not the only one who needs to recover from the birth.

Many babies do little else besides sleep at first. Most newborns spend 14–18 hours a day sleeping—although not all at once. Short stretches of sleep broken up by brief alert periods are normal. But again, it depends on the baby. Some newborns sleep less and are fussy when they wake up. Others sleep for long stretches and are quiet and calm when they are awake.

What Happens to Your Baby Next

When you are ready to part with your new baby, the nurse will weigh and measure the baby, give him a bath, slip identification bands around the baby's ankle and wrist, and perhaps take handprints and footprints. For the next few hours, the doctor and nurses will make sure the baby is in good health.

Medical Care

Your baby will receive a complete physical exam in the hospital. A doctor or nurse will look your baby over from head to toe, listen to the breathing and heartbeat, check the pulse, feel the belly, and look for normal newborn reflexes. Other steps will be taken to help prevent health problems:

• *Vitamin K shot*—A newborn's body can't make vitamin K on its own for a few days, so vitamin K routinely is given by an injection. Vitamin K is needed for the blood to clot after a cut. The vitamin K shot also helps protect against a rare but severe bleeding disorder.

* **Antibiotic** *ointment or solution in the baby's eyes*—This treatment protects against infection from germs that can get into the eyes during birth.

* *Immunizations against* **hepatitis B virus (HBV)**—Babies can get HBV from their mothers during birth so this vaccine is given as a precaution. Left untreated, HBV can lead to severe illness and liver damage.

Tests
Before the baby leaves the hospital, a few tests will be done to check for certain health conditions:

* *Hearing test*—There are two kinds of hearing tests for newborns. Both are painless and take about 10 minutes. In one test, a tiny speaker and microphone are put in the baby's ear. The speaker makes soft clicking sounds. The ear's response to the sounds is measured by the microphone. In the other test, soft earphones are placed over your baby's ears. Then three special sensors are attached to the baby's head. The earphones play soft clicks. The sensors measure brain-wave responses to the sounds. If the screening test shows there might be hearing loss, the doctor will refer your baby to a hearing specialist for further testing.

* *Blood test*—A small blood sample will be taken and checked for certain diseases, such as phenylketonuria and **hypothyroidism** (low thyroid hormone). Both conditions can cause mental retardation. Complications usually can be avoided if these conditions are found and treated early. The blood also will be tested for hypoglycemia (low blood sugar), sickle cell anemia, and many rare metabolic conditions. Which tests the baby receives depends on which state you live in. You and your pediatrician also can request that additional tests be done, but these tests may not be covered by your insurance.

Circumcision
If you and your partner have decided to have your baby boy circumcised, it will be done by your ob-gyn or other health care provider soon after birth, before the baby leaves the hospital. The procedure should be performed with a local anesthetic. Circumcision for religious reasons can be done outside the hospital (see Chapter 7, "Month 8 [Weeks 29–32]," for more discussion).

Postpartum: The First Week

If you had a normal vaginal delivery, you will be discharged from the hospital soon after the baby is born, once it is established that your condition is stable. How long you stay depends on your health. However, your insurance policy may have limits as to how long they will cover hospitalization postpartum. How long you stay after a *cesarean delivery* can depend on why the cesarean delivery was done and how much time you need to resume normal functions.

Before you are discharged, you will be given instructions to follow in case of problems or an emergency. You should arrange for a follow-up exam for you and your newborn. You health care provider will want to check you about 2–6 weeks after the birth. Your baby generally should be evaluated within 1–2 weeks unless there are issues that need to be addressed sooner. He probably will be examined by a doctor once a month for the first 3 months.

You also may receive a tetanus–diphtheria–pertussis (Tdap) shot before leaving the hospital. The American College of Obstetricians and Gynecologists recommends that women who have never received Tdap get this immunization if 2 or more years have elapsed since their last tetanus and diphtheria (TD) booster. The TD booster is the "tetanus shot" that you get every 10 years or when you have an injury. It protects against both tetanus and diphtheria. The Tdap vaccine adds pertussis vaccine to this booster shot (the "a" in "Tdap" stands for "acellular," a type of pertussis vaccine). Pertussis, commonly known as whooping cough, can be a serious and sometimes life-threatening illness in newborns. The immediate family is most often the source of the infection for infants. One Tdap shot currently is recommended for people who will be in contact with infants younger than 12 months. Family members younger than 64 years who will be in contact with the baby also should receive a Tdap shot if they have not already had one.

Bleeding

Once your baby is born, your body sheds the blood and tissue that lined your uterus. This vaginal discharge is called *lochia*. For the first few days after delivery, lochia is heavy and bright red. It may have a few small clots. You should wear sanitary pads during this time—not tampons.

As time goes on, the flow gets lighter in volume and color. A week or so after birth, lochia often is pink or brown. Bright red discharge can come back, though. You may feel a gush of blood from your vagina during breastfeeding, when your uterus contracts. By 2 weeks postpartum, lochia often is light brown or yellow. After that, it slowly goes away. How long the discharge lasts differs for each woman. Some women have discharge for just a couple of weeks after their babies are born. Others have it for a month or more.

Uterine Contractions

For a few days after giving birth, you will feel your uterus contract and then relax as it shrinks back to its normal size. These cramps are sometimes called afterbirth pains. While you wait for these cramps to ease, you can find some relief by taking an over-the-counter pain reliever.

Perineal Pain

Your **perineum** is the area between your **vagina** and **rectum**. If you have stitches in this area from an **episiotomy** or tear, you'll likely have a few weeks of swelling and pain as the perineum heals. To help ease the pain and heal quicker, try these tips:

* Apply cold packs or chilled witch-hazel pads to the area.
* Do **Kegel exercises** a day or so after birth.
* Ask your doctor about using a numbing spray or cream to ease pain.
* If sitting is uncomfortable, sit on a pillow.
* Sit in a bathtub of warm water just deep enough to cover your buttocks and hips (called a sitz bath).

Painful Urination

In the first days after delivery, you may feel the urge to urinate but can't pass any **urine**. You may feel pain and burning when you urinate. That's because during birth, the baby's head put a lot of pressure on your **bladder**, your **urethra** (the opening where urine comes out), and the muscles that control urine flow. This pressure can cause swelling and stretching that gets in the way of urination.

To lessen swelling or pain, try a warm sitz bath. When you are on the toilet, spray warm water over your **genitals** with a squeeze bottle. This can help trigger the flow of urine. Running the tap while you are in the bathroom may help too. Be sure to drink plenty of fluids as well. This pain usually goes away within days of delivery.

Many new mothers have another problem: involuntary leakage of urine, or urinary incontinence. With time, the tone of your pelvic muscles will return and the incontinence will go away in most cases. You may feel more comfortable wearing a sanitary pad until the problem goes away. Doing Kegel exercises (see p. 28) also will help tighten these muscles sooner.

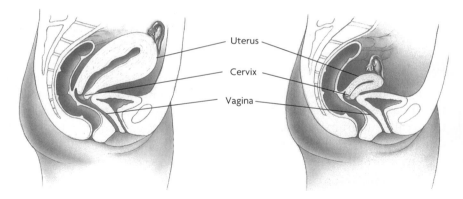

Uterus

Cervix

Vagina

The uterus before and after birth. Just after birth, the uterus measures about 7 inches long and weighs about 2½ pounds (*left*). In 6 weeks, it has returned to normal size (*right*). The normal size is about 3 inches long, weighing about 2 ounces.

Abdomen

Right after delivery, you will still look like you are pregnant. During pregnancy, the abdominal muscles stretched out little by little. They won't just snap back into place the minute your baby is born.

Give your body time to go back to normal. Exercise will help. Ask your doctor when it is safe to start exercising. Doing a few exercises at least three times per week will get you started.

Hemorrhoids

If you had varicose **veins** in your **vulva** or hemorrhoids during pregnancy, they may get worse after delivery. These sore, swollen veins also can show up for the first time now because of the intense straining you did during labor. In time, hemorrhoids and vulvar varicosities will get smaller or go away. For relief, try medicated sprays or ointments, dry heat (from a heat lamp or hairdryer turned on low), sitz baths, and cold witch-hazel compresses. Also, try not to strain when you have a bowel movement because this can make hemorrhoids worse.

Bowel Problems

It may be hard to have bowel movements for a few days after delivery. There are lots of reasons for this: stretched abdominal muscles, sluggish bowels as a result of surgery or pain medication, and an empty stomach after not eating during labor. You also may be afraid to move your bowels because of pain from an episiotomy or hemorrhoids. If you have constipation and painful gas, try these tips to help the problem:

- Take short walks as soon as you can.
- Eat foods high in fiber and drink plenty of fluids.
- Ask your doctor about taking a stool softener.

You may find that the urge to have a bowel movement may not feel the way it used to. In some cases, you may not be able to control your bowel movements. Loss of normal control of the bowels is called fecal incontinence. It can be caused by the stretching and tearing of nerves near the rectum during birth. You may pass gas when you do not mean to or do not expect it. If you have lost the normal control of your bowels, tell your doctor about your symptoms. Much can be done to help you regain control of your bowels.

Postpartum: Week 2 Through Week 12

In the weeks following your baby's birth, your body will change as it adjusts to not being pregnant. You also will be caring for a newborn. It can be a very stressful time. Taking care of your physical and mental well-being is key. Having people nearby for support may also help ease your transition into your new role.

Your Changing Body

While you were pregnant, your body worked round-the-clock for 40 weeks to help your baby grow. Now that your baby is here, there's more work to be done as your body recovers from pregnancy, labor, and delivery. It will take time for things to get back to normal.

Swollen Breasts
Your breasts fill with milk about 2–4 days after delivery. When this happens, they may feel very full, hard, and tender. The best relief for this engorgement is breastfeeding. Once you and your baby settle into a regular nursing pattern, the discomfort will go away. Severe engorgement should not last more than about 36 hours.

Women who do not breastfeed may experience discomfort from engorgement. When the breasts are not stimulated to produce more milk, this feeling will gradually subside, but it often takes about 7–10 days. In the meantime, try the following measures:

- Wear a well-fitting support bra or sports bra. Do not bind your breasts, which can make your pain worse.

- Apply ice packs to your breasts to reduce swelling.
- Don't express any milk. This sends a signal to your breasts to make more.
- Take pain medication, such as ibuprofen, if you need it.

Fatigue

You are going to be tired. You just finished a very hard task—childbirth. Your new baby will cause you and your partner many sleepless nights for a while until she gets into a regular sleeping schedule.

You can't really avoid fatigue, but there are steps you can take to make sure you're not totally exhausted from the job of being a new mom:

- *Ask for help*—Your family and friends are more than likely eager to pitch in. Let them. Be specific when others want to know what they can do. Ask a friend to bring something for dinner, stop at the grocery store, start a load of laundry, or watch the baby or an older child for a couple of hours so you can take a nap.

- *Sleep when your baby sleeps*—Use your baby's nap time to rest—not to tackle household chores.

- *Suggest quiet play*—If you have an older child, set him or her up with a few puzzles, picture books, or other quiet activities so you and the baby can rest.

- *Take it easy*—Only do what must be done and keep trips out of the house short.

- *Limit visitors*—If you are feeling tired, it's perfectly fine to say no to family and friends who want to stop by. Don't feel guilty. There will be plenty of time for people to meet your new baby when you are feeling rested.

- *Eat a healthy diet*—It may be hard to find time to eat when you are caring for a new baby. Even so, it's vital that you do. Foods rich in protein and iron help fight fatigue.

Sweating

In the weeks after birth, many new mothers find themselves drenched with sweat. This happens most often at night. Don't worry about it. Your body is adjusting to changing hormone levels. To keep your sheets and pillow dry at night, you can sleep on a towel until the sweating eases.

Return of Menstrual Periods

If you are not breastfeeding, your period may return about 6–8 weeks after giving birth. It could start even sooner. If you are breastfeeding, your men-

THE POSTPARTUM PERIOD • 219

strual periods may not start again for months. Some breastfeeding mothers don't have a menstrual period until their babies are fully weaned.

After birth, your **ovaries** may release an **egg** before you have your first menstrual period. This means you can get pregnant before you even know you are fertile again. If you don't want another baby right way, start using a birth control method, such as a condom, as soon as you resume having sex.

Once **menstruation** returns, it may not be the same as before you were pregnant. Menstrual periods may be shorter or longer, for instance. Chances are, they'll slowly return to normal. Some women notice that menstrual cramps are less painful than they were before they got pregnant.

Postpartum Danger Signs

Postpartum discomforts are normal. However, some discomforts may be a sign that there is a problem. Call your doctor if you have any of these symptoms:

- Fever more than 100.4°F
- Nausea and vomiting
- Pain or burning during urination
- Bleeding that's heavier than a normal menstrual period or that increases
- Severe pain in your lower abdomen
- Pain, swelling, and tenderness in your legs
- Chest pain and cough or gasping for air
- Red streaks on your breasts or painful new lumps in your breasts
- Pain that doesn't go away or that gets worse from an episiotomy, perineal tear, or abdominal incision
- Redness or discharge from an episiotomy, tear, or incision
- Vaginal discharge that smells bad
- Feelings of hopelessness that last more than 10 days after delivery

Postpartum Sadness and Depression

Feeling sad after having a baby is actually very common. In fact, about 70–80% of new mothers have these feelings that are known as the "baby blues" or "maternity blues." But for about 13% of women, these feelings are more intense and don't go away in a few weeks. This can signal a more serious condition called **postpartum depression.**

Baby Blues
Many new mothers are surprised by how fragile, alone, and drained they feel after the birth of a child. Their feelings don't seem to match their expectations. They wonder, "What have I got to be depressed about?" Also, they fear that

having these feelings means they are bad mothers. These emotions, however, are very normal. Many women feel sad after giving birth. Most often, these blue feelings are mild and will go away on their own within a couple of weeks.

When you feel blue, remind yourself that you have just taken on a huge job. Feeling sad, anxious, or even angry doesn't mean you are a failure as a mother. It also doesn't mean you are mentally ill. It simply means that your body is adjusting to the normal changes that follow the birth of a child.

Keep in mind, too, that things will soon start looking up again. Until then, do the following things to help you conquer the blues:

• Talk to your partner or a good friend about how you feel.
• Get plenty of rest.
• Ask your partner, friends, and family for help.
• Take time for yourself. Get out of the house each day, even if it's only for a short while.

Postpartum Depression
Postpartum depression is marked by feelings of despair, severe anxiety, or hopelessness that get in the way of daily life. It is more likely to occur in women who have had one or more of the following conditions:

• Mood disorders before pregnancy
• Postpartum depression after a previous pregnancy
• Recent stress, such as losing a loved one, family illness, or moving to a new city

If you are depressed, your depression can affect your baby. Getting treatment is important. Talk to your doctor right away if you have any of these signs of depression:

• Feeling restless or moody
• Feeling sad, hopeless, and overwhelmed
• Crying a lot
• Having no energy or motivation
• Eating too little or too much
• Sleeping too little or too much
• Having trouble focusing or making decisions
• Feeling worthless and guilty
• Losing interest or pleasure in activities you used to enjoy
• Withdrawing from friends and family
• Having headaches, aches and pains, or stomach problems that don't go away

If you or your partner notice any of these signs and symptoms, you need to contact your health care provider. Often a woman is unaware that she is depressed, and it is a family member who notices the signs and symptoms. Your health care provider can figure out if your symptoms are caused by depression or something else. If you are diagnosed with depression, it can be treated. Treatment can include talking to a therapist or psychologist, taking antidepressant medications, or both. Most antidepressant drugs are safe to use while breastfeeding.

Getting Back Into Shape

The demands of being a mother may have left you feeling too tired to exercise. The extra effort is worth it, though. Working out boosts your energy level and your sense of well-being. It also restores muscle strength and helps you get back in shape.

Most women can start exercising as soon as they feel up to it. However, talk to your doctor about when you can get started. If you had a **cesarean delivery** or problems after delivery, it may take a little longer to feel ready for exercise. For safety's sake, follow the same guidelines you did for a healthy lifestyle when you were pregnant.

If you stayed fit during pregnancy, you'll have a head start. Even so, don't attempt hard workouts right away. If you didn't do much exercise before, take it slowly now. Start with easy exercises and work up to harder ones.

Walking is a very good way to ease back into fitness. Take a brisk walk as often as you can—every day if possible. This will help prepare you for more intense exercise when you feel up to it. Walking is a great activity. It's easy to do, and you don't need anything except comfortable shoes. You can even take the baby with you in a stroller or carrier, so you don't need to hire a baby sitter. It may do you both good to get fresh air and see other people.

Swimming is another great postpartum exercise. There also are exercise classes designed just for new mothers. To find one, check with local health and fitness clubs, community centers, and hospitals.

No matter what sort of exercise you do, design a program that meets your needs. You may want to strengthen your heart and lungs, tone your muscles, lose weight, or do all three.

Also try to choose a program you'll keep doing. Staying fit over the long haul is more important than getting into shape right after birth. Your doctor can suggest forms of exercise that will help you meet your fitness goals.

Exercises for the Postpartum Period

The following exercises are designed to tone and strengthen your abdominal muscles. Start slowly, and if you have had a cesarean delivery, be careful of your incision.

- **Head Lifts**—When you can do 10 head lifts at a time, proceed to shoulder lifts.
  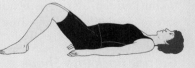
  1. Lie on your back with your knees bent, your feet flat on the floor, and your arms along your sides.
  2. Inhale and relax your belly.
  3. Exhale slowly as you lift your head off the floor.
  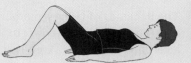
  4. Inhale as you lower your head again.

- **Shoulder Lifts**—When you can do 10 shoulder lifts at a time, proceed to curl-ups.
  1. Lie on your back with your knees bent, your feet flat on the floor, and your arms along your sides.
  2. Inhale and relax your belly.
  3. Exhale slowly and lift your head and shoulders off the floor. Reach with your arms so that you do not use them for support. If this bothers your neck, place both hands behind your head.
  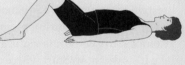
  4. Inhale as you lower your shoulders to the floor.
  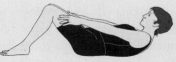

- **Curl-Ups**
  1. Lie on your back with your knees bent, your feet flat on the floor, and your arms along your sides.
  2. Inhale and relax your belly.
  3. Exhale. Reach with your arms, and slowly raise your torso until it is half-way between your knees and the floor (about a 45-degree angle). If you need more support for your neck and head, place your hands behind your head.
  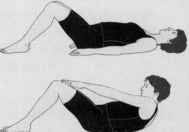
  4. Inhale as you lower your torso to the floor.

- **Kneeling Pelvic Tilt**—Tilting your pelvis back toward your spine helps strengthen your abdominal muscles.
  1. Kneel on your hands and knees with your back straight.
  2. Inhale.
  3. Exhale and pull your buttocks forward, rotating the pubic bone upward.
  4. Hold for a count of three.
  5. Inhale and relax.
  6. Repeat five times. Add one or two repetitions a day if you can.

- **Leg Slides**—This simple exercise tones abdominal and leg muscles. It is safe to do after a cesarean delivery, because it does not put much strain on your incision. Try to do leg slides a few times a day.
  1. Lie flat on your back and bend your knees slightly.
  2. Inhale, and slide your right leg from a bent to a straight position.
  3. Exhale, and bend it back again.
  4. Keep both feet on the floor and relaxed.
  5. Repeat with your left leg.

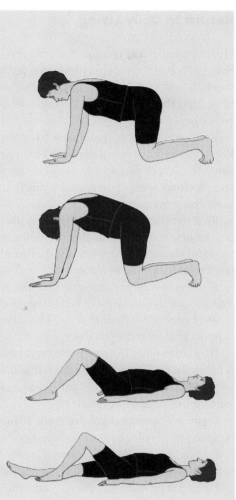

Return to Daily Living

Having a baby will change the way you live your daily life. Your relationship with your partner will be affected. Your old routines may no longer work. If you know this in advance and try to accept these changes rather than fight them, you'll be a lot more relaxed as you start your life with the new baby.

Keep in mind, too, that a new baby touches the lives of the whole family. Each person has a role and should take part in the baby's care. There will be some tension as you all adjust to having a baby around. Talk about it. Share your feelings with your partner, your parents, and your children. Listen to their concerns as well.

Talk to other new moms, too. Just hearing that your family isn't the only one feeling the effects of the birth of a baby can help you cope during this stressful time. The support of other mothers also can make you feel more comfortable in your new role.

If the stress of parenting seems like too much to handle, get some help. Talk to your doctor or call a local crisis hotline. All new parents reach the end of their rope from time to time. This is even truer if you don't have a lot of support or if your baby is fussy.

No matter what triggers them, never take out your emotions on your child. A baby can get injured easily, even if you don't intend to hurt him. Shaking a baby for just a few seconds, for instance, can do enough harm to cause life-long brain damage or even death.

If you ever fear that you are going to lose control and hurt your baby, hand him to your partner or another loved one and walk away. If you are alone, put your baby in a safe place, such as the crib. Then go into another room (if you can, one that's out of earshot of your baby's cries) until you calm down.

Once the episode has passed, ask yourself what you can do to prevent it from happening again. Tell your partner you need more help, for instance. Ask friends and relatives for help when you have been on baby duty for too long without a break. Find out what sort of community services, such as counseling or financial help, are available to you.

Nutrition

It's common to lose as many as 20 pounds in the month after delivery. Although it may be tempting to follow up this weight loss with a crash diet so you can squeeze back into your old clothes, don't do it. Dieting can deny your body vital nutrients and delay healing after birth. If you are breastfeeding, strict dieting will deprive your baby of the calories and nutrients he needs.

Instead, try to be patient. Keep up the good eating habits you began in pregnancy. If you do, you'll be close to your normal weight within a few months. Combining healthy eating with exercise will help the process.

Lifestyle Changes

The healthy lifestyle habits you developed while you were pregnant shouldn't stop once the baby is born. If you smoked but stopped during pregnancy, don't start up again. If you need help quitting, see your health care provider. Secondhand smoke has been linked to an increased risk of **sudden infant death syndrome** in newborns. Babies exposed to secondhand smoke also are more likely to develop lung problems, such as asthma, allergies, and ear infections than babies who are not exposed to secondhand smoke. If you are breastfeeding, be aware that the nicotine and other chemicals in cigarettes can be passed along to your baby (although there is no conclusive evidence that these chemicals can harm the baby). Not smoking is one of the best things that you can do for your own health as well as your baby's.

Postpartum Visit

Arrange a visit to see your health care provider 4–6 weeks after your baby's birth. (If you had a cesarean delivery, you may be seen about 2 weeks after surgery to check the incision.) The goal of this checkup is to make sure that your body has recovered from pregnancy and birth and that you are not having any problems.

During the visit, the health care provider will check your weight, blood pressure, breasts, and abdomen. He or she also will do a pelvic exam to make sure a tear or episiotomy has healed and that your vagina, *cervix*, and uterus have returned to their normal state. If you had gestational diabetes mellitus, you may need to have a blood *glucose* test at this visit (see Chapter 19, "Diabetes Mellitus").

Use this time to bring up any questions or concerns you have about the healing process, breastfeeding, birth control, weight loss, sex, or your emotions. To help you remember everything to talk about, jot down any questions you have and bring them with you to this visit.

Sex After Childbirth

Your health care provider will tell you when you and your partner can begin having sex again after the baby is born. Although there is no set time limit, most likely you will have to wait at least 4–6 weeks to be sure you've healed completely. However, it is perfectly normal if even after these weeks have passed that you find you don't have much interest in sex. There are many reasons for this:

- *Fatigue*—Once you get your baby to sleep, all you or your partner may want to do is sleep too.

- *Stress*—Coping with your baby's demands can leave you with little desire for sex.

- *Fear of pain*—Your breasts may be tender and your perineum may be sore. If you are breastfeeding, low **estrogen** levels may make your vagina dry. This can make sex uncomfortable.

- *Lack of desire*—Hormone levels decrease after birth. As a result, so does your desire for sex.

- *Lack of opportunity*—Sex takes energy, time, and focus. When you are a new parent, these all tend to be in short supply.

During the weeks that you may not feel up to sexual intercourse, try to be intimate with your partner in other ways, such as hugging and kissing. When you do feel comfortable and ready to have sex again, it's a good idea to keep the following things in mind:

- Spend private time with your partner when you talk only about each other—not the baby or household problems.

- Find a time for sex when you are not rushed. Wait until the baby is sound asleep or you can drop him off with a friend or a relative for a couple of hours.

- Use a water-soluble lubricant cream or jelly to help with vaginal dryness.

- Try different positions to take pressure off the sore area and to control penetration.

- If sex isn't comfortable yet, there are many other ways to give and receive sexual pleasure, such as mutual **masturbation** or oral sex.

- If you have concerns about sexual problems, be honest and discuss them with your partner.

Birth Control

If you and your partner are ready to start having sex again, it is important to use birth control. Birth control can allow your body to heal before having another baby and allow you to plan your family. Even if you want your children to be close in age, it's best to wait at least 12 months before getting pregnant again. It is believed that babies conceived less than 6 months (or more than 5 years) after you give birth have a higher risk of **preterm** birth, low birth weight, and small size. Babies born soon after their siblings may have these problems because the mother's body has not had time to replace nutritional stores. Postpartum stress also is a factor. It is unclear why the longer time between pregnancies may affect fetal health. Of course, each family has different needs and desires when it comes to child spacing. Discuss the issue with your partner and your health care provider.

If you are not breastfeeding, your fertility can return within weeks of giving birth. If you are breastfeeding, it can be hard to tell when fertility returns. Keep in mind, too, that if you used fertility drugs to get pregnant the first time, it doesn't mean you can't get pregnant without them.

To be on the safe side, choose a form of birth control before you have sex for the first time. Today, there's a wide array of birth control methods for both women and men. Each has pros and cons. Before choosing one, talk about it with your health care provider.

Certain types of birth control may interfere with breastfeeding. If you are breastfeeding, choose a method that's compatible. Also, if you want more children, make sure the method you choose is easily reversible.

Hormonal Methods

Hormonal methods work by preventing **ovulation**. You will still have your menstrual period each month with some types of hormonal birth control.

Birth Control Pills

Oral contraceptives are the most common method of hormonal birth control. Taken as directed, the pill also is one of the most effective forms of birth control. Less than 1 out of 100 women will get pregnant each year if they take the pill each day as directed. Combination pills contain estrogen and **progestin**. If you are breastfeeding, estrogen can cut down on your milk supply. For this reason, you should not use combination pills while breastfeeding.

More effective

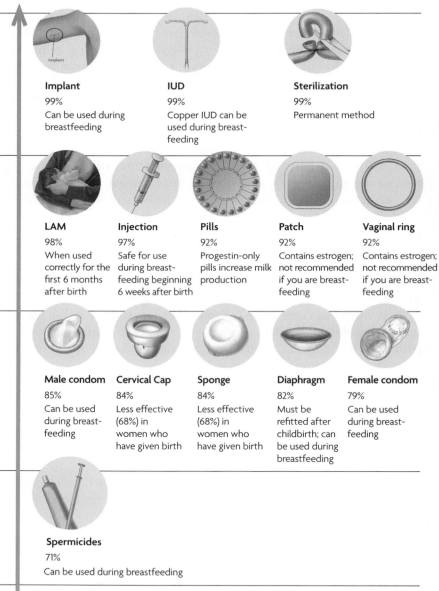

Implant
99%
Can be used during breastfeeding

IUD
99%
Copper IUD can be used during breast-feeding

Sterilization
99%
Permanent method

LAM
98%
When used correctly for the first 6 months after birth

Injection
97%
Safe for use during breast-feeding beginning 6 weeks after birth

Pills
92%
Progestin-only pills increase milk production

Patch
92%
Contains estrogen; not recommended if you are breast-feeding

Vaginal ring
92%
Contains estrogen; not recommended if you are breast-feeding

Male condom
85%
Can be used during breast-feeding

Cervical Cap
84%
Less effective (68%) in women who have given birth

Sponge
84%
Less effective (68%) in women who have given birth

Diaphragm
82%
Must be refitted after childbirth; can be used during breastfeeding

Female condom
79%
Can be used during breast-feeding

Spermicides
71%
Can be used during breastfeeding

Less effective

Effectiveness of birth control methods. This chart shows methods of birth control arranged from the least effective to the most effective. It's important to choose a method that's both effective and fits your lifestyle. The method of birth control that you used before having a baby may not be as suitable for you after having a baby.

Another option for breastfeeding moms is the so-called "minipill." These pills contain progestin only. They are a better choice if you are breastfeeding because there is no estrogen to affect the milk supply. Minipills also can be used by some women who cannot take estrogen for other reasons. The dose of progestin is even lower than that found in low-dose birth control pills. Unlike other birth control pills, each minipill pack consists of 28 tablets of active hormone that you need to take every day at the same time of day.

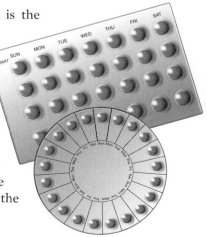

Birth control pills

Birth Control Injections
Birth control injections are given by your doctor in your arm or buttock every 3 months. As long as your injections are up-to-date, you don't have to do anything else to prevent pregnancy. Progestin-only injections can be used if you are breastfeeding.

Implant
The birth control implant is a single rod, about the size of a matchstick, that is inserted under the skin of the upper arm. It releases progestin. Because it doesn't contain estrogen, the implant can be used during breastfeeding. It's also highly effective, doesn't require you to remember anything, and works for 3 years. Its main drawback is that it can cause irregular bleeding, which usually goes away in 6–9 months, or a lack of menstrual periods altogether.

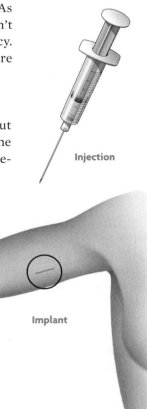

Injection

Implant

Birth Control Patch
The contraceptive patch is a small, square patch that sticks to your skin—usually on your lower abdomen, buttocks, or upper body. It releases doses of estrogen and progestin through your skin. Because it con-

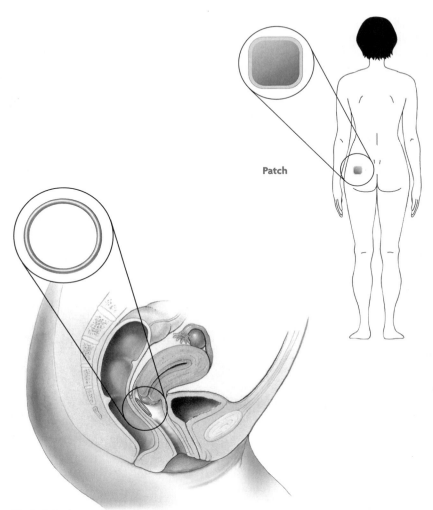

Patch

Vaginal ring

tains estrogen, it's not recommended if you are breastfeeding. A new patch is placed on the skin once a week for 3 weeks in a row, followed by a patch-free week. You will have a period during the patch-free week.

Vaginal Ring

This flexible, plastic ring is placed in the upper vagina and releases both estrogen and progestin. Because it contains estrogen, it is not a good choice for breastfeeding moms. You insert a new ring each month and keep it in place for 3 weeks. During the week it is out, you will have your menstrual period.

Intrauterine Devices

The **intrauterine device (IUD)** is a small, T-shaped device that is inserted into the uterus by your doctor. It prevents pregnancy by blocking sperm from joining with an egg or preventing a fertilized egg from implanting in the uterus.

There are two brands of IUDs available in the United States: the hormonal IUD (Mirena) and the copper IUD (ParaGard). The hormonal IUD releases a small amount of progesterone into the uterus and is effective for 5 years. The copper IUD releases a small amount of copper and is effective for 12 years. Both types of IUDs are very effective. Both can be easily removed at any time if you want to get pregnant or switch to another form of birth control.

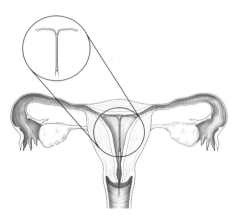

Intrauterine device

Barrier Methods

Barrier methods work by keeping sperm from reaching the egg. If you choose a barrier method, be sure to use it each time you have sex.

Spermicides

Spermicides are chemicals that destroy sperm before they can fertilize the egg. Spermicides come in various forms, including creams, gels, foams, and vaginal suppositories. Spermicides are placed in the vagina, close to the cervix, before sex.

Spermicide

Diaphragm

A diaphragm is a dome-shaped device that fits inside the vagina and covers the cervix. It can be inserted 1–2 hours before you have sex and is used with a spermicide. If you used a diaphragm before, you must be refitted after giving birth.

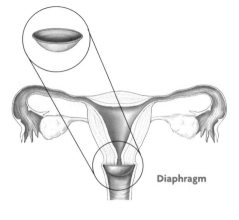

Diaphragm

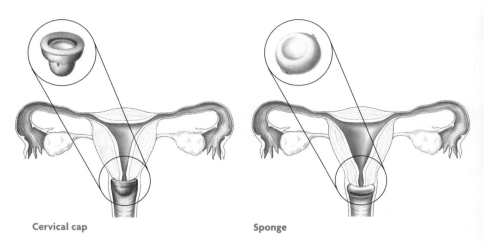

Cervical cap   Sponge

Cervical cap

The cervical cap is smaller than a diaphragm and fits more tightly over the cervix. It stays in place by suction. It is used with spermicide. Like the diaphragm, it must be fitted and prescribed by a doctor. Also like the diaphragm, it needs to be refitted after having a baby. It may be less effective in women who have given birth (68% effective) than in women who haven't (84% effective).

Sponge

The sponge is a doughnut-shaped device made of soft foam with spermicide. It is inserted into the vagina and covers the cervix. The sponge is convenient because it's available over the counter. However, it is less effective in women who have given birth—the effectiveness rates are the same as those for the cervical cap.

Male Condom

The male condom is a thin rubber sheath worn over a man's penis, which blocks his ejaculate from entering the vagina. Latex condoms are the most effective way to protect yourself against **sexually transmitted diseases**, including **human immunodeficiency virus (HIV)** infection and **acquired immunodeficiency syndrome (AIDS)**.

Female Condom

The female condom is a plastic pouch that lines the vagina. It is held in place by a closed inner ring at the cervix and an open outer ring at the entrance of the vagina.

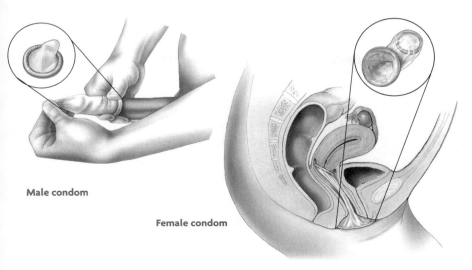

Male condom

Female condom

Lactational Amenorrhea Method

The Lactational Amenorrhea Method (LAM) is a temporary method of birth control that is based on the natural infertility that occurs when a woman is breastfeeding. When an infant suckles regularly, it suppresses the release of hormones that stimulate ovulation and menstruation. If a woman does not ovulate, she cannot become pregnant. The method is highly effective if used correctly.

For this method to work, a woman must follow certain breastfeeding guidelines. LAM is most effective when a woman is fully breastfeeding, which means that the infant receives no other liquid or food, not even water, in addition to breast milk. Although giving other liquids or formula on occasion may be fine, it may make ovulation more likely. Also, the time between feedings should not be longer than 4 hours during the day or 6 hours at night.

An important part of LAM is knowing when to start using another form of birth control to prevent pregnancy. To determine this time, a woman can ask herself three questions:

1. Has my period returned?
2. Am I supplementing regularly with formula or other food or liquids or allowing long periods without breastfeeding, either during the day or at night?
3. Is my baby more than 6 months old?

If you answer yes to any of these questions, your risk of pregnancy is increased, and you should use another form of birth control. However, you can still continue to breastfeed your baby if you choose a form of birth control that is compatible with breastfeeding.

Emergency Contraception

If you and your partner have unprotected sex or your birth control method fails during sex, you can use emergency contraception to prevent pregnancy.

One type of emergency contraception available in the United States is known as Plan B. It can prevent pregnancy if taken within 120 hours (5 days) of sex. Plan B contains progestin and consists of two pills that are taken 12 hours apart; or they can be taken at the same time. It reduces the chance of pregnancy by up to 89% and can be purchased from your pharmacist without a prescription. Another type, called Plan B One-Step, consists of a single pill. It also can be purchased without a prescription.

Your doctor also can insert a copper IUD as a form of emergency contraception. Both Plan B and the IUD work by preventing ovulation, blocking *fertilization*, or keeping a fertilized egg from implanting in the uterus.

Permanent Birth Control

Sterilization is an option if both you and your partner are sure you don't want any other children. Sterilization is more than 99% effective, and, in most cases, it's permanent.

Female Sterilization

Female sterilization can be performed during a surgical procedure or with a nonsurgical procedure called a *hysteroscopy*.

Tubal Ligation. Surgical sterilization is called **tubal ligation** or "having your tubes tied." During the procedure, the **fallopian tubes** are cut and tied to stop the egg from going from the ovary to the uterus. It also blocks sperm from reaching an egg. Tubal ligation won't affect your menstrual periods or your pleasure of sex. Some women choose to get sterilized right after their babies are born, while they are still in the hospital. The surgery is easier then because the uterus is still enlarged and pushes the fallopian tubes up in the abdomen. If you want to be sterilized after giving birth to your baby, talk to your health care provider about it well ahead of time. In some cases, it can be done a few minutes after the birth, with the same anesthesia used for the delivery. Women are immediately sterile after having this procedure.

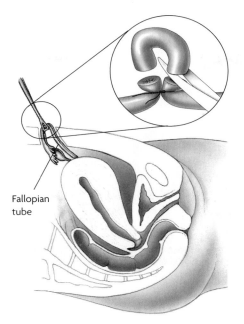

Postpartum tubal ligation. A small vertical or horzontal cut is made near the navel, and each fallopian tube is pulled through the incision. The tube is closed off with sutures or with a clamp device (not shown). The section between the closed-off section is removed.

Hysteroscopic Sterilization. Another method of sterilization, called hysteroscopic sterilization, also is available. This procedure can be performed in a health care provider's office or clinic, and it does not require an abdominal incision or *general anesthesia*. It can be done beginning 3 months after childbirth. Two kinds of hysteroscopic sterilization have been approved for use in the United States: the Essure System and the Adiana Permanent Contraception System.

Hysteroscopic sterilization involves inserting an instrument called a hysteroscope into the uterus though the vagina, and placing a small device into each fallopian tube. The devices cause scar tissue to form, which blocks the fallopian tubes and prevents the egg from being fertilized. It takes about 3 months after the procedure for the tubes to become completely blocked. During this time, you can become pregnant, and you will need to use another form of birth control. At the 3-month mark, you will have a *hysterosalpingography*, an X-ray procedure, to make sure that the fallopian tubes are blocked.

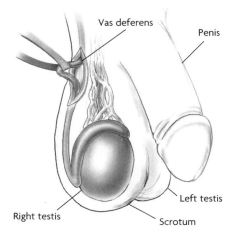

Vasectomy. One or two small cuts are made in the skin of the scrotum. Each vas is pulled through the opening until it forms a loop. A small section is cut out of the loop and removed.

Male Sterilization

Male sterilization is called **vasectomy**. It involves cutting or tying the **vas deferens** (tubes through which sperm travel) so no sperm is released when a man ejaculates. Vasectomy does not affect a man's ability to get erections or have orgasms. The procedure is done quickly and the man can go home the same day. However, it may take up to 3 months for a man to become sterile after the procedure. Beginning a few weeks after a vasectomy, a man will have periodic tests of his semen to see if there are any sperm.

Although there is surgery to reverse sterilization, it doesn't always work. Also, the operation to reverse female sterilization is major surgery.

Returning to Work

If, when, and how you go back to work after having a baby are personal choices. Paid maternity-leave policies vary from state to state and from employer to employer. The federal Family and Medical Leave Act guarantees women up to 12 weeks of unpaid leave after giving birth.

Beyond your recovery from birth, there are other factors to take into account. You have to think about how much money you make and how long your family can do without it. You have to look at the costs of and options for child care too. If you are breastfeeding, you should give yourself time to establish a good nursing relationship with your baby. You also will want to decide about continuing breastfeeding when you go back to work.

Be careful to build in some leeway for yourself. In other words, you can't predict for sure what will happen. You may not know how you'll feel about work until after your baby is born. For instance, some women plan to scale back on work or even put their careers on hold for a few years. Then they find that they miss the excitement and self-esteem they get from their jobs. Other women plan to go back to work full-time shortly after giving birth. Once their babies arrive, though, they are less sure about being both a mother and a full-time worker.

Working mothers have a number of options these days. A growing number of employers let new mothers work part-time, work from home 1 or 2 days a week, job share, condense their work weeks, or work flexible hours. Also, some companies offer on-site child care, which is a real bonus for new mothers. They can bring their babies to work with them and visit them during breaks and lunch hours and continue to breastfeed.

There are many things to consider when searching for good child care for your newborn. Will you use a day care center or a nanny? Finding child care for a young infant can be an anxious time for any couple. But be patient and make your selection only when you're most at ease (see page 144 for more tips on finding good child care).

Part III
Nutrition

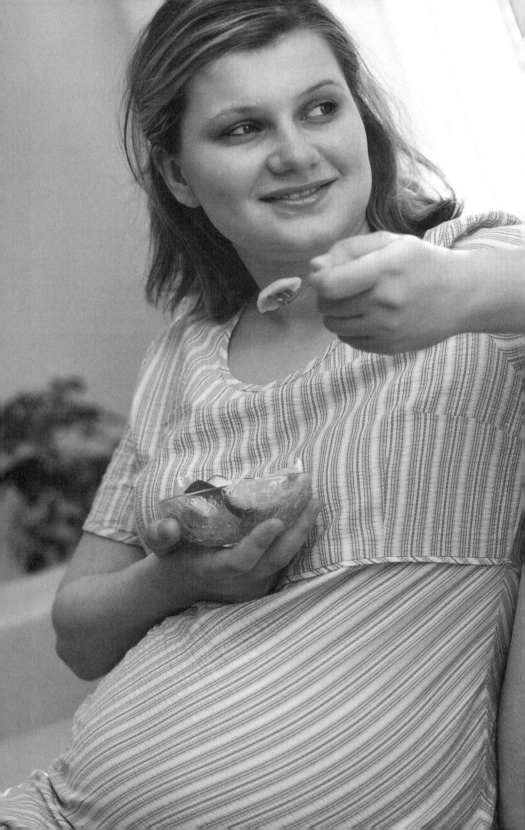

Chapter 13
Nutrition During Pregnancy

A well-balanced, healthy diet is crucial during pregnancy. Good nutrition is needed to meet the added demands on your body, as well as those of your growing baby. The old adage "You're eating for two" is still true—to a point. It doesn't mean that you can eat twice as much. Finding a balance between getting enough nutrients while maintaining a healthy weight is important for you and your baby's future health. A pregnant woman who is of a normal weight before pregnancy needs only about 300 extra calories a day—the amount that's in a glass of skim milk and half a sandwich.

Healthy eating during pregnancy may take a little effort, but it will be a major benefit for you and your baby. If you already eat a balanced diet, all you have to do is add a few extra well-chosen calories. If you haven't been eating a healthy diet, pregnancy is a great time to change old habits and develop healthy new ones. Breastfeeding mothers need to pay careful attention to their diets as well (see Chapter 14, "Feeding Your Baby").

Planning a Healthy Diet

The U.S. Department of Agriculture has designed an online interactive diet-planning program called the "My Pyramid Plan for Moms" specifically for women who are pregnant or breastfeeding (see Resources). This program gives you a personalized plan that includes the kinds of foods in the amounts that you need to eat for each trimester of pregnancy. Another tool, called "Menu Planner for Moms" allows you to see whether your daily food

choices are meeting your nutrient requirements and calorie recommendations. You also can use the Menu Planner to plan meals and snacks.

Getting Started

The My Pyramid Plan for Moms may make eating a healthy diet easier. To
get the most from it, you should understand a few key principles.

Every diet should include proteins, carbohydrates, vitamins, minerals,
and fats. These nutrients fuel your body and help your baby grow. The best
sources of nutrients are foods. While you're pregnant, it's important to eat a
variety of healthy foods in order to get all the necessary nutrients that both
you and your growing baby will need in the months to come.

The My Pyramid Plan for Moms is based on specific food groups: vegetables, fruits, milk, grains, and meat and beans. Also included is a discretionary
group of foods that don't fall into any of these groups. This group contains
the extras that aren't essential to our diets, such as high-fat or sugary foods,
or extra amounts of the foods in the other food groups. Fats and oils make up
another group.

The amount of food that you need to eat each day is calculated according
to your height, prepregnancy weight, due date, and how much you exercise
during the week. The recommendations are given in standard sizes that most
people are familiar with, such as cups and ounces.

Nutrients You Need

Nutrients are the building blocks of the body. They are used to build bones,
muscles, and organs. During pregnancy, you not only need to maintain your
own body, but you also need to support the growth of your baby's body. Getting enough nutrients during pregnancy safeguards your own health and
contributes to your baby's normal development (see Table 13-2 on page 244).

Protein
Protein provides the nutrients your body needs to grow and repair muscles and other tissues. During pregnancy, protein also is the building
block for your baby's cells. Most pregnant women need 71 grams of protein per day. Animal-based foods, such as meat, fish, poultry, and dairy
products, are high in protein:

- Beef, pork, and fish
- Chicken
- Low-fat milk
- Eggs

What Is a Dietary Reference Intake?

Dietary reference intakes are recommended amounts an individual should consume daily of certain nutrients, vitamins, and minerals (see Table 13-1). They are intended to be used as a guide for good nutrition and are the basis of the nutrition guidelines in the U.S. Department of Agriculture's My Pyramid Plan. You'll also see the words "daily value" on most food labels. The daily value is the amount of a nutrient that an average person should eat every day. Daily values are derived, in part, from dietary reference intakes.

Don't worry about eating the dietary reference intake for each nutrient every day. Your body stores nutrients for later use. Just try to eat a variety of foods and eat the recommended amounts from the basic food groups. If you do, chances are good that your diet is healthy and that your baby is getting the right amount of nutrients.

Table 13-1 Dietary Reference Intakes for Women

	Pregnant Women			Breastfeeding Women		
	14–18 Y	19–30 Y	31–50 Y	14–18 Y	19–30 Y	31–50 Y
Protein (g)	71	71	71	71	71	71
Calcium (mg)	1,300	1,000	1,000	1,300	1,000	1,000
Phosphorus (mg)	1,250	700	700	1,250	700	700
Magnesium (mg)	400	350	360	360	310	320
Iron (mg)	27	27	27	10	9	9
Zinc (mg)	12	11	11	13	12	12
Iodine (microgram)	220	220	220	290	290	290
Selenium (microgram)	60	60	60	70	70	70
Vitamin A (microgram)	750	770	770	1,200	1,300	1,300
Vitamin C (mg)	80	85	85	115	120	120
Vitamin D (microgram)*	5	5	5	5	5	5
Vitamin E (mg)[†]	15	15	15	19	19	19
Vitamin K (microgram)	75	90	90	75	90	90
Thiamin (mg)	1.4	1.4	1.4	1.4	1.4	1.4
Riboflavin (mg)	1.4	1.4	1.4	1.6	1.6	1.6
Niacin (mg)[‡]	18	18	18	17	17	17
Vitamin B$_6$ (mg)	1.9	1.9	1.9	2.0	2.0	2.0
Folic acid (microgram)	600[§]	600[§]	600[§]	500	500	500
Vitamin B$_{12}$ (mg)	2.6	2.6	2.6	2.8	2.8	2.8

Abbreviations: Y = years

*In the absence of adequate exposure to sunlight. Value is vitamin D as cholecalciferol. 1 microgram cholecalciferol = 40 international units vitamin D.

[†] As α-tocopherol.

[‡] As niacin equivalents. One mg of niacin = 60 mg of tryptophan.

[§] As dietary folate equivalents. One dietary folate equivalent = 1 microgram food folate = 0.6 microgram of folic acid from fortified food or as a supplement consumed with food = 0.5 microgram of a supplement taken on an empty stomach.

Reprinted with permission from Dietary reference intakes: vitamins; Dietary reference intakes: elements; Dietary reference intakes: Macronutrients. Courtesy of the National Academies Press, Washington, D.C. These tables can be accessed at the Institute of Medicine of the National Academies web site www.iom.edu/CMS/54133.aspx.

Table 13-2 Key Nutrients in Pregnancy

Nutrient	Source
Protein	Meat, fish, eggs, beans, dairy products
Carbohydrates	Bread, cereal, rice, potatoes, pasta
Fat	Meat, eggs, nuts, peanut butter, margarine, oils
Vitamins	
A	Green leafy vegetables, deep yellow or orange vegetables (carrots and sweet potatoes), milk, liver
Thiamin (B₁)	Whole-grain or enriched breads and cereals, fish, pork, poultry, lean meat, milk
Riboflavin (B₂)	Milk, whole-grain or enriched breads and cereals, liver, green leafy vegetables
B₆	Beef liver, pork, ham, whole-grain cereals, bananas
B₁₂	Animal foods, such as liver, milk, poultry (vegetarians should take a supplement)
C	Citrus fruit, strawberries, broccoli, tomatoes
D	Fortified milk, fish liver oils, sunshine
E	Vegetable oils, whole-grain cereals, wheat germ, green leafy vegetables
Folic acid	Green leafy vegetables; dark yellow or orange fruits and vegetables; liver, legumes and nuts; fortified breads, cereals, rice, and pastas
Niacin	Meat, liver, poultry, fish, whole-grain or enriched cereals
Minerals	
Calcium	Milk and dairy products; sardines and salmon with bones; collard, kale, mustard, spinach, and turnip greens; fortified orange juice
Iodine	Seafood, iodized salt
Iron	Lean red meat, liver, dried beans, whole-grain or enriched breads and cereals, prune juice, spinach, tofu
Magnesium	Legumes, whole-grain cereals, milk, meat, green vegetables
Phosphorus	Milk and dairy products, meat, poultry, fish, whole-grain cereals, legumes
Zinc	Meat, liver, seafood, milk, whole-grain cereals

Plant products such as grains and legumes also are good sources of protein. For strict vegetarians (called vegans), getting enough protein can be a challenge, but it can be done with good meal planning and knowing which plant foods contain the most protein.

Carbohydrates
Carbohydrates (food sugars) are the body's main source of energy. There are two types of food sugars: simple sugars and starches.

> ## Whole Grains and Refined Grains
>
> There are two types of grains: whole grains and refined grains. Whole grains contain the entire grain kernel. Examples of whole grains are brown rice, bulgur, oatmeal, and whole-wheat flour. Refined grains have been processed to remove the outer covering of the grain kernel. This processing also removes some of the fiber and other nutrients. Examples are white rice and white bread. It's recommended that whole grains make up at least one half of the grains that you eat daily.

Simple sugars provide a quick energy boost because they are ready to be used by the body right away. Simple sugars are found in table sugar, honey, syrup, fruit juices, hard candies, and many processed foods.

Starches are a more complex form of sugar. It takes your body longer to process them, so starches provide longer-lasting energy than simple sugars. Starches are found in bread, rice, pasta, fruits, and starchy vegetables such as potatoes and corn.

Starchy foods also contain fiber. Your body doesn't use fiber the same way it uses other nutrients. Fiber helps flush out your digestive system and helps prevent constipation. It also helps rid your body of excess fat and cholesterol. The following foods are good sources of fiber:

- Fruits (especially dried fruits, berries, oranges, and apples and peaches with the skin)
- Vegetables (such as dried beans and peas)
- Whole-grain products (such as whole-wheat bread or brown rice)

It's important to have a balance of fruits, vegetables, and grains. Not all starches offer the same benefits, so choose a variety of foods from this group. Because they have other nutrients, fruits and vegetables are better sources of carbohydrates than bread and grains.

Try to limit simple sugars. They have more calories than they have nutrients, and the energy they provide is used up quickly. Eating a candy bar might give you a brief "sugar high." It doesn't offer much nutrition, though, and you'll soon feel tired again. The right kinds of starches have lots of nutrients and fiber. They also give you longer-lasting energy.

Fats

Many people have come to think of fat as bad. Although too much fat isn't good for you, the body needs a certain amount of fat to function normally.

Fat helps your body use vitamins A, D, E, and K as well as proteins and carbohydrates.

Fat also is very high in calories. Ounce for ounce, fat has more than double the calories as the same amount of protein or carbohydrates. Fat that your body doesn't need right away is stored as fat tissue. This tissue is converted into energy when your body needs more calories than you eat. These fat stores play an important role in making breast milk for your newborn. If you do not use these calories, the fat stores accumulate. Excess body fat can lead to several health problems, including *diabetes mellitus*, heart disease, and joint problems.

You should be aware of different types of fats in your diet:

- Saturated fats come mainly from meat and dairy products. They tend to be solid when chilled—like butter and lard, for instance. Palm oil and coconut oil also are saturated fats.

- Trans fats are a kind of saturated fat. Trans fats are made when liquid oils are turned into solid fats like shortening and hard margarine. This is done to make foods last longer and give them better flavor. Vegetable shortenings, some margarines, crackers, cookies, and snack foods like potato chips contain trans fats.

- Unsaturated fats tend to be liquid and come mostly from plants and vegetables. Olive, canola, peanut, sunflower, and fish oil are all unsaturated fats.

Too much saturated fat and trans fat can increase your cholesterol level and lead to heart disease. They should make up less than one third of the total fat in your diet, or no more than 10% of the calories you eat each day. The other two thirds of the fat in your diet, or about 20% of your daily calories, should come from unsaturated fat.

Fat is found in many foods—from meat and baked goods to non-dairy coffee creamer. You can reduce the fat in your diet by changing the way you prepare foods:

- Broil, bake, poach, or steam your food instead of frying or sauteing it.
- Skim liquid fat from soups.
- Trim all fat from meats.
- Remove skin from poultry.
- Cut back on butter, margarine, cream, oil, and mayonnaise.
- Choose unsaturated fats over saturated fats and trans fats as often as you can.

Vitamins and Minerals
Vitamins and minerals are natural chemicals found in foods that perform important functions in the body. You need a certain amount of vitamins and

minerals each day to keep your body running efficiently and to support your growing baby. Some vitamins and minerals play key roles in prenatal development, including iron, calcium, folic acid, and vitamin D.

Iron. Iron is used to make hemoglobin. This protein in red blood **cells** carries oxygen to your organs, tissues, and baby. Just like the other cells in your body, blood cells die and are replaced in a constant process. The iron from blood cells is used to make more hemoglobin.

When you become pregnant, you may not have enough iron stored in your body to make the extra blood you and your baby need, causing **anemia**. Women need more iron in their diets during pregnancy to support the growth of the baby and to produce extra blood. The recommended daily amount of iron you should consume while pregnant is 27 milligrams.

Eating certain foods will give you extra iron. Lean beef and pork, organ meats, dried fruits and beans, whole grains, and dark leafy greens are all high in iron. Some women may need extra iron in the form of an iron supplement. If your health care provider recommends an iron supplement, follow these tips:

- Vitamin C helps your body absorb the iron in food. It's a good idea to take your iron pill with a glass of fruit juice that's high in vitamin C.

- **Calcium** can block iron absorption. If you also are taking a calcium supplement, take your iron supplement in the morning and take calcium at night.

- Iron supplements can cause constipation and bloating when you first start taking them. Your body should adjust to the extra iron in a few days.

- Keep iron supplements away from children (as with all medication).

Folic Acid. Folic acid is used to make the extra blood your body needs during pregnancy. Not getting enough folic acid in your diet before pregnancy and in the early weeks of pregnancy increases the risk of birth defects such as **neural tube defects** (defects of the spine and skull). Lack of folic acid also may increase the risk of certain other birth defects.

Folic acid is added as a supplement to certain foods (breads, cereal, pasta, rice, and flour). It also is in some foods, such as leafy dark-green vegetables, citrus fruits, and beans. However, because it may be difficult to get all of the folic acid you need from food sources alone, it is recommended that all women of childbearing age take a multivitamin supplement containing 0.4 milligrams of folic acid a day.

Some women may need increased amounts of folic acid. Women who are pregnant with twins, have certain medical conditions, or are taking certain medications have increased folic acid needs. If you have had a child with a neural tube defect or other birth defects, you will need 4 milligrams daily—10 times the amount recommended for most women. The increased amount of folic acid should be taken separately, not as part of a multivitamin supplement. Otherwise, you would get too much of the other vitamins. Your health care provider will prescribe this high-dose folic acid supplement. For more information about folic acid, see page 23.

Calcium. Calcium is used to build your baby's bones and teeth. If you don't get enough of this mineral from food, your baby will get the calcium it needs from your bones. Calcium deficiency can lead to **osteoporosis** (fragile bones). It also may cause you to lose teeth.

Pregnant women should get 1,000 mg of calcium each day (1,300 mg for those younger than 19 years). Drinking about 3 cups of milk a day will fill this quota if you are older than 19 years. Milk and other dairy products, such as cheese and yogurt, are the best sources of calcium. These foods also are good sources of calcium:

• Fortified orange juice
• Nuts and seeds
• Sardines
• Salmon with bones
• Collard, kale, mustard, spinach, and turnip greens

If you are **lactose intolerant** (you have trouble digesting milk products), you can get calcium in other ways. You may try pills or drops with an enzyme that helps your body break down milk sugar. Taking a daily antacid made with calcium is another simple way to boost your calcium intake. Also, many stores carry low-lactose milk and cheese. Iron prevents calcium from being absorbed, so do not take calcium with iron.

Vitamin D. Vitamin D helps build your baby's bones and teeth. You need about 200 international units of vitamin D daily—about what is in a few glasses of vitamin D fortified milk. Fish liver oils and fatty fish, such as salmon, are good sources of vitamin D. Also, exposure to sunlight converts a chemical in the skin to vitamin D. Despite these natural vitamin D sources, many people are vitamin D deficient. If your health care provider thinks that you may be deficient in vitamin D, a test can be done to check the level of vitamin D in your blood. If it is below normal, you may need to take vitamin D supplements.

Food Groups

To get the nutrients you need, you should eat a variety of foods. To make meal planning easier, the My Pyramid Plan for Moms breaks foods down into the following groups:

1. *Vegetable group*—This group provides vitamins such as A, C, and folic acid, and minerals such as iron and magnesium. Vegetables are low in fat and high in fiber. When you're planning your meals, choose a wide array of vegetables, which will help ensure that you get a variety of nutrients. Women who are worried about pesticides may want to think about buying vegetables and fruits that are grown without chemicals (organic). Some of the pesticide that has been applied can be removed from fruits and vegetables by washing them with warm water and a small amount of soap and rinsing them. Eat a mixture of these kinds of vegetables:

   - Dark-green vegetables (spinach; romaine lettuce; cooked greens, such as kale, collards, turnip greens, and beet greens)
   - Orange vegetables (carrots, sweet potatoes, pumpkin)
   - Starchy vegetables (potatoes, winter squash, beets)
   - Dry beans (navy, pinto, kidney beans) and peas
   - Other vegetables (tomatoes and tomato sauces, peppers, broccoli, cauliflower, lettuce)

The Top 12 Fruits and Vegetables With the Highest Levels of Pesticides

According to the Environmental Working Group, the following fruits and vegetables are those with the highest levels of pesticides:

1. Peaches	7. Cherries
2. Apples	8. Kale
3. Bell peppers	9. Lettuce
4. Celery	10. Grapes (imported)
5. Nectarines	11. Carrots
6. Strawberries	12. Pears

When possible, buy the organic versions. Organic fruits and vegetables can be more expensive than conventional produce. If you are on a budget and need to limit your organic purchases, buying just organic milk is a very good choice. Organic milk contains no **hormones** or **antibiotics**. Many people think it also tastes better.

2. *Fruit group*—This group provides vitamins A and C, potassium, and fiber. Choose fresh, frozen, canned, or dried fruit. Eat plenty of citrus fruits, melons, and berries. Although fruit juices also provide nutrients, you should try to eat whole fruits whenever possible. Here are some examples:

- Cantaloupe
- Honeydew melon
- Mangoes
- Prunes or prune juice
- Bananas
- Apricots
- Oranges or orange juice
- Red or pink grapefruit
- Avocados

3. *Milk group*—Milk and products made from milk are a major source of protein, calcium, phosphorus, and vitamins. Calcium is a key nutrient during pregnancy and breastfeeding. If you don't like the taste of milk, eat yogurt, cottage cheese, or sliced cheese. Choose fat-free (skim) or low-fat (1%) items as often as you can.

4. *Grains group*—This group provides complex carbohydrates (starches). Grains are a good source of energy, vitamins, minerals, and fiber. Try to make at least one half of the grains that you eat each day whole grains. Examples include the following foods:

- Cooked cereals (such as oatmeal)
- Ready-to-eat cereals
- Bread
- Rice
- Pasta

5. *Meat and beans group*—This group provides B vitamins, protein, iron, and zinc. Your baby needs plenty of protein and iron to develop. Choose lean meats and trim off the fat and skin before cooking. Examples from this group include:

- Cooked dry beans and peas
- Nuts and seeds (sunflower seeds, almonds, hazelnuts, pine nuts, peanuts, and peanut butter)
- Lean beef, lamb, and pork
- Poultry
- Eggs
- Shrimp, clams, oysters, and crab

- Halibut, cod, rainbow trout, herring, sardines, rockfish, and yellowfin tuna (You should avoid eating shark, swordfish, king mackerel, and tilefish—which have high levels of mercury—while you are pregnant or breastfeeding. See p. 86 for more details about the safety of eating fish during pregnancy.)

In addition to these food groups, there is an extra food group that contains extra fats and sugars that we eat daily. Fats and oils are another separate group. Most of the fat and oil in your diet should come from plant sources (olive oil, nut oils, and grapeseed oil). Limit fats derived from animal sources, such as butter and lard.

How Much Should You Eat?

In the past, you were told to eat a certain number of servings from each food group. The problem with the term "serving" is that few people know what a serving of a specific food is. To make things easier, the My Pyramid Plan for Moms gives amounts in familiar measurements like cups and ounces. To get an idea of what an ounce is, 1 pound equals 16 ounces. If you have bought a half a pound of beans, you have 8 ounces. A quarter pound is 4 ounces. If you want to be really precise, you can get a kitchen scale, but it's not necessary. The plan gives recommendations about how much to eat of different kinds of foods to meet your daily requirements.

Putting It All Together

To get an idea of how the Plan works, the following table (Table 13-3) provides guidelines for a pregnant woman of normal weight who gets less than 30 minutes of exercise a day. The guidelines are different for each trimester because nutritional needs tend to change throughout pregnancy. In the first trimester, morning sickness can affect your eating habits. You may crave certain foods or not feel like eating. In the second and third trimesters, your appetite usually increases. Also, it is recommended that most of your weight gain occur during the second and third trimesters of pregnancy. The total number of calories recommended for each trimester gradually increases to reflect this gradual weight gain. The 300 extra calories that a pregnant woman needs is averaged out over the three trimesters of pregnancy.

Knowing how to read food labels will help you with meal planning. Remember to factor in snacks, which are a good way to get needed nutrition and extra calories. Pick snacks that have the right nutrients and that are low in fat and sugar. Fruit, cereal, and yogurt are healthier than candy, soda, or potato chips.

Table 13-3 Sample Dietary Guidelines

These guidelines are for a pregnant woman who is a normal weight who gets less than 30 minutes of exercise a day. They show the recommended daily food intake.

	First Trimester	Second Trimester	Third Trimester	Comments
Total calories per day	1,800	2,200	2,400	
Grains*	6 ounces	7 ounces	8 ounces	1 ounce is one slice of bread, ½ cup of cooked rice, ½ cup of cooked pasta, 3 cups of popped popcorn, or five whole wheat crackers
Vegetables†	2 ½ cups	3 cups	3 cups	2 cups of raw leafy vegetables count as 1 cup
Fruits	1 ½ cups	2 cups	2 cups	One large orange, one large peach, one small apple, eight large strawberries, or ½ cup of dried fruit count as 1 cup
Milk	3 cups	3 cups	3 cups	Two small slices of swiss cheese or ⅓ cup of shredded cheese count as 1 cup
Meat and beans	5 ounces	6 ounces	6 ½ ounces	½ cup of cooked beans, 25 almonds, 13 cashews, or nine walnuts count as 2 ounces
Extras	290 calories	360 calories	410 calories	These extra calories come from high-fat and high-sugar foods, or higher amounts of foods from the five food groups
Fats and oils	6 teaspoons	7 teaspoons	8 teaspoons	Some foods are naturally high in fats and oils, such as olives, some fish, avocados, and nuts

*Make one half whole grain.

†Make sure that you get a mixture of dark green, orange, starchy, and other vegetables, including dry beans and peas.

You may find it easier to eat six smaller meals spread out over the day rather than to try to consume your necessary nutrients and calories in three larger meals. To make these minimeals, just divide the daily recommended amount of foods from each of the food groups into small portions. Milk and half a sandwich made with meat, fish, peanut butter, or cheese with lettuce

Calories: Amount of energy the food supplies in each serving.

Total Fat: The amount of fat in one serving. Fats are often broken down into trans fats and saturated fats. The amounts of these two types of fats should be limited in a healthy diet.

Nutrients: A list of the nutrients the product contains. Nutrients often listed here are total fat, cholesterol, sodium, total carbohydrate, and protein.

Serving Size: The amount served and eaten. The numbers on the label refer to this amount of food.

% Daily Value: For each nutrient listed, a percentage of the Daily Value that the food supplies is shown. % Daily Value is based on a 2,000 calorie diet. If you eat less than 2,000 calories a day, the percentage would be lower. If you eat more than 2,000 calories, the percentage would be higher.

Footnote: The footnote gives detailed information about the amount of nutrients that are needed in a 2,000 calorie and 2,500 calorie diet.

Nutrition Facts

Serving Size: 1 package (28g)
Servings Per Container: 1

Amount Per Serving

Calories 100	Calories from Fat 10

	% Daily Value*
Total Fat 1g	2%
Saturated Fat .5g	2%
Trans Fat 0g	
Cholesterol 0g	0%
Sodium 450mg	19%
Total Carbohydrate 22g	7%
Dietary Fiber 2g	8%
Sugars 0g	
Protein 3g	

Vitamin A 0%	•	Vitamin C 0%
Calcium 0%	•	Iron 3%

*Percent Daily Values are based on a 2,000 calorie diet. Your daily values may be higher or lower depending on your calorie needs:

		Calorie	2,000	2,500
Total Fat	Less than		65g	80g
Sat. Fat	Less than		20g	25g
Cholesterol	Less than		300mg	300mg
Sodium	Less than		2,400mg	2,400mg
Total Carbohydrate			300g	375g
Dietary Fiber			25g	30g

Calories per gram:
Fat 9 • Carbohydrate 4 • Protein 4

All packaged foods must be clearly labeled with nutrition information. Reading all food labels can help you make smart food choices. The label will tell you how many grams of fat and how many calories are in each serving.

and tomato make an excellent minimeal. Other ideas are low-fat milk and fresh fruits, cheese and crackers, and soups.

Keep in mind that this sample plan is one designed for a woman of average weight who gets little exercise. If you are overweight or underweight, your plan will be different. Overweight women will not need as many extra calories, while underweight women will need more. Exercise also is a factor. Those who exercise more will need more calories.

Weight Gain During Pregnancy

Pregnant women need to gain a certain amount of weight during pregnancy (see Table 13-4). A woman who gains too few pounds is more likely to have a small baby (less than 5½ pounds). These babies often have health problems after birth. Women who gain too much weight also are at risk for health problems. These problems include **gestational diabetes mellitus**, high blood pressure, and a baby that's too large (**macrosomia**).

The amount that you should gain is based on your pre-pregnancy weight. Body mass index (BMI) is a measure of body fat based on height and weight (see Appendix A for a BMI chart). A BMI of 18.5–24.9 is normal. A BMI of 25–29.9 means you are overweight. A person with a BMI of 30 or higher is considered obese. See the table for the amount of weight you should gain during pregnancy depending on your BMI.

You should gain weight gradually throughout pregnancy, with most of your weight gain occurring in the second and third trimesters. You will have your weight checked at each **prenatal care** visit, and your health care provider will keep track of how much weight you have gained. If you are gaining weight too fast, you may be told to slow down. Try cutting down on the "extra" calories that you consume—the extra fats and sugars, as well as large portions and second helpings, before cutting calories from the five major food groups. If you aren't gaining enough weight, do the opposite—try eating more than the recommended amounts from the five food groups. Don't double up on the extras.

Obesity and Pregnancy

Obesity is a major health problem in the United States. Women who are overweight or obese may have problems during pregnancy, such as gestational diabetes mellitus or macrosomia. Obesity can be related to other health problems for women also, such as high blood pressure. Chapter 17, "Obesity and Eating Disorders," gives more information about obesity and pregnancy and how it is managed.

Table 13-4 Weight Gain During Pregnancy

Prepregnancy Body Mass Index	Recommended Total Weight Gain During Pregnancy (in Pounds)	Rate of Weight Gain in the Second and Third Trimesters* (Pounds per Week)
Underweight (BMI less than 18.5)	28–40	1–1.3
Normal weight (BMI 18.5–24.9)	25–35	0.8–1
Overweight (BMI 25–29.9)	15–25	0.5–0.7
Obese (BMI more than 30)	11–20	0.4–0.6

Abbreviation: BMI, body mass index

*Assumes a first-trimester weight gain between 1.1 pounds and 4.4 pounds.

Data from Institutes of Medicine (US). Weight gain during pregnancy: reexamining the guidelines. Washington, DC: National Academies Press; 2009.

Pregnancy and Eating Disorders

Anorexia nervosa and **bulimia nervosa** are serious eating disorders that starve a woman's body of key nutrients. In women with anorexia nervosa or bulimia nervosa, the normal weight gain that occurs in pregnancy and her changing body can cause anxiety and cause her condition to worsen. Eating disorders that were under control before pregnancy may start again during pregnancy. Counseling and medication may help control the emotional aspects of eating disorders. If you have an eating disorder or have had one in the past, tell your health care provider. Chapter 17, "Obesity and Eating Disorders," discusses eating disorders in more detail and how they are treated during pregnancy.

Prenatal Vitamin Supplements

The best nutrient sources are foods. Except for iron, folic acid, and possibly calcium, a well-rounded diet should supply all of the nutrients you need during pregnancy. To get these extra nutrients, a prenatal vitamin supplement is recommended for most women. Take prenatal vitamin supplements only as directed. Large doses of anything—even a good thing—can be harmful. Don't take more than the dietary reference intake for any vitamin or mineral, especially vitamins A and D, without getting your health care provider's approval. Very high levels of vitamin A have been linked to severe birth defects. Your prenatal multivitamin supplement should contain no more than 5,000 international units of vitamin A. If you are already taking a multivitamin supplement, let your health care provider know.

Special Nutrition Concerns

For most women, careful meal planning and a daily prenatal vitamin supplement will provide all their nutritional needs. But some mothers-to-be have special nutritional issues that they will need to address during pregnancy.

Vegetarian Diets

If you are a vegetarian, it is still possible to get all of the nutrients you and your baby need during pregnancy. It just takes extra planning. Tell your health care provider at your first prenatal care visit that you are a vegetarian and ask whether he or she has a recommended diet plan for you to follow. The advice in this section also can be helpful when planning your meals and factoring in the extra calories and nutrients you will need during pregnancy.

There are several types of vegetarians. Lacto-ovo vegetarians eat milk products and eggs but no meat or fish. Semivegetarians eat poultry and fish but no red meat, such as beef or pork. Vegans eat no animal products, including milk, eggs, and honey.

Because animal products usually are high in protein and iron, getting enough of these nutrients may be a challenge for vegetarians. Lacto-ovo vegetarians can get adequate protein from dairy products and eggs. Vegans need to search out non-animal protein and iron sources. Beans and tofu are protein-rich, non-animal foods, and blackstrap molasses is a good source of iron. Cooking in an iron skillet can also introduce more iron into your diet. To increase your absorption of iron, it's helpful to consume a food high in vitamin C—a natural enhancer of iron absorption—at the same meal as a food high in iron. An iron supplement may be needed to ensure that you're getting enough of this mineral.

Vegans also need to make sure that they are getting enough calcium. Dark leafy greens, calcium-enriched tofu, and other calcium-enriched products (soy milk, rice milk, orange juice) are all high in calcium. Vitamin D—found in animal foods, such as salmon, tuna, and milk—is needed to promote absorption of calcium. Although Vitamin D is generated naturally in the body through sun exposure, vegetarians often are deficient in this vitamin. Your health care provider can measure your vitamin D levels. If you are found to be vitamin D deficient, you may need to take a daily supplement.

Other nutrients that vegans should pay close attention to are folic acid, vitamin B_{12}, and zinc:

- *Folic acid*—Vegans and other vegetarians need to make sure that they are getting enough folic acid in their diets to decrease the risk of having a child with a neural tube defect. Many women have a hard time getting the recommended amount—0.4 milligrams per day—from food sources alone. A daily vitamin containing this amount of folic acid is recommended for all women of childbearing age.

- *Vitamin B_{12}*—Vitamin B_{12} plays a key role in fetal development. Because it readily crosses the placenta, a regular source is needed to maintain a constant level in the body. Good sources are meat substitutes, fortified cereals, and fortified nutritional yeast.

- *Zinc*—Zinc is a mineral that is important to the baby's growth and development. Nuts and nut butters are good sources of zinc and also provide protein and vitamin B_{12}.

Keep in mind that it may be more difficult to gain weight while eating a vegan diet. Snacks are a good way to get in those extra calories, as are calorie-dense food like nuts and soy products.

Low Stores of Nutrients

Pregnancy demands a lot from your body. Having more than one pregnancy in a short time can wipe out some of the nutrients your body needs to help nourish you and your baby. Iron and calcium, for instance, are minerals that may be at low levels in a woman who has pregnancies close together.

If you have been pregnant more than twice in 2 years, including pregnancies that ended in abortion or miscarriage, you may not have had a chance to replace the nutrients your body has lost. Your stores also may be low if you had complications in a pregnancy, if you had a *low-birth-weight* baby, or if you are very thin.

If any of these scenarios fit your situation, you may benefit from consultation with a nutritionist. A nutritionist can help you design a diet plan that includes all of the necessary nutrients and can help you track your progress throughout pregnancy.

Unusual Cravings

Pregnant women often have food cravings. Most often, giving in to these cravings does no harm. Cravings can cause problems if you eat only a few types of food for long periods. They also can be less than healthy if you indulge your cravings for one type of food, for example, and neglect the rest of your diet.

Pica is a strong urge some women feel to eat nonfood items such as laundry starch, clay, or chalk. If you feel these urges, don't indulge in them. Eating nonfood items can be harmful and prevent you from getting the nutrients you need.

Women With Certain Diseases

Aside from the health problems they cause, some diseases can cause nutrition problems as well. Medications that are used to keep a disease under control may affect how your body absorbs food. Conditions such as kidney disease, diabetes mellitus, and phenylketonuria, in which a woman lacks an enzyme needed to process certain foods, call for special diets. For women who have such conditions, it can be hard to eat a balanced diet. Your health care provider may change your medication, advise another diet, or take other steps to help you get the nutrients you need.

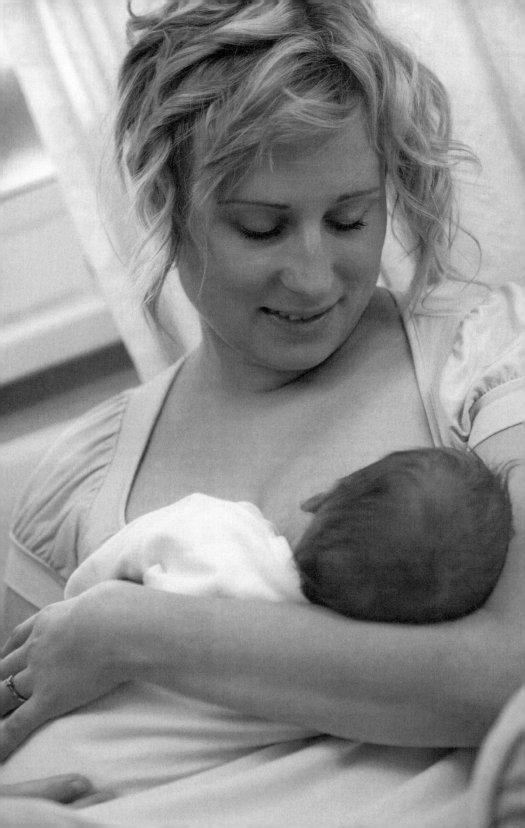

Chapter 14
Feeding Your Baby

Whether to breastfeed or bottle-feed your baby with formula is an important decision parents-to-be must make. Medical experts, such as the Centers for Disease Control and Prevention (CDC), the American College of Obstetricians and Gynecologists, and the American Academy of Pediatrics (AAP), say breastfeeding is the best choice for feeding your baby because of the many nutritional benefits found in breast milk. However, breastfeeding may not be the right option for all women (see box "When You Should Not Breastfeed"). For many new mothers, the choice of whether to breastfeed or bottle-feed is based on their lifestyle or specific medical conditions they might have.

If you are having a difficult time deciding which way is best for you, it may help to talk to your or your baby's health care provider, your partner, or your friends who have breastfed their babies. Remember, though, that the decision to breastfeed or bottle-feed your baby is a very personal one. But there are some things you may want to consider as you decide which is best for you and your new baby.

Breastfeeding and Bottle-feeding: A Comparison

Both babies and mothers gain many benefits from breastfeeding:

• *Good for the baby*—Your baby will get many benefits from breast milk:
  —Breast milk is the most complete form of nutrition for infants. It has the right amount of fat, sugar, water, and protein that is needed for a baby's growth and development.

When You Should Not Breastfeed

As good as breastfeeding is, it is not for every woman. There are some situations in which a woman should not breastfeed her baby:

- *Infections*—If you have certain infections, they can be passed to your baby through breast milk. You should not breastfeed if you have **human immunodeficiency virus (HIV)** or active **tuberculosis**. If tuberculosis is treated, and you are no longer contagious, the baby can be breastfed. If you have hepatitis B virus infection, your baby should be immunized within the first few hours after birth.

- *Chronic Illnesses*—Although many women with certain chronic diseases are able to breastfeed, often it's not the illness itself that causes concern, it's the medications a woman takes to control the health problem.

Certain prescription and over-the-counter medications can pass through breast milk and harm the baby. In such cases, your health care provider may advise you to switch to another medicine, take the medication just after breastfeeding, or lower your dose until your baby is no longer breastfeeding. Most of the time, medications are not harmful.

There are some drugs that you should not take while nursing. Prescription drugs that can pass into breast milk and harm a baby include ergotamine (used to treat migraine headaches), lithium (used to treat mental illness), some drugs used to treat high blood pressure, and chemotherapy drugs (used to treat cancer). Be sure any health care provider treating you knows that you are breastfeeding. If you have a chronic illness or take medication for an ongoing health condition, talk to your health care provider about breastfeeding before your baby is born. Also, if you need to be treated for an illness or health condition after giving birth, be sure to tell the health care provider that you are breastfeeding.

— Breast milk is easier than formula for babies to digest. Infants who are breastfed have less gas, fewer feeding problems, and often less constipation than those given formula.
— It contains **antibodies** that can protect infants from bacterial and viral infections, including ear infections, diarrhea, pneumonia, and respiratory infections.
— Premature babies do better when breastfed than premature babies who are fed formula.

- *Good for you*—New mothers also get many benefits from breastfeeding their babies:
  — Breastfeeding uses up extra *calories*, making it easier to lose the weight you gained during pregnancy. It also helps the *uterus* return to its original size and decreases the amount of bleeding you may have after giving birth.
  — Research shows that women who breastfeed may have lower rates of certain breast and ovarian cancers.
  — Breastfeeding, especially exclusive breastfeeding (no supplementing with formula), delays the return of normal *ovulation* and menstrual cycles. (However, you should still talk with your health care provider about birth control choices.)
  — Breastfeeding saves time and money. You do not have to purchase, measure, and mix formula.
  — The physical contact of breastfeeding helps you bond with your baby. It can help them feel more secure and comforted.

If you are unable to breastfeed or decide not to, you will need to bottle-feed:

- Commercially prepared infant formulas are a nutritious alternative to breast milk and even contain some vitamins and nutrients that breastfed babies need to get from supplements.

- Bottle-feeding is convenient because either parent (or another caregiver) can feed the baby a bottle at any time. But keep in mind that babies also can be bottle-fed with breast milk that you pump and store.

- Because formula digests more slowly than breast milk, formula-fed babies usually need to eat less often than do breastfed babies.

- Mothers who bottle-feed don't have to worry about what they eat or drink or what medications they are taking that could affect their babies.

Whether you breastfeed or bottle-feed, it is recommended that all babies get 400 international units of vitamin D a day to ensure strong, healthy bone growth. Vitamin D is available in liquid form that you give your baby with a dropper. Babies who are fed formula mostly likely are getting the recommended amount of vitamin D per day, but check the label on your baby's formula to make sure.

Choosing to Breastfeed

If you've decided to breastfeed, it might be a good idea to take a breastfeeding class from a certified *lactation* specialist before your baby is born. These classes are offered at many hospitals and parents' centers and can teach you what you need to know to get started. They also can help you avoid some common problems many mothers face when they first start to breastfeed.

If you aren't able to take a class, there is plenty of information available on the Internet or just a phone call away. La Leche League International provides support and education to mothers who wish to breastfeed and can answer any of your questions and concerns (see Resources).

After the Baby Is Born

Right after you give birth, someone in the delivery room can help you find a good position and put your baby to your breast (see box "Good Breastfeeding Positions"). Placing the baby next to your skin helps maintain the baby's body temperature and is a great way to start breastfeeding your new baby. This also is the time that your newborn is most alert and ready to suck. Later, your baby may be too sleepy to nurse well.

During the first few days after birth, your breasts initially produce *colostrum*, a thin, yellowish fluid. This is the same fluid that leaks from some women's breasts during pregnancy. The colostrum that your breasts produce for the first few days after birth helps your newborn's digestive system grow and function. It is rich in protein and is all your baby needs for the first few days of life. It is especially high in antibodies that help make your baby immune to diseases.

Within 3 or 4 days your body sends a signal to your breasts to start making milk. At first this milk is thin, watery, and sweet. It quenches the baby's thirst and provides sugar, proteins, minerals, and the fluid the baby needs. Over time, the milk changes. It becomes thick and creamy. This milk will satisfy hunger and give your baby the nutrients he needs to grow.

When your baby is breastfeeding, the nerves in your nipples send a message to your brain. In response, your brain releases *hormones* that tell the ducts in your breasts to let down their milk so that it flows through your nipples. This is called the let-down reflex. Some women barely notice let-down. Others have a pins-and-needles feeling in their breasts 2–3 minutes after their babies start nursing.

Sometimes, let-down is slowed if you are in pain or feeling anxious or stressed. Other times, it is triggered simply by looking at your baby, thinking about your baby, or hearing your baby cry. For some women, hearing any

Good Breastfeeding Positions

Finding a good position will help the baby latch on. It also will help you relax and be comfortable. Use pillows or folded blankets to help support the baby.

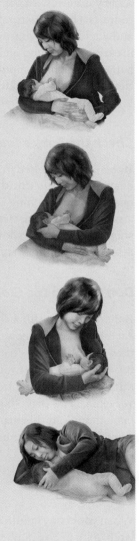

- *Cradle Hold*—Sit up as straight as you can and cradle your baby in the crook of your arm. The baby's body should be turned toward you and his belly should be against yours. Support the baby's head in the bend of your elbow so that he is facing your breast.

- *Cross-Cradle Hold*—As in the cradle hold, nuzzle your baby's belly against yours. Hold the baby in the arm opposite the one you are using to nurse. For instance, if the baby is nursing from your right breast, hold him or her with your left arm. Place the baby's bottom in the crook of your left arm and support the baby's head and neck with your left hand. This position gives you more control of the baby's head. It's a good position for a newborn who is having trouble nursing.

- *Football Hold*—Tuck your baby under your arm like a football. Hold the baby at your side, level with your waist, so he is facing you. Support the baby's back with your upper arm and hold his head level with your breast. The football hold is good for nursing twins. It's also good if you had a cesarean delivery because the baby doesn't lie on your abdomen.

- *Side-Lying Position*—Lie on your side and nestle your baby next to you. Place your fingers beneath your breast and lift it up to help your baby reach your nipple. This position is good for night feedings. It's also good for women who had a cesarean delivery because it keeps the baby's weight off the incision. Rest your head on your lower arm. You may want to tuck a pillow behind your back to help hold yourself up.

baby cry will trigger the let-down reflex. When your milk lets down, your breasts will feel full, and you will want to breastfeed very soon.

Get the Baby Latched On

A baby is born with the instincts he needs to nurse. For instance, the rooting reflex is a baby's natural instinct to turn toward the nipple, open his mouth, and suck. When you and your baby are ready to begin nursing, cup your breast in your hand and stroke your baby's lower lip with your nipple. The baby will open his mouth wide (like a yawn). Quickly center your nipple in the baby's mouth, making sure the tongue is down, and pull him close to you. You need to bring your baby to your breast—not your breast to your baby.

Check the Baby's Technique

If the baby is latched on correctly, he will have all of your nipple and a good deal of the *areola* (the dark area around the nipple) in his mouth. The baby's nose will be touching your breast. The baby's lips also will be curled out around your breast. The baby's sucking should be smooth and even. You should hear him swallow. You may feel a slight tugging. You may feel a little discomfort for the first few days. You shouldn't feel any severe pain, though.

Don't Watch the Clock

Experts used to think that newborns should nurse for just a few minutes at each breast. They now know that this may make babies stop eating before they are full. Cutting back on nursing time also keeps your breasts from making enough milk. Let your baby set his own nursing pattern. Many newborns nurse for 10–20 minutes on each breast. (A baby who wants to nurse for a very long time—say, 30 minutes on each side—may be having trouble getting enough milk. If this happens each time you breastfeed, tell your health care provider.) When your baby is full, he will let go of your breast. If not, gently break the suction.

Switch Sides

When your baby empties one breast, offer the other. Don't worry if he doesn't latch on to it. You don't have to nurse at both breasts in one feeding. You may want to put a safety pin on your bra strap to mark the side your baby nursed from last. At the next feeding, offer the other breast first.

FEEDING YOUR BABY • 265

Nurse on Demand

When your baby is hungry, he will nuzzle against your breast, make sucking motions, or put his hands to his mouth. Crying is a late sign of hunger. (Rooming in with your baby at the hospital will help you pick up on these cues.) Follow your baby's signals—not the clock. Using a schedule for feeding times will deprive your baby of nourishment and tell your body to make less milk. During the first few weeks, your baby should be fed at least 8–12 times in 24 hours (every 2–3 hours). Some newborns are happy to go 3 hours between feedings. Others need to nurse once an hour for the first few weeks. Over time, you and your baby will set your own schedule.

The Challenges

Some new mothers breastfeed without any problems. But it's perfectly normal for minor problems to arise at first, especially if it is your first time breastfeeding. The good news is that most problems can be overcome with a little help and support. If you need help, don't hesitate to call your health care provider or see a lactation specialist.

Sore Nipples

Breastfeeding should not hurt. There may be some tenderness at first, but it should gradually go away as the days go by. Poor latch-on and positioning are the major causes of sore nipples because the baby is probably not getting enough of the areola into his mouth and is sucking mostly on the nipple. Check the positioning of your baby's body and the way he latches on and sucks. To minimize soreness, make sure that your baby's mouth is open wide, with as much of the areola in his mouth as possible. You should find that it feels better right away once the baby is positioned correctly. If you have sore nipples, you are more likely to postpone feedings because of the pain, but this can lead to overly full or engorged breasts, which can then lead to plugged milk ducts in the breast. If your baby is latched on and sucking correctly, he should be able to nurse as long as he likes without causing any pain. If it hurts, take the baby off of your breast and try again. Ask for help if it is still painful for you.

Engorgement

Engorgement may occur when your milk comes in a few days after delivery. Engorged breasts feel full and tender. You may even run a low fever. If the fever exceeds 101°F or if you are in severe pain, call your health care provider. If your breasts are very engorged, it can be hard for your baby to latch on.

Once your body figures out just how much milk your baby needs, the problem should go away. This often takes a week or so. In the meantime, you can do the following things:

- Feed the baby more often to help drain your breasts.
- Express a little milk with a pump or by hand to soften your breasts before nursing.
- To help your milk flow, massage your breasts, take hot showers, or apply hot packs to your breasts before feedings.
- After feedings, apply cold packs to your breasts to relieve discomfort and reduce swelling.

Inverted or Flat Nipples
It is very common for a woman to have one or both nipples that do not protrude fully. In most cases, women with flat or inverted nipples can breastfeed.

During the first feedings after birth is the time when inverted or flat nipples are most likely to present problems. It may be hard for the baby to latch on at first. Ask for help from your health care provider or a lactation expert. You may be advised to use a breast pump just before breastfeeding or to stimulate the nipple in other ways. Breastfeeding will be easier as the baby grows bigger and stronger.

Blocked Ducts
If a duct gets clogged with unused milk, a hard, tender knot will form in your breast. Call your health care provider if the knot doesn't go away within a few days or if you run a fever. In the meantime, try these tips:

- Let your baby nurse long and often on the breast that is blocked.
- Offer the breast with the blocked duct first.
- If there's any milk left in your breast after a feeding, pump it out or hand express it.
- Take a hot shower or apply a hot pack to the lump before nursing.
- Massage the lump while your baby nurses to help the milk drain.

Mastitis
If a blocked duct doesn't drain, it may become inflamed and a breast infection—called mastitis—can result. If you have this condition, you may have flu-like symptoms, such as fever, aches, and fatigue. Your breasts also will be swollen, painful, streaked with red, and feel hot to the touch.

If you think you have mastitis, call your health care provider right away. He or she will prescribe an ***antibiotic*** to treat the infection. You should feel

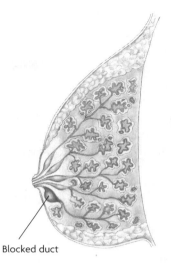

Blocked duct

Blocked duct. This condition occurs when a duct becomes clogged with milk.

better within a day or two of starting treatment, but keep taking the treatment for the full prescription.

Until then, do the same things you'd do to treat a blocked duct. Get plenty of rest and drink lots of fluids. Your health care provider may suggest you take ibuprofen to ease your discomfort. In the meantime, do not stop breastfeeding. Breastfeed your baby often to help drain your breast (the baby cannot catch the infection). If you stop breastfeeding, the clogged duct will get more inflamed, your milk supply will go down, and recovery will take longer.

Common Questions

How long should I breastfeed my baby?

The AAP and the American College of Obstetricians and Gynecologists recommend that a mother should breastfeed for the baby's first 6 months. Beyond that, the AAP and the College encourage breastfeeding until at least 12 months, and longer if both the mother and baby are willing. According to the CDC, many mothers are trying to follow this 6-month rule. In 2005, for instance, 74% of new mothers started breastfeeding their babies, and 43% were still breastfeeding at 6 months.

Keep in mind that you can breastfeed for as long as you and your child want. Any amount of breastfeeding, even a few days, is good for the baby. But, the longer you stick with it, the better off your baby will be.

When you want to stop breastfeeding, there are a few ways to do it. Some women slowly drop feedings as their baby eats more food and starts drinking from a cup. This can be a long process. It's a gradual change for both of you.

Other women decide to wean their baby when he reaches a certain age. In this case, it's still best to take it slow. A sudden stop in breastfeeding can cause you physical pain as your breasts fill with unused milk. It also can be hard for your baby.

One approach is to replace one nursing session with a bottle or cup-feeding every few days. Start by cutting out the feedings your baby seems to enjoy the least. Slowly work your way up to the more important ones. Most often, the feeding before bedtime is the last to go and the hardest to give up. As you reduce the amount you nurse, your milk supply will decrease slowly.

Is my baby getting enough milk?

When an infant is fed formula, it's simple to figure out how much he is drinking. All you have to do is add up those empty bottles. Not so with breastfeeding. There are other ways to tell if your baby is well nourished:

- Your baby nurses often. A newborn should nurse at least 8–12 times in 24 hours. The bigger your baby is, the more his stomach will hold and the less often he will need to eat. Even so, a newborn shouldn't go more than 3 hours without nursing (even at night). Each nursing session should last 20–45 minutes.

- Your baby is full after nursing. A baby who's just had a good meal will be drowsy and content.

- Your breasts fill and empty. Your breasts should feel full and firm before feedings. After, they should be less full and feel softer.

- The baby goes through lots of diapers. After your milk comes in, your baby should soak at least six diapers per day. His **urine** should be nearly clear. During the first month, your baby should have at least three bowel movements per day. In fact, most breastfed newborns pass a stool after each feeding. The stool should be soft and yellow.

- Your baby is gaining weight. Most newborns lose a little weight at first. After 2 weeks, your baby should be back up to his weight at birth. The health care provider will weigh your baby at each visit and let you know if he isn't gaining enough weight. If you are worried that your baby isn't getting enough milk, tell the health care provider.

What kind of diet should I have?

When you are pregnant, your body stores extra nutrients and fat to prepare you for breastfeeding. Even so, once your baby is born, you need more food and nutrients than normal to fuel milk production. During breastfeeding, you need about 200 calories per day more than you did during pregnancy. That's 500 calories more than you needed before you got pregnant. You'll also need to drink lots of liquids during the day because breastfeeding uses up lots of fluid. You need at least eight glasses of liquid per day. If you get dehydrated, it can affect your milk supply.

Breastfeeding moms need 1,000 milligrams of calcium per day. You can get this amount by eating plenty of dairy products like milk, yogurt, and cheese. If you can't digest milk products, ask your health care provider about taking a calcium supplement. Be sure to get folic acid each day too. This will help you maintain good health and ensure that you have plenty of folic acid stores. Your health care provider may suggest that you keep taking a daily prenatal vitamin supplement until your baby is weaned.

Some nursing infants are sensitive to certain foods in their mothers' diets. If your baby acts fussy or gets a rash, diarrhea, or congestion within a couple hours of nursing, let his health care provider know. This can signal a food allergy. The most common culprits are foods made from cow's milk (cheese, yogurt), peanuts, soy, wheat, eggs, and corn. Try eliminating any food that you suspect is causing the baby's reaction for a few days and see if your baby seems better. You also may want to keep a food diary. Keeping a diary will help you spot links between what you eat and how your baby reacts.

Now that I'm no longer pregnant, is it OK for me to smoke cigarettes and drink alcohol again?

It's important to keep in mind that when you breastfeed, everything you put into your body still goes to your baby, just like when you were pregnant. If you smoke, the times when you are pregnant and breastfeeding are the best times to quit. And although quitting smoking is the best thing you can do for your health and that of your baby, the AAP does still believe that breast milk remains the ideal food for a baby, even if you smoke.

Whether it's OK to drink alcohol and breastfeed depends on how much and when you drink. Although alcohol passes freely into a mother's milk, an occasional glass of wine or cocktail doesn't appear to harm a nursing baby in the long run. If you're going to have an occasional alcoholic beverage or have more than one drink, wait at least two hours per drink before nursing your baby to give the alcohol a chance to dissipate from your body. If you drink alcohol heavily (more than two drinks per day on a regular basis), however, research shows it can harm your baby, including causing drowsiness, weakness, and abnormal weight gain.

I've had breast surgery. Can I still breastfeed?

Surgery to remove cysts and other benign breast lumps rarely causes problems with future breastfeeding. If you have had surgery on your breasts, talk to your pregnancy health care provider or surgeon before your delivery date to help plan for breastfeeding.

Many women who have had their breasts enlarged are able to nurse their babies; however, some women with breast implants may have problems if the implants rupture. A rupture may cause scarring that affects milk production and release. If you are worried about your breast implants, talk to your health care provider.

Likewise, women who have had surgery to reduce the size of their breasts may have breastfeeding problems. Breast-reduction surgery can cut into milk ducts and prevent a nursing mother from making enough milk. If you have had this surgery, talk with your health care provider to be sure your nipples, areolas, and ducts were left intact.

I've heard about breast milk banks. What are they?

Breast milk banks collect donated breast milk from nursing mothers and make it available to premature and critically ill babies in hospitals across the country. Breastfeeding mothers who have an abundant milk supply can become donors at any of the nation's milk banks. Once a mother becomes a donor, she sends frozen breast milk to the breast milk bank to help babies in need. If you're interested in donating to or using breast milk from a bank, your health care provider or breastfeeding instructor may be able to give you information about banks in your area.

Going Back to Work

You can continue feeding your baby breast milk even after you return to work. It just takes extra time and planning.

Tell Your Employer

If you are returning to work once your planned maternity leave comes to an end, notify your boss that you are breastfeeding and will need to take breaks throughout the day to pump your milk to give to your baby later. If you are lucky enough to have on-site day care, you can simply breastfeed your baby at regular intervals.

Discuss with your boss where you can pump at work if you don't have your own private office. Make sure it is a clean, private, quiet area. You'll need a chair, a small table, and an outlet if you are using an electric pump. If your boss cannot help you with your needs, make your requests to your human resources department. Also make sure you have somewhere to store the milk (see box "Storing Breast Milk").

Your boss may have some concerns about how you plan to fit pumping into your workday. You can plan to pump your breast milk during lunch or other breaks. You could offer to make up work time for time spent pumping milk. During an 8-hour workday you should be able to pump enough milk during morning, lunch, and afternoon breaks. Using a double pump—which pumps both breasts at the same time—is even quicker. By double pumping, you may be able to pump in 10–15 minutes rather than 20–30 minutes.

Storing Breast Milk

- After pumping, you can refrigerate your milk, place it in a cooler, or freeze it for the baby to be fed later. Many breast pumps come with carrying cases that have a section to store your milk with ice packs. Don't leave breast milk at room temperature for more than 8 hours because the enzymes will begin to digest the fat.

- Store breast milk in clean glass or plastic bottles or special milk-collection bags. Store it in small amounts (2–4 ounces) to avoid wasting it. Mark the bottles or bags with the date the milk was pumped. If you are going to freeze it, leave a 1-inch space at the top of the container.

- You can keep breast milk in the refrigerator (40°F or below) for up to 2 days. Do not store milk in the door of the refrigerator because the temperature can vary there. If you need to store milk longer than 2 days, you can keep it in a deep freeze (0°F or below) for up to 3 months.

- Never thaw frozen milk at room temperature. To thaw frozen milk, hold it under cool running water. Once it has begun to thaw, use warm running water to finish. You also can let frozen milk slowly thaw in the fridge. Once milk is thawed, use it within 24 hours. Never refreeze milk that has been thawed.

- You can add freshly expressed milk to breast milk that was pumped before. Always cool the fresh milk first.

- Warm chilled breast milk by placing it in a bowl of very warm water. Don't heat bottles on the stove or in the microwave. This destroys breast milk's disease-fighting qualities.

Know Your Rights

Many states have passed laws that require employers to allow you to breastfeed at your job. These laws say your employer must provide a space for you to breastfeed or allow paid or unpaid time for mothers who are breastfeeding or both. To find out if your state has passed a breastfeeding law for employers, check the La Leche League International's web site (see Resources).

Pumping Milk

There are a few basics steps that you should know about pumping your milk:

- *Get a good pump.* There are many different kinds of breast pumps available. Some are more portable than others, are quieter, and may be more expensive. Manual (hand-operated) breast pumps range in price from $14 to $50. The newer automatic electric pumps designed for mothers who need to regularly pump their milk cost more than $200 and include a carrying case and an insulated section for storing milk containers. Some pumps can be purchased at baby supply stores or general department stores. However, high-quality automatic pumps may be purchased or rented from a lactation consultant, at a local hospital, or from a breastfeeding organization. You'll see them listed as "single-user pumps." You should never borrow or share another mother's breast pump because of the risk of contamination.

- *Be sterile.* It is best to wash your hands before pumping your breast milk and to make sure the table or area where you are pumping also is clean. Each time you are done pumping, it is best to thoroughly wash your pumping equipment with soap and water and let it air dry. This helps prevent germs from getting into the breast milk.

- *Relax.* Pumping milk takes about the same time as breastfeeding, unless you are using a double automatic breast pump. The let-down reflex is important during pumping in order to express a good amount of milk. It may help to have a picture of your baby closeby. You also can try other things to stimulate the let-down reflex, like applying a warm, moist compress to the breast, gently massaging the breasts, or just sitting quietly and thinking of a relaxing setting. Once you begin expressing your milk, think about your baby.

Choosing to Bottle-feed

If you have decided that bottle-feeding is a better option for you, rest assured that formulas on the market today will give your baby the right nutrients he needs to grow.

Picking a Formula

There are different types of infant formula to choose from, so talk to your baby's pediatrician for recommendations on picking the best one. There are three major types available:

1. *Cow's milk formulas*—Most infant formula is made with cow's milk that has been changed to give it the right balance of nutrients, such as those found in breast milk.

2. *Soy-based formulas*—Soy-based infant formulas are an option for babies who can't digest or are allergic to cow's milk formula or to lactose, a sugar naturally found in cow's milk. However, babies who are allergic to cow's milk also may be allergic to soy milk.

3. *Protein hydrolysate formulas*—These are meant for babies who have a family history of milk or soy allergies. Protein hydrolysate formulas are easier to digest and less likely to cause allergic reactions than are other types of formula. They also are called hypoallergenic formulas.

Once you choose the type of formula to feed your baby, you'll have to decide which form to buy as well. Infant formulas come in three forms:

1. Powdered formula is the least expensive. Each scoop of powdered formula must be mixed with water.

2. Liquid concentrated formula also must be mixed with water.

3. Ready-to-use formulas do not need to be mixed with water but are the most expensive.

Bottles

You may have heard about a chemical called bisphenol-A (BPA) that is used in some plastic bottles, including baby bottles, and in the lining of canned foods. Results of some research suggest that BPA can disrupt the body's hormones and may lead to problems such as infertility and cancer. Research results also suggest that *fetuses*, infants, and children exposed to BPA may have toxic effects on the brain, nerves, and prostate gland. Because BPA crosses the *placenta*, infants can be exposed to BPA indirectly before birth. After birth, infants can be exposed through eating food stored or given in plastic bottles. Bisphenol-A also has been found in breast milk.

After reviewing the current research, the U.S. Food and Drug Administration (FDA) has stated that the levels of BPA to which infants and children are exposed are well below those that can cause harmful effects. However, the FDA also concluded that more research into BPA needs to be done, and it also is reviewing the existing research on the behavioral and nervous system effects of BPA. Parents who wish to take precautions against BPA can use glass or non–BPA-containing plastic bottles, which are now available in many stores and online.

The Challenges

As with breastfeeding, mothers who bottle-feed their babies also have to cope with a few challenges. Meeting these challenges requires time and planning.

Preparation
You will have to have enough formula on hand at all times, and you must prepare the bottles. The powdered and condensed formulas must be prepared with sterile water, which needs to be boiled until the baby is at least 6 months old.

Some parents warm bottles up before feeding the baby, although this often isn't necessary. The microwave should never be used to warm a baby's bottle because it can create dangerous hot spots.

Instead, run refrigerated bottles under warm water for a few minutes if the baby prefers a warm bottle to a cold one. Another option is to put the baby's bottles in a pan of hot water (away from the heat of the stove) with the temperature tested by squirting a drop or two of formula on the inside of the wrist.

Sterilization
Bottles and nipples need to be sterilized before they are used the first time. You then must wash them after each time you use them. Bottles and nipples can transmit bacteria if they aren't cleaned properly, as can formula if it isn't stored in sterile containers.

Refrigeration

If bottles are left out of the refrigerator longer than 1 hour, the formula must be thrown out. Prepared bottles of formula should be stored in the refrigerator for no longer than 24–48 hours (check the formula's label for complete information).

Part IV
Special Considerations

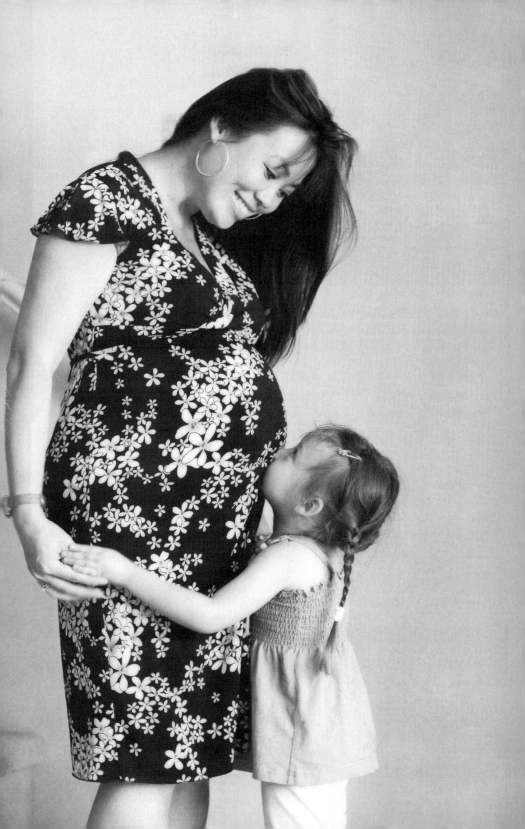

Chapter 15
Having Another Baby: What to Expect the Second Time Around

Congratulations! You're pregnant again! Now that you've been through it once, you already know a lot about what to expect in the coming trimesters and during labor and delivery. The changes that your body will experience during pregnancy won't be such a surprise this time around. You may even find that you don't have the roller coaster of emotions that you did with your first pregnancy. You're a pro at this now.

It is important, though, to remember that every pregnancy is different. You may not have changed much, but this pregnancy may not be like your first one.

How Will It Be Different?

There are some things that tend to change after your first pregnancy, and some that tend to remain the same. But when it comes down to it, there really is no way of knowing what your second (or third) pregnancy will be like.

Some things are likely to be different this time:

- *You'll be more tired this time*—One thing that is almost always true of a later pregnancy is that you will have more fatigue. There are a few reasons for this. First, you're older than you were during your first pregnancy. You may not have had a chance to get back in shape after giving birth. Second, you have another child (or children) to take care of, which can be tiring even when you aren't pregnant. Add in work and other obligations, and you will no doubt feel much more tired than you did the first time around.

- *You'll show earlier*—In fact, you may need to start wearing maternity clothes before your fourth month of pregnancy. That's because your abdominal muscles were stretched by your prior pregnancy and they may not have regained their former strength. As a result, these muscles won't hold the growing **uterus** in or up as well as they did during the first pregnancy.

- *You'll feel the baby move sooner*—Chances are, you'll feel this baby move a few weeks earlier than you felt your first baby. The baby isn't really moving sooner. You just know what to look for this time.

- *You'll notice Braxton Hicks contractions sooner*—**Braxton Hicks contractions** may show up during the second trimester rather than the third trimester, for instance.

- *Your breast changes are different*—They may not be as tender or grow as much as they did before. If you breastfed your first baby, your breasts may begin to leak earlier in pregnancy, too.

Possible Problems

Although every pregnancy is different, you'll likely have at least some of the other discomforts you had in your first pregnancy. Knowing this can help motivate you to take proactive steps to lessen them or possibly prevent them altogether. For example, if you had constipation or hemorrhoids last time, you can try to prevent these problems early on by eating plenty of fiber or taking a fiber supplement, drinking plenty of water, and exercising regularly.

Besides these types of normal pregnancy symptoms, if you're a healthy woman and had no serious problems the first time around, your risk for complications now is low. If, however, you have certain medical conditions, such as high blood pressure, depression, or **diabetes mellitus**, they can cause problems during pregnancy. Your health care provider will want to be sure these conditions are under control as this pregnancy progresses.

Also, if you had any pregnancy complications during your first pregnancy, such as **preterm** birth, hypertension, **preeclampsia**, or **gestational diabetes mellitus**, you may be at an increased risk for these complications in subsequent pregnancies. Keep in mind, though, that just because you had a problem in a past pregnancy doesn't mean it will happen again.

If you had one of the following complications, it's a good idea to see your health care provider early in this pregnancy. You can discuss your risks of developing complications and find out how to possibly recognize signs and symptoms earlier. There also may be steps you can take to reduce your risks:

- *Preterm birth*—If you have had a preterm birth (delivery before 37 weeks of pregnancy), especially in the second trimester, you're at a higher risk of it happening with this pregnancy as well. Preterm birth can result from early contractions (preterm labor), preterm **premature rupture of the membranes** (PROM), or problems with your ***cervix*** (cervical insufficiency). If you have a history of preterm birth, you should talk to your doctor early in pregnancy. You may be advised to avoid strenuous physical activity and watch for the signs and symptoms of infection. Additional testing, such as measurement of cervical length by **ultrasound**, may be offered, and you may receive certain treatments, depending on your situation (see Chapter 23, "Preterm Labor, Preterm Birth, and Premature Rupture of Membranes").

- *Preterm PROM*—The risk of preterm PROM (a condition in which the membranes that hold the ***amniotic fluid*** rupture before 37 weeks of pregnancy) happening in another pregnancy if you have had it before is between 16% and 32%. However, PROM can happen even when there are no known risk factors (see Chapter 23).

- *Depression*—You are at greater risk for **postpartum depression** if you had it in a previous pregnancy. Talk to your health care provider about what steps you can take to decrease your risk this time around. It may be recommended that you try behavioral therapy or take an antidepressant medication. Also, getting enough rest and exercise during your pregnancy has some benefits.

- *Gestational diabetes mellitus*—If you had gestational diabetes mellitus before, or if you had a very large baby, you are at increased risk of having it again. In addition, women who have had gestational diabetes mellitus have a higher chance of developing diabetes mellitus later in life. Because of the problems this condition can cause, your health care provider will discuss ways to lower your risks through diet, exercise, and possibly medication (see Chapter 19, "Diabetes Mellitus").

- *Preeclampsia*—Preeclampsia is most often a problem during first pregnancies, but you can be at risk for having it again if it was a problem before (see Chapter 18, "Hypertension").

- *Intrauterine growth restriction*—In some pregnancies, the unborn baby does not grow and develop normally, a condition called intrauterine growth restriction. Women who previously have given birth to a smaller than normal infant are more at risk for this condition in their next pregnancies, so your doctor may order ultrasound exams during your pregnancy to monitor your baby's growth (see Chapter 27, "Growth Problems").

I'm Just Thinking About Getting Pregnant Again

You're not pregnant yet, but you are having thoughts of wanting another child. The timing of when to plan your next pregnancy is a decision for both you and your partner. Only you two can decide what you are ready to handle—physically, emotionally, and financially.

You may want to talk to your doctor about your plans to have another baby. Your doctor can give you an idea about what the ideal spacing is between children. Even if you want your children to be close in age, it's best to wait at least 12 months before getting pregnant again. Doctors believe that babies conceived less than 6 months (or more than 5 years) after you give birth have a higher risk of preterm birth, low birth weight, and small size. Babies born soon after their siblings may have these problems because the mother has not had time to recover from childbirth or replenish her body's nutrients.

It also is helpful to await the return of regular menstrual cycles because a regular menstrual cycle will help you determine when you become pregnant earlier and help establish a more accurate estimated date for delivery. Having as accurate a due date as possible is particularly helpful if you have had an early delivery in a prior pregnancy or if unexpected complications occur later in this pregnancy

When you do decide to become pregnant again, schedule a prepregnancy checkup with your doctor to make sure you are as healthy as possible. As part of your visit, your doctor will ask about your diet and lifestyle.

For example, if you haven't had much success getting back to your prepregnancy weight since having your first baby, your doctor may tell you that now is the time to try harder. Results of some studies show that gaining too much weight between pregnancies may lead to complications, such as high blood pressure and gestational diabetes mellitus.

To help control your weight between pregnancies, start exercising for at least 30 minutes on 3 days a week. Put the baby in a stroller and take walks around the neighborhood or around a nearby shopping mall. Work out with an exercise DVD if leaving home is difficult. Also, stick to a healthy diet to control the number of calories you eat each day.

Overall, as you plan your next pregnancy, it is a good idea to start the healthy habits you had during your first pregnancy. It's never too early to get your body in the best possible shape.

Telling Your Other Children

You may wonder when is the best time to tell your other children that you are going to have another baby. You know your children best, so it's really your decision when to tell them. It depends both on how old your children are and how you think they will handle the news.

Some experts suggest that you should wait until sometime after your first trimester, when the risk of miscarriage decreases. You may want to wait until after a healthy pregnancy is confirmed by listening for the baby's heartbeat or by ultrasound exam. With young children, it's also a good idea to wait until you're starting to show. Your children may have a hard time imagining that there's a baby growing inside you if your body still looks the same. It is easier to explain what you're talking about once you have a little bump.

Whenever you do give the news, be sure to remind your children that you love them and that the new baby won't change that. Also reassure your children that delivering the baby won't harm you. Let them know that even though you will be in the hospital, it's not because you're sick.

To prevent your children from feeling left out, involve them in your pregnancy as much as you can. The relationship between siblings is one of the longest and most important ones in life. These tips can help promote the bond right from the start:

- Take your children shopping and let them pick out items for their new brother or sister.
- Let them suggest the baby's name they like best and take part in the decision.
- Tell your children about the role they can play in helping you with the new baby.
- Read books together about pregnancy and on being a big brother or sister.
- Show your children some photos of what you looked like when you were pregnant with them. And show them their own baby pictures.

It's also a good idea to set up the baby's room early. If you need to move your children out of a crib or into a different room, do it as early as possible so that they don't feel displaced by the new baby. As your due date gets near, it may help them to hear stories of how you were proud to have your own sibling sleep in your crib or wear your clothes when you were little. Ask them to help pick a few of their old toys to give to the baby.

Remember that welcoming another baby into the family will likely bring both happiness and anxiety for your other children. Just do your best to plan ahead for the new arrival to help make the transition as easy as you possibly can.

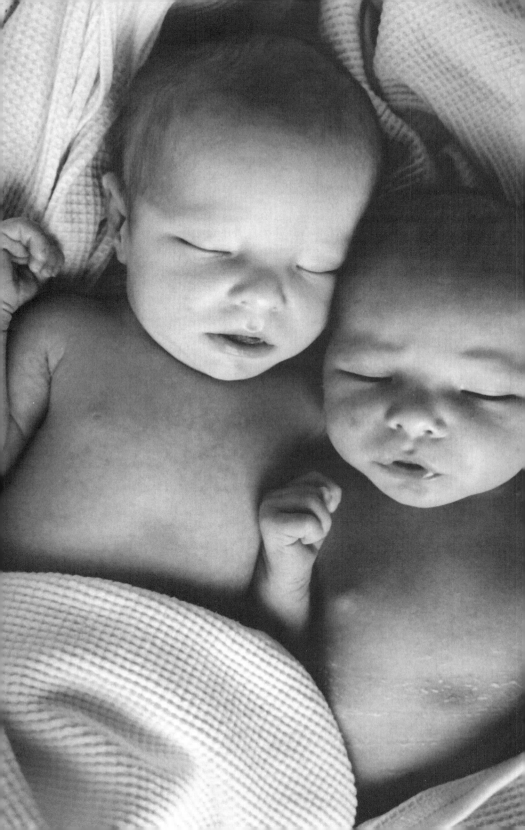

Chapter 16
Multiples: When It's Twins, Triplets, or More

When a woman is carrying more than one baby, it is called a ***multiple pregnancy***. In the past 20 years, multiple pregnancies have become more common in the United States. In fact, according to the National Center for Health Statistics, between 1980 and 2003, the number of twin births increased by two thirds (66%), and the number of mothers having triplets or more than three babies (called higher-order multiples) increased fourfold.

Today, more than 3% of babies are born in sets of two, three, or more, and about 94% of these multiple births are twins. Some of this increase in multiple pregnancies is because more women older than 35 years are having babies, and women in this age group are at a higher risk of having twins.

However, all experts agree that what's led to the increase in the number of multiple pregnancies more than anything else is that more women are undergoing fertility treatments to become pregnant. These treatments increase the risk of multiple pregnancy. It is important to discuss the risks of multiple pregnancy, and possible ways to prevent it, with your doctor if you are having fertility treatments (see box "Fertility Treatments and Multiple Pregnancy").

Making Multiples

Multiple births occur when more than one fertilized egg implants and grows in the uterus. This process can occur naturally, or it can be induced artificially during fertility treatments.

Fertility Treatments and Multiple Pregnancy

Fertility treatments are a major factor in the increase in multiple pregnancies over the past 20 years. Although all fertility treatments increase the risk of multiple pregnancy, it is most common in women who use fertility drugs to induce *ovulation*. Several drugs can be used to stimulate ovulation. When a drug called clomiphene citrate is used, 5–12% of the pregnancies that are achieved are twins, and less than 1% are triplets or greater. When drugs called gonadotropins are used, 20% of the pregnancies achieved are multiple pregnancies. Most of these are twin pregnancies, but up to 5% are triplets or greater.

With *assisted reproductive technologies*, *eggs* are fertilized outside of the body. The eggs can be from a donor, or they can be generated by the woman herself with fertility drugs. The resulting *embryo* or embryos are transferred to a woman's *uterus* or *fallopian tube*. The risk of multiple pregnancy increases as the number of embryos transferred increases. About 45% percent of pregnancies aided by assisted reproductive technologies result in twins and about 7% in triplets or more.

Because of the risks associated with multiple pregnancy, the American Society for Reproductive Medicine recommends taking a preventive approach when fertility treatments are used. If you and your partner are considering fertility treatments, your fertility specialist will talk with you about the risks of having a multiple pregnancy and how you may avoid having more than one baby. For example, with assisted reproductive technologies, you may choose to limit the number of embryos that are transferred to the uterus. It's less likely that you will become pregnant with triplets or more if only one or two embryos are transferred. With ovulation induction, *ultrasound* can be used to monitor the number of eggs that are developing in the *ovaries,* and blood tests can measure *hormone* levels. If the ultrasound exam reveals a large number of developing eggs, or if the blood test results show a high level of hormones, it may be recommended that you do not attempt pregnancy during that cycle to avoid the risk of multiple pregnancy.

Fraternal or Identical Twins?

The most common kind of multiple pregnancy is twins, and twins come in two types—fraternal and identical:

- *Fraternal twins*—Most twins are fraternal. Each fraternal twin grows from a separate fertilized *egg* and *sperm*. Each fraternal twin has its own

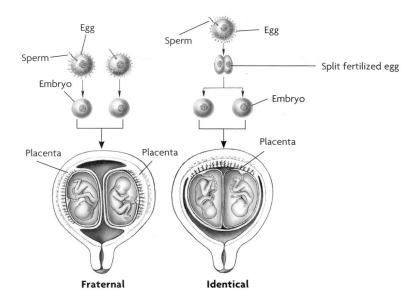

Egg

Sperm

Sperm

Egg

Embryo

Split fertilized egg

Embryo

Placenta

Placenta

Placenta

Placenta

Fraternal

Identical

Types of twins. Fraternal twins are formed from two eggs and each has a placenta. Identical twins are formed from one egg that splits into two. They share the same placenta and sometimes the amniotic sac.

placenta and *amniotic sac*. Because each twin grows from the union of a different egg and a different sperm, these twins are similar only in the same way any brother and sister are. The twins can be both boys, both girls, or one of each.

• *Identical twins*—When one fertilized egg splits early in pregnancy and grows into two or more *fetuses*, identical twins are formed. Identical twins share a placenta, but often each has its own amniotic sac. Because identical twins share the same genetic material at the start, they are the same sex and have the same blood type, hair color, and eye color.

Three or More Babies

A pregnancy with three or more babies can be formed by more than one egg being fertilized, a single fertilized egg splitting, or both processes occurring in the same pregnancy. This higher-order pregnancy rarely happens naturally—only 1 of about 3,000 births—and is most often the result of fertility treatments.

How to Know When It's More Than One Baby

Years ago, mothers in labor who just gave birth to their baby were often surprised to hear the doctor yell, "There's one more baby coming!" But luckily, these types of surprises rarely happen these days because most mothers-to-be learn they're carrying multiples fairly early. An ultrasound examination can detect most multiples by your 12th week of pregnancy.

Before an ultrasound exam is done, however, there are other signs that can alert your doctor that you are pregnant with more than one baby:

• Rapid weight gain during the first trimester
• Severe morning sickness
• Abnormal results on the quadruple screening test done around 16 weeks of pregnancy to check for certain birth defects (see p. 354)
• Hearing more than one heartbeat during a prenatal exam
• Your uterus being larger than expected during a prenatal exam

The Risks

The risk of problems during pregnancy increases with the number of babies. That is, there is a higher risk of problems with twins than with a single baby and a higher risk of problems with triplets than with twins.

A multiple pregnancy can affect your health as well as your babies' health. However, with proper prenatal care, your doctor can diagnose and manage the complications and help protect you and the babies from more serious problems (see box "What Kind of Doctor Should You See"). You should be aware of the complications that are more likely with a multiple pregnancy.

Preterm Birth

Preterm birth—birth before 37 weeks of gestation—is the most common problem of multiple pregnancies. More than 50% of twins and more than 90% of triplets are born preterm. The number of weeks you will be pregnant decreases with each additional baby (see Table 16-1).

When babies are born preterm, they often have problems breathing and eating. Serious, long-term problems also can occur, including cerebral palsy and other neurologic problems, vision problems, problems with the digestive system, and developmental delays. Because prematurity is so common in multiple pregnancies, it is important to be prepared for the possibility that your babies may have these problems. The risk of these problems increases the earlier the babies are born.

What Kind of Doctor Should You See?

Many mothers who are expecting multiples wonder if they need to see a maternal–fetal medicine subspecialist during their pregnancy. These subspecialists, also called perinatologists, are obstetricians who specialize in caring for pregnant women who may be at high risk for special health problems. But having a multiple pregnancy does not mean you need a subspecialist. If you are healthy, you can choose to see an obstetrician who has experience caring for women with multiple pregnancies. If you have other conditions that put you at risk for complications or if you have a history of pregnancy problems, your obstetrician may refer you to a subspecialist. The maternal–fetal medicine subspecialist will usually help take care of you and your babies, along with your regular obstetrician.

Keep in mind that being referred to a maternal–fetal medicine subspecialist does not mean your doctor expects your pregnancy will be difficult. Usually, the referral is done to give extra protection for you and the babies and to put your mind at ease.

Table 16-1 Duration of Multiple Pregnancies

Type of Pregnancy	Average Gestational Age at Time of Delivery	Average Birth Weight
Singleton	40 weeks	7 lb (3,300 grams)
Twin	35 weeks	5.5 lb (2,500 grams)
Triplet	33 weeks	4 lb (1,800 grams)
Quadruplet	29 weeks	3 lb (1,400 grams)

From Multiple pregnancy and birth: twins, triplets, and higher order multiples: a guide for patients. Patient Information Series. Birmingham, AL: American Society for Reproductive Medicine; 2004.

If you go into labor before 34 weeks and it is detected early enough, your doctor may be able to delay delivery for a few days. Postponing the birth for even a few more days can make a big difference. You also may receive a steroid medication that can help the babies' lungs mature.

It's important to be able to recognize preterm labor if you are pregnant with more than one baby and to call your health care provider if you have any of these signs or symptoms:

- Change in vaginal discharge (becomes watery, mucus-like, or bloody)
- Increase in amount of vaginal discharge
- Pelvic or lower-abdominal pressure
- Constant, low, dull backache

- Mild abdominal cramps, with or without diarrhea
- Regular or frequent contractions or uterine tightening, often painless (four times every 20 minutes or eight times an hour for more than 1 hour)
- Ruptured membranes (your water breaks, whether a gush or a trickle)

Preeclampsia

Preeclampsia is a condition of pregnancy in which there is high blood pressure and protein in the **urine**. The risk of the condition is more than double for women carrying twins compared to women having only one baby.

Preeclampsia can be mild or severe. It can reduce the blood flow to the babies, limiting their oxygen and nutrients. The babies may need to be delivered early if your blood pressure becomes too high. Preeclampsia can progress to seizures in the mother, a life-threatening condition called **eclampsia**. The only treatment for eclampsia is prompt delivery, no matter the **gestational age** of the babies.

Growth Problems

Women carrying multiple babies are at increased risk for growth problems in one or more babies. For example, twins are more likely to be smaller than average size compared with a single baby. Ultrasound typically is used to check the growth of each baby and the amount of **amniotic fluid** about every 3–4 weeks throughout pregnancy.

Twins are called **discordant** if one is much smaller than the other. Discordant twins are more likely to have problems during pregnancy and after birth. Twins may be discordant because of poor functioning of the placenta, genetic problems, or **twin–twin transfusion syndrome**.

Twin–twin transfusion syndrome can develop when identical twins share a placenta. The blood passes from one twin to the other through their shared placenta. The twin that gives the blood will be very small and have too little amniotic fluid. The other twin can have too much blood and amniotic fluid. Some of the extra fluid may need to be removed. If twin–twin transfusion syndrome is severe, the twins may have to be delivered early or treated with laser surgery.

Gestational Diabetes Mellitus

Women carrying multiple babies are at increased risk of **gestational diabetes mellitus**—a pregnancy-related form of **diabetes mellitus**. This condition can cause the baby to grow especially large, increasing the risk of injuries during vaginal delivery. Babies born to women with gestational diabetes mellitus also may have breathing difficulties and other problems during the newborn period.

What to Expect

Women who are carrying more than one baby may need special care during pregnancy, labor, and delivery. You may need to see your health care provider more often than a woman carrying one baby. You also may need to adjust your diet and exercise routine.

Eating More

When pregnant with multiple babies, you will need to eat more than if you were carrying one baby. Eating well is important for your health and the health of your babies. During pregnancy, you need to eat about 500 more calories per day for a total of about 2,700 calories per day for twins. If you are pregnant with triplets, or higher order of multiples, you will have to increase the amount of calories per day accordingly.

In addition to a prenatal vitamin supplement, your doctor may prescribe extra vitamin and mineral supplements to help your babies grow. *Anemia* is more common in women who are pregnant with twins, so it's especially important to take your prenatal vitamin and iron supplements as prescribed. Folic acid also is important for twins, so you should take a prenatal vitamin supplement that contains folic acid.

Gaining More Weight

Along with eating well, gaining the right amount of weight is very important for the health of your babies. You will need to gain more weight when carrying more than one baby than if you were having only one.

If you're expecting twins, you should gain between 37 pounds and 54 pounds. If you were overweight, however, before pregnancy, you should gain between 31 pounds and 50 pounds. If you were obese (a body mass index of 30 or greater), you should gain between 25 pounds and 42 pounds (see Appendix A). Gaining the necessary pounds during your pregnancy should be done gradually. With twins, your doctor will advise you to gain about 1 pound per week in the first half of pregnancy. In the second half of pregnancy, you should aim to gain a little more than 1 pound each week.

Careful Exercise

Getting regular exercise is important in every pregnancy. When you're carrying multiple babies, though, you'll have to use some caution. Your doctor may advise you to stay away from high-impact exercise, such as aerobics and running. Better choices for you to remain active during your pregnancy are sports that are lower-impact, such as swimming, prenatal yoga, and walking.

More Monitoring

You will need special *prenatal care* when having a multiple pregnancy. You'll be scheduled to see your health care provider for prenatal checkups more often and will need some extra monitoring to check the well-being of your babies.

Your health care provider may use some or all of these techniques:

- Have you count your babies' movements (called *kick counts*) at home
- Examine your *cervix* by physical exam or ultrasound exam for changes that may indicate that you are at risk for preterm labor
- Repeat ultrasound exams to check the babies' growth
- Measure the babies' heart rate in response to their own movements (called a *nonstress test*)
- Perform a *biophysical profile*, which includes checking the babies' heart rate, body movement, muscle tone, and the amount of amniotic fluid by ultrasound exam

Restrictions and Bed Rest

Although bed rest and restricted activity often is prescribed for women carrying multiple babies, it hasn't been studied enough to prove that it results in healthier babies or a healthier mom. The same holds true for routine hospitalization for women with higher-order multiple pregnancy. However, results of studies of routine hospitalization of women carrying twins have shown that it does not prolong the pregnancy.

Your Delivery

The chance of needing a *cesarean delivery* is higher when you're pregnant with twins than when you're pregnant with one baby. However, you have a good chance of having a normal vaginal delivery if both babies are in a head-down position and there are no other complications. If you are carrying three or more babies, your doctor will most likely recommend a cesarean delivery because it is safer for the babies.

How your babies are born depends on certain factors, including:

- Position of each baby
- Weight of each baby
- Your health
- Health of the babies

Sometimes both a vaginal delivery and cesarean delivery may be needed to deliver twins. When the lower twin is in the head-down position but the higher twin is not, once the first twin is born, the other twin can sometimes be turned or delivered with feet or buttocks first. When this can't be done, the second twin is delivered by cesarean delivery.

Labor, especially the pushing stage, may take longer with twins. Babies usually are born several minutes apart in a vaginal delivery, but it can take longer.

Preparing Yourself

Having more than one baby can be both an exciting time and an overwhelming one. It is important for you and your partner to be as prepared as possible for the coming adventure of being new parents to more than one baby. It may be helpful to talk with other parents who have multiple babies. Although it's impossible to be prepared for every contingency, the following challenges are those that many families of multiple babies encounter:

- *High health care costs*—Because multiple babies often are born with health problems, they may require short-term and long-term specialized health care. Have a financial plan in place to deal with these health care costs. If you have health insurance, make sure that it will cover the costs of this specialized care.

- *Extra help*—You will need some extra hands to help care for your babies, so be sure to line up your volunteers well before your due date. Also, make sure that at least some of your helpers are in for the long haul. You will most likely need helpers for several weeks to months, depending on how many babies you have.

- *Stress and fatigue*—Caring for multiples is stressful. Preterm babies need smaller, more frequent feedings, and sleep can be in short supply for the parents. One parent most likely will need to stay at home to care for multiple infants.

It's a good idea to enroll in a childbirth class that is especially for parents expecting twins or more. Plan to take the classes during your fourth month to sixth month of pregnancy when you are more likely to be most comfortable. Your health care provider or nurse should be able to help you find a class.

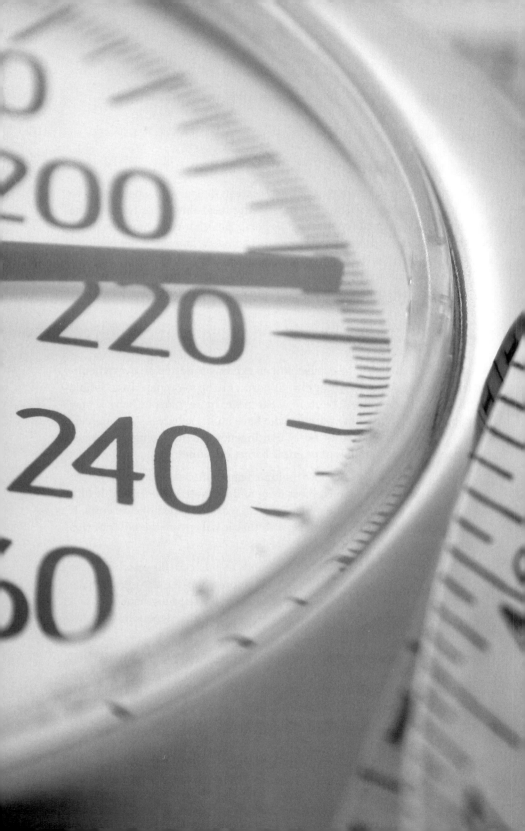

Chapter 17
Obesity and Eating Disorders

Obesity and eating disorders are common in women. Both can affect pregnancy. If you have either of these conditions, you need to be aware of the risks that they pose. Your health care provider and you can work together to manage your pregnancy and avoid some of these risks.

Obesity and Pregnancy

The number of obese women in the United States has increased a great deal during the last 20 years. Research has shown that about one third of adult women are now obese, and obesity is one of the country's fastest-growing health problems.

When a woman is obese during pregnancy, the risk of problems for both her and the baby is higher. With proper care, however, many obese moms-to-be are able to have completely safe pregnancies and healthy babies.

Are You Obese?

You are considered obese if your body mass index (BMI) before pregnancy is 30 or higher (use the chart in Appendix A to determine your BMI). Body mass index measures your body fat based on your height and weight. Including obesity, the BMI has three different categories of weight:

1. Normal weight—BMI of 18.5–24.9
2. Overweight—BMI of 25–29.9
3. Obese—BMI of 30–39.9

When a person's BMI is 40, doctors consider it morbid obesity, meaning you are at a much greater risk for life-threatening health problems.

What Are the Risks?

As with any other time in your life, being obese during pregnancy poses extra health risks. While you are pregnant, the extra weight you are carrying increases the chance of problems for you and your baby. Your doctor will monitor you during your prenatal visits to help catch these possible complications if they arise:

- *High blood pressure*—High blood pressure during pregnancy is 10 times more likely if you are obese. When high blood pressure during pregnancy is not treated, it can lead to health problems for mother and baby.

- *Preeclampsia*—This condition occurs only during pregnancy. **Preeclampsia** is characterized by high blood pressure and protein in the urine. It can lead to serious complications for the mother. The baby may need to be delivered early.

- *Gestational diabetes mellitus*—High blood **glucose** levels caused by **gestational diabetes mellitus** increase the risk of having a very large baby and possible **cesarean delivery** (see Chapter 19, "Diabetes Mellitus").

- *Cesarean delivery*—If your baby needs to be delivered by cesarean delivery, your risk of complications from the procedure is higher if you are obese.

- *Birth defects*—Babies born to obese mothers have an increased risk of having birth defects, especially **neural tube defects**.

- *Labor and delivery complications*—Having too much body fat can make it difficult for your doctor to use **ultrasound** to check your baby's weight and position in your **uterus**. It also is harder to hear your baby's heartbeat.

Before You Become Pregnant

If you are obese, the best course of action is to lose weight before becoming pregnant. Shedding excess weight puts you in the best physical condition for pregnancy and will benefit both you and your baby.

Try to Lose Weight

If your BMI is more than 30 and you are planning to get pregnant, talk to your doctor. Your doctor can help you work out a healthy plan to get closer to your ideal weight before you become pregnant. Losing a few pounds can help to lower your chances of a high-risk pregnancy.

Have You Had Bariatric Surgery?
Many women who have undergone bariatric (weight loss) surgery wonder how it will affect them when they become pregnant. Research shows that having these types of surgical procedures doesn't affect your pregnancy in any harmful way. In fact, if you have had bariatric surgery and have lost weight, you are less likely to have problems in pregnancy, such as gestational diabetes mellitus and high blood pressure, than obese women who haven't had surgery.

You should, however, delay getting pregnant for the 12–24 months after surgery. This is the time when you will have the most weight loss. If you had problems such as *polycystic ovary syndrome*, lack of *ovulation*, or irregular menstrual periods before your surgery, these problems may resolve on their own as you rapidly drop the excess weight. It's important to be aware of this possibility because the increase in fertility may lead to an unintended pregnancy. It's also important to note that if you've had gastric bypass surgery, it may affect how medication, including *oral contraceptives*, is absorbed into your body. You may need to switch to another form of birth control.

When you do become pregnant, there are a few things you'll need to do to make sure you stay as healthy as possible:

• You may have certain vitamin deficiencies, so you will need to take your daily prenatal vitamin supplement and maybe more vitamin sup-

Types of Bariatric Surgery

Bariatric surgery is performed on part of the digestive tract to treat morbid obesity. The two most common types of bariatric surgery done today are gastric bypass surgery and the banding procedure:

1. In gastric bypass surgery, a small pouch is created from the stomach, restricting the amount of food you can eat. The remaining part of the stomach is sealed off with staples. The small intestine is also reconfigured so that food bypasses the main absorbing parts of the digestive tract.

2. In the banding procedure, a fluid-filled band is placed around the stomach, which reduces the amount of food it can hold. The size of the band can be adjusted, if needed.

plements for iron, vitamin B$_{12}$, folic acid, and **calcium.** It is recommended that you get these vitamins as separate supplements, rather than in a daily multivitamin supplement. An excess of the other vitamins in multivitamin supplements, such as vitamin A, can be harmful during pregnancy.

- Make sure you know how much weight you should gain each month, and watch your weight closely. Weight gain recommendations are based on your prepregnancy BMI. See page 25 for these recommendations.

- If you've had lap band surgery, have the doctor who performed your surgery monitor you during pregnancy. Some women may have nutrient deficiencies as a consequence of this surgery. Adjustments can be made to the band during pregnancy to help improve nutrition in pregnant women.

When You Are Pregnant

If your BMI is more than 30, the latest guidelines from the Institute of Medicine state that you should gain between 11 pounds and 20 pounds while you're pregnant. If your BMI is 40 or greater, your health care provider may suggest that you gain less weight, gain no weight, or possibly lose a modest amount of weight during your pregnancy. This weight loss should not be drastic and should be individualized for your particular situation. You should not attempt to lose weight during pregnancy unless you are under a health care provider's close supervision.

Throughout your pregnancy, you more than likely will have more tests done than an average-weight mom-to-be. For instance, at your early prenatal visits, your doctor will give you a blood glucose test to check for gestational diabetes mellitus. You may be given the test again in your later months too.

As your due date approaches, your health care provider may explain that you need special care if you have a cesarean delivery. Obese women may need extra attention before, during, and after the procedure to decrease the risk of certain problems, such as ***deep vein thrombosis***.

Eating Disorders and Pregnancy

Each year in the United States, 10 million women struggle with an eating disorder. Some women with eating disorders may experience a temporary remission of their symptoms when they become pregnant. For other women, eating disorders that were under control before pregnancy may start again during pregnancy. And sometimes, an eating disorder may begin during pregnancy.

Do You Have an Eating Disorder?

Anorexia nervosa and *bulimia nervosa* are two types of eating disorders. They often have different warning signs and result in different health problems.

Anorexia Nervosa

A person with anorexia nervosa diets to extremes because she feels she is too fat even when she is not. Most women with anorexia nervosa have an intense fear of being fat. They want to be thin so badly that they may starve themselves—sometimes to death.

You should be aware of the symptoms of anorexia nervosa and tell your health care provider if you have them:

- You diet nonstop (even when thin), refuse to eat except in small portions, or want to eat alone.
- You have lost a lot of weight and still think you are fat.
- Your menstrual periods stop.
- You exercise excessively.
- You have fine hair growing on your face and arms.
- You are losing hair from your head.
- Your skin is dry, pale, and yellowed.

Bulimia Nervosa

Women with bulimia nervosa binge eat—which means they eat large amounts of food in a short time. They then purge the excess food by vomiting; using *laxatives,* diuretics (water pills), or emetics (pills that cause vomiting); or fasting.

Signs that you may have bulimia are listed as follows:

- Swelling around the jaw
- Bloating
- Bloodshot eyes
- Problems with teeth and gums
- Weakness and fatigue
- Mood swings and a feeling of being out of control

How Eating Disorders Can Harm You and Your Baby

Having an eating disorder can affect your pregnancy in many ways. When you don't eat, neither does your baby. If you do not gain enough weight while you're pregnant, it can lead to a number of problems for both of you. Some of the problems are listed as follows:

* Miscarriage
* *Preterm* birth
* *Low birth weight*
* *Depression*
* Slow growth of the baby
* Gestational diabetes mellitus
* Preeclampsia

The laxatives, diuretics, and other medications you take to purge your meals also can harm your baby. These substances take away nutrients and fluids before they are able to feed and nourish the baby.

Getting Help

If you are living with an eating disorder, tell your health care provider right away. The sooner you can resolve your problem, the better. The good news is that many women with eating disorders can have healthy babies. Also, it is not uncommon for women with eating disorders who are underweight to have problems conceiving. With a return to normal weight, fertility often returns as well.

Have your health care provider refer you to a trained professional who can help treat your disorder and any other concerns. It's a good idea to try both individual and group therapy. You may need medication as well.

As you work to overcome the negative effects of anorexia nervosa or bulimia nervosa, there are steps you can take to put you on a path to a healthy pregnancy. First, ask your health care provider to refer you to a nutritionist who can help you learn about healthy eating. Once you have an eating plan in place, try to gain the recommended weight during your pregnancy. The right amount of weight gain is crucial to having a healthy baby. If you need more support, ask for it.

If You Have a History of Eating Disorders

Some women who have had an eating disorder and have received treatment may experience a return of the signs and symptoms of their eating disorder during pregnancy. Pregnancy raises body-image issues for just about every woman. For a woman with a past eating disorder, these issues can trigger the return of the disorder.

If you have a history of an eating disorder, it is important to tell your health care provider early in pregnancy. Together, you can monitor your feelings and be alert to any signs that the disorder has returned. It may be a good idea to continue counseling or seek out a counselor when you become pregnant.

Part V
Medical Problems During Pregnancy

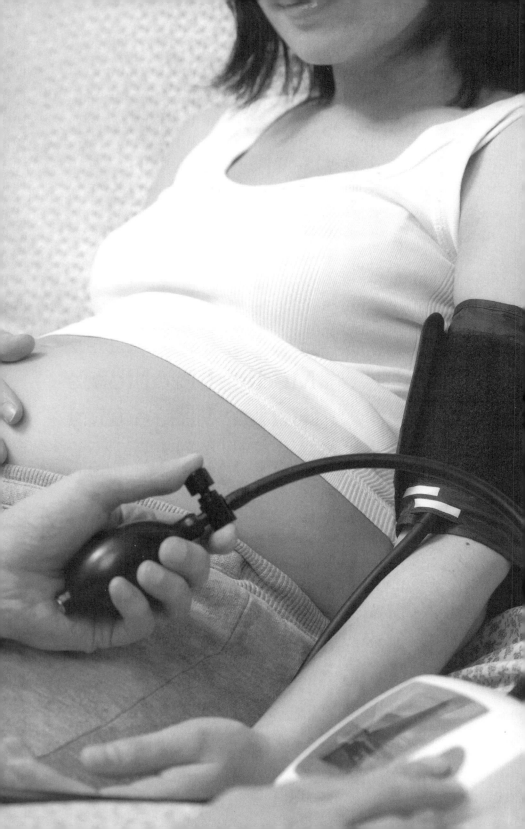

Chapter 18
Hypertension

B lood pressure is the pressure the blood exerts against the blood vessel walls as the heart pumps. The pressure increases when the heart contracts and pushes blood into the vessels and decreases when the heart relaxes.

Blood pressure is recorded as two numbers: the systolic pressure (as the heart beats) over the diastolic pressure (as the heart relaxes between beats). When a blood pressure reading is taken, the higher number represents the systolic pressure and the lower number represents the diastolic pressure. For instance, 120/80 (120 over 80) means the systolic pressure is 120 and the diastolic pressure is 80.

Your blood pressure goes up and down all day long—even from one minute to the next. It changes based on your activity level, body temperature, diet, emotions, and any medications you might take. If your health care provider finds that your blood pressure is higher than normal during one of your prenatal visits, another reading will be taken again later to see if it has gone back to a normal level.

If, after several readings, your systolic blood pressure is 140 or greater, your diastolic pressure is 90 or greater, or both, you have high blood pressure or hypertension. Hypertension is a "silent disease," because it does not in itself

Your Blood Pressure Reading

110 = systolic = pressure in arteries when heart contracts

80 = diastolic = pressure in arteries when heart relaxes

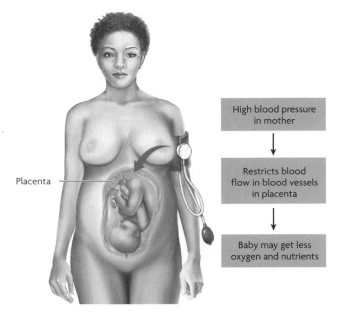

Placenta

High blood pressure
in mother

↓

Restricts blood
flow in blood vessels
in placenta

↓

Baby may get less
oxygen and nutrients

Hypertension. Hypertension during pregnancy can decrease the amount of oxygen and nutrients the baby receives.

cause symptoms. However, hypertension needs to be controlled because it can lead to serious health problems, such as heart failure, kidney failure, or stroke.

Chronic Hypertension

When high blood pressure has been present for some time before pregnancy, it is known as chronic hypertension. Chronic hypertension also may be diagnosed during pregnancy if a woman has high blood pressure before 20 weeks of pregnancy or if she has high blood pressure later in pregnancy and the condition lasts for longer than 12 weeks after the birth of the baby.

Risks During Pregnancy

Chronic hypertension can cause problems during pregnancy. The baby receives all of its nutrients and oxygen from the mother's blood flowing through the ***placenta.*** Hypertension can restrict the flow of blood, resulting in an increased risk of the following problems and conditions:

* ***Preterm*** birth
* Growth problems

- *Placental abruption* (a condition in which the placenta detaches from the uterine wall)
- *Cesarean delivery*
- Fetal death

Hypertension in pregnancy also may affect the pregnant woman. Pregnancy increases the amount of blood in the body. In a woman with hypertension, this increase in blood volume places added stress on the heart and **kidneys**. In addition, hypertension in pregnancy may mask a condition called **preeclampsia**.

The Importance of Prepregnancy Evaluation

Ideally, if you have had chronic hypertension for several years, you should see your health care provider before becoming pregnant. The purpose of this pre-pregnancy evaluation is to determine whether your hypertension is under control and whether it has affected your health. Because hypertension may affect the heart and kidneys, you may be given tests to check the function of these organs.

The information gained from these tests is used to assess the risks that pregnancy will have on your future health. If you have severe hypertension, you may be at risk for serious complications, such as kidney or heart failure. However, most pregnant women with mild chronic hypertension have perfectly normal pregnancies without any long-term effects.

In addition to tests, you and your health care provider can discuss steps that you can take to help make your pregnancy safer. The goal of these actions is to lower your blood pressure before pregnancy:

- If you are overweight, lose weight through diet and exercise.
- Take your blood pressure medication as prescribed.
- Stop smoking.

Managing Hypertension in Pregnancy

Women with chronic hypertension may receive additional testing during pregnancy to monitor their condition and that of their baby. These tests enable your health care provider to detect potential problems soon after they occur.

Women with mild hypertension usually do not require treatment with antihypertensive medications during pregnancy. Some women who take medication when they are not pregnant can stop taking medication during pregnancy. Other women, usually those with severe hypertension, need to continue treatment during their pregnancies. Talk to your health care provider about the best treatment for you. In some cases, a woman may need to switch to a different medication that still helps control her blood pressure but is safer to use during pregnancy.

Gestational Hypertension

When high blood pressure first occurs during the second half of pregnancy, it is known as gestational hypertension. This type of high blood pressure goes away soon after the baby is born. If you develop gestational hypertension, you may need to see your health care provider more often to have your blood pressure checked. About one quarter of women with gestational hypertension develop preeclampsia.

Preeclampsia

Preeclampsia is a condition that occurs only during pregnancy. It is characterized by high blood pressure and increased amounts of protein in the urine. It usually starts after the 20th week of pregnancy and can affect all organs of the body. Preeclampsia causes stress on the kidneys and also can affect the liver and brain.

Preeclampsia usually is detected by urine tests or high blood pressure readings. Some symptoms of this condition include the following:

- Headaches
- Vision problems
- Rapid weight gain
- Upper abdominal pain

Doctors do not know why some women develop preeclampsia, but they do know that some women are at higher risk than others. You are more likely to get preeclampsia if the following conditions apply to you:

- You are pregnant for the first time.
- You are pregnant with more than one baby (twins, triplets, or more).
- You have had preeclampsia in a previous pregnancy.
- You have a history of chronic hypertension.
- You are older than 35 years.
- You have certain medical conditions, such as **diabetes mellitus,** kidney disease, and **lupus.**
- You are obese.
- You are African American.

If you develop preeclampsia, a decision will need to be made about whether to deliver the baby. If you have mild preeclampsia, you will be monitored closely with frequent visits to your health care provider and tests to check your and the baby's health. You may have to stay in the hospital for a few days at first. If all remains well, you should be able to have your baby at term (at least 38 weeks).

If you have severe preeclampsia, but your baby would not survive if delivered, you will be closely monitored and have frequent tests. Daily testing may be recommended in some cases, and you may need to stay in a hospital. Severe preeclampsia is best managed by an obstetrician who has experience caring for women with pregnancy complications, such as a maternal–fetal medical subspecialist. The decision to deliver the baby is based on *gestational age* and the condition of the mother or baby. Early delivery depends in part on whether the hospital is equipped with a neonatal intensive care unit, a specialized department that cares for preterm babies. If it is not, the pregnant woman may be transported to a different hospital that has a neonatal intensive care unit to give birth.

Eclampsia

Eclampsia is defined as the onset of seizures in a pregnant woman for several days to weeks after delivery. It can occur in a woman who has preeclampsia or gestational hypertension, or it can be the first sign of hypertension. Eclampsia is a life-threatening condition. When eclampsia occurs during pregnancy, the baby must be delivered regardless of gestational age. Women with this condition require special care to control their high blood pressure and prevent additional seizures so that delivery can be safely accomplished. When eclampsia occurs after birth, it is treated with medications to control seizures and decrease blood pressure.

Hemolysis, Elevated Liver Enzyme Levels, and Low Platelet Count Syndrome

Some pregnant women with high blood pressure also develop a condition known as HELLP syndrome. HELLP stands for **H**emolysis, **E**levated **L**iver enzyme levels, and **L**ow **P**latelet count. It is a rare illness, but a serious one. Women with HELLP syndrome may have bleeding, liver, and blood pressure problems that may put her life at risk. Treatment usually is delivery of the baby, regardless of the gestational age.

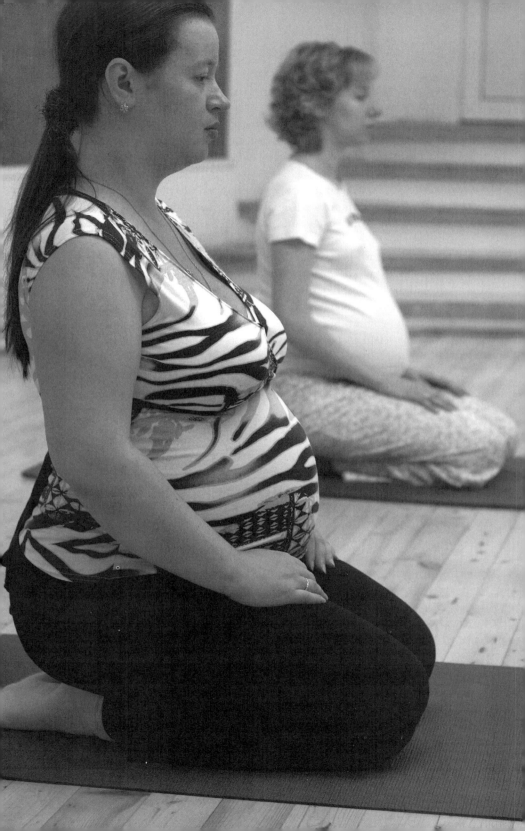

Chapter 19
Diabetes Mellitus

Diabetes mellitus is a disease in which the body does not make or properly use **insulin**. Insulin is a **hormone** that converts **glucose** (sugar) into energy. It is made by **cells** in the pancreas. When the body does not make enough insulin or does not use it correctly, glucose cannot get into cells and instead stays in the blood. Over time, high blood sugar levels can damage your heart, eyes, and **kidneys**.

There are three types of diabetes mellitus: type 1 diabetes mellitus, type 2 diabetes mellitus, and **gestational diabetes mellitus**. In type 1 diabetes mellitus, the body makes little or no insulin on its own. In type 2 diabetes mellitus, the body makes enough insulin but the body's cells are insulin resistant. It takes more than the normal amounts of insulin to manage the blood sugar level. Gestational diabetes mellitus is diabetes mellitus that occurs during pregnancy.

Pregestational Diabetes Mellitus

If you have type 1 or type 2 diabetes before you become pregnant, it is known as pregestational diabetes mellitus. About 1 in 100 women have this condition.

Risks to Your Pregnancy

Women with poorly controlled pregestational diabetes are at risk for several pregnancy complications. However, the risk of developing the following complications can be significantly reduced if a woman controls her blood glucose levels before and during pregnancy:

- *Birth defects*—Birth defects, most often involving the heart, brain, and skeleton, can occur. These defects have been linked to high blood sugar levels early in pregnancy, when these organs are developing.

- *Miscarriage and stillbirth*—Both **miscarriage** and **stillbirth** are more common in pregnant women with poorly controlled diabetes.

- *Hydramnios*—**Hydramnios** is a condition in which there is too much **amniotic fluid** in the **amniotic sac** that surrounds the baby. It can lead to **preterm** labor and delivery.

- *Preeclampsia*—**Preeclampsia** occurs only during pregnancy and typically includes high blood pressure and increased levels of protein in the urine. The baby may need to be delivered early. Severe preeclampsia can lead to seizures and kidney or liver problems and is a common cause of preterm birth.

- *Macrosomia*—**Macrosomia** is a condition in which a baby is significantly bigger than average. Women with a macrosomic fetus are more likely than women with a normal-sized fetus to experience difficult labor and higher rates of cesarean birth. Risk factors for macrosomia include maternal diabetes and pregnancy prolonged past the due date by more than 2 weeks. Macrosomia can be very difficult to predict accurately.

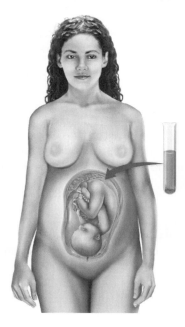

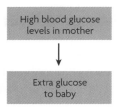

High blood glucose levels in mother

↓

Extra glucose to baby

Diabetes during pregnancy. During pregnancy, high blood glucose levels can cause the developing baby to receive too much glucose. As a result, the baby can grow too large.

- *Respiratory distress syndrome*—This syndrome can make it harder for the baby to breathe after birth. The risk for **respiratory distress syndrome** is greater in babies of mothers with diabetes.

Preconception Care

If you have diabetes and are planning a pregnancy, it is important for you to see your doctor before you become pregnant. During this preconception visit, you will learn how to take steps before pregnancy that can minimize the risk of complications later. You should plan the timing of your pregnancy while working with an obstetrician, a maternal–fetal medicine subspecialist, or other doctor to get your blood glucose levels under very tight control. Beginning your pregnancy in this way increases the likelihood of a healthy baby and successful pregnancy. It also will prepare you for the extra work that you will need to do to keep your glucose levels under tight control throughout pregnancy.

Many women with diabetes who have never been pregnant are surprised at how low the recommended blood sugar level is for pregnancy. Your doctor likely will recommend that you frequently check your blood glucose levels in order to achieve a fasting level below 100. The recommended goal for 1 hour after eating is a level below 140. A blood test called a hemoglobin A_{1C} may be used to track your progress. This test gives an estimate of how well your blood glucose level has been controlled over the prior 4–6 weeks. Once your hemoglobin A_{1C} level is below 7, the risk of miscarriage and stillbirth is very close of that of women without diabetes. At that point, it is reasonable to consider getting pregnant.

Preconception care also allows your doctor to diagnose and treat any medical problem you may have because of your diabetes. In addition to monitoring your blood glucose levels and adjusting your medication, it is important to try to attain a near normal body weight through a healthy diet and exercise. Your health care provider can give you information about how to plan a healthy diet and exercise program, or you may be referred to a nutritionist or other expert.

Gestational Diabetes Mellitus

Pregnancy causes a natural form of insulin resistance that is designed to increase the mother's blood glucose level slightly in order to make more fuel available for the baby. About 4% of women, however, cannot produce enough insulin to maintain a normal blood glucose level to offset the increased food intake, body weight, and insulin resistance. These women develop gestational diabetes. This form of diabetes occurs at the beginning of the last third of pregnancy, when the baby begins to put on the most weight.

Risk Factors

Some women are at higher risk of developing gestational diabetes, especially those who have the following conditions:

- Are overweight
- Have had gestational diabetes mellitus before
- Have a close relative with diabetes mellitus
- Had problems in a previous pregnancy, such as stillbirth
- Are Native American, Asian, Hispanic, African American, or Pacific Islander
- Have had a very large baby
- Have a condition called *polycystic ovary syndrome*

If you have any of these risk factors, your health care provider may test you for gestational diabetes during one of your early prenatal visits. If you do not have risk factors, you may be tested between 24 weeks and 28 weeks of pregnancy.

How It Can Affect Your Pregnancy

In women with gestational diabetes, high blood glucose levels increase the risk of having a very large baby and possible *cesarean delivery*. Preeclampsia also is more common in women with gestational diabetes.

Once tests show that you have gestational diabetes, your health care provider will monitor you closely. Gestational diabetes usually disappears after the baby is born, but about one half of women with this condition will develop type 2 diabetes later in life. For this reason, in the future, it is important to tell all of your health care providers that you have had gestational diabetes so that you can continue to be monitored.

Managing Your Diabetes

Diabetes must be controlled during pregnancy. Whether you have pregestational diabetes or gestational diabetes, managing diabetes during pregnancy takes a lot of work and commitment. Doing so requires daily tracking of glucose levels, healthy eating, regular exercise, and, sometimes, medication.

Prenatal care also is important. If you have diabetes, you will see your doctor more often while you are pregnant.

Tracking Glucose Levels

Women with pregestational diabetes and gestational diabetes will need to monitor their blood glucose levels frequently. Only by knowing your glucose levels throughout the day will it be possible to appropriately adjust your diet, exercise, and medication to keep your glucose levels in the normal range. Your health care provider will tell you how often you should perform these checks. If you get sick, you may need to check your levels more often. Late in pregnancy, you also may need to check more often.

Your health care provider will show you how to check your glucose with a glucose meter. Checking your glucose level is an important part of keeping it within the normal range. For the best results, follow the schedule your health care provider gives you. Keep accurate notes and report your levels at each prenatal visit.

Healthy Eating

A balanced diet is a key part of any pregnancy. Your baby depends on the food you eat for its growth and nourishment. Diet is even more important if you have diabetes—as important as medication. Not eating properly can cause glucose levels to go too high or too low.

The number of calories you need depends on your weight, stage of pregnancy, age, and level of activity. In most cases, the diet will include special meals. Meals and snacks will be spread throughout the day and before bedtime. You may be asked to keep a log of what you eat. Changes may be needed to improve glucose control or to meet the needs of the growing baby.

Exercise

For all women, but especially those with diabetes, exercise is important. Exercise helps keep glucose levels in the normal range. You should get at least 30 minutes of exercise daily. Discuss your exercise program first with your health care provider.

Medications

Women with pregestational diabetes who took insulin before pregnancy usually will need to increase their insulin dosage while they are pregnant.

This increase is needed for three reasons:

1. A tighter level of glucose control is recommended during pregnancy in order to prevent some of the complications of diabetes mellitus.

2. The recommended daily calorie intake is higher during pregnancy, so higher insulin doses are needed.

3. During pregnancy, a pregnant woman's body becomes increasingly resistant to insulin, requiring greater doses of insulin to achieve the same level of blood sugar control for the same amount of glucose.

Insulin is safe to use during pregnancy and does not cause birth defects. It is important to work with your health care provider and diabetic educator in order to appropriately adjust the amount, types, and timing of your insulin doses. If you used an insulin pump before you became pregnant, you probably will be able to continue in most circumstances. Sometimes, it will be recommended that a woman taking insulin shots switch instead to pump therapy, or switch from pump therapy to insulin shots.

Some women with either gestational diabetes or type 2 pregestational diabetes can control their blood glucose levels with diet and exercise alone. However, if these measures don't keep blood glucose levels in the normal range, medication may need to be added. Oral medications that work to increase the effectiveness of the body's own insulin often can successfully keep blood glucose levels under control. These medications often are used to treat type 2 diabetes. The dosage typically needs to increase as pregnancy progresses. If oral medications do not keep glucose levels under control, it may be necessary for women with pregestational type 2 diabetes or gestational diabetes to be switched to insulin shots.

Prenatal Care

Prenatal care helps monitor your health as well as that of the baby. You may need special tests that can help your doctor be aware of any problems and take steps to correct them. An **ultrasound** exam often is performed at 18–22 weeks of pregnancy in women with diabetes to check for the presence of birth defects. However, ultrasound is not a perfect test. Women with diabetes are at increased risk of having a baby with congenital heart disease, among others, and ultrasound is an imperfect test for these conditions. If you are very overweight, ultrasound may not be as helpful. Ultrasound also is used in a pregnancy in which the mother has diabetes to monitor fetal growth, in order to plan for the birth.

Toward the end of pregnancy, you may have a weekly test (or more often) to make sure your baby is doing well—either a **nonstress test** or a *biophysical profile*. Daily *kick counts* according to your doctors' directions late in pregnancy are important as well.

Additional tests that you might have are extra urine tests to check for urinary tract infection and complications, such as kidney disease or preeclampsia. Hemoglobin A_{1C} levels may be repeated. Your health care provider may recommend tests of your kidney function.

Delivery

For most women with diabetes that has been controlled well throughout pregnancy, it is safe to allow labor to happen on its own. Early delivery (before 40 weeks of pregnancy) may be recommended for women whose diabetes is poorly controlled, who have had a prior stillbirth, or who are experiencing complications such as kidney disease. In these cases, tests for fetal lung maturity, which involves undergoing *amniocentesis*, are performed. Depending on the test results, medications called *corticosteroids* can be given to help the baby's lungs mature.

Most women are able to have a vaginal birth. If there is evidence that the baby is very large, a cesarean delivery may be recommended. Women with diabetes will need tracking of their glucose levels and close monitoring of the baby during labor.

If your glucose levels were well controlled during your pregnancy, your baby is less likely to have problems after birth. Some babies, though, may need to spend time in a special care nursery if they have breathing problems, low glucose levels, or *jaundice* (yellow skin).

Postpartum Care

Fifty percent of women with gestational diabetes will develop type 2 diabetes later in life. The risk can be reduced if you maintain a healthy weight through diet and exercise after the baby is born. In addition, women who have gestational diabetes usually are tested for diabetes 6–12 weeks after they give birth. Even if the test results are normal, the American Diabetes Association recommends that you should still be tested for diabetes every 3 years.

If you have pregestational diabetes, you will be able to go back to your prepregnancy insulin dosage very soon after birth. If you breastfeed, you will need to eat extra calories and monitor your blood glucose levels frequently. Talk to your health care provider or a lactation consultant about the amounts and types of foods that you should eat to get these extra calories.

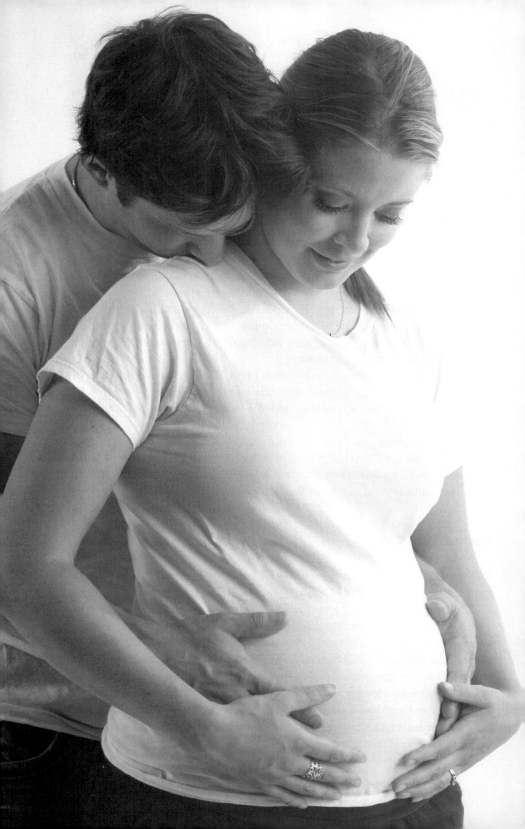

Chapter 20
Other Chronic Conditions

Pregnancy puts many new demands on your body. For women with an existing medical condition, becoming pregnant may change the way their condition is managed. Most women with medical problems can have healthy babies. It just takes special care and more effort. Some medical conditions may need closer monitoring during pregnancy in order to prevent problems for both the woman and her baby.

If you have a medical problem, you may need to have extra tests, see your health care provider more often, or get special treatment. You may be able to monitor your condition from home; in some cases, you may need to stay in a hospital.

Often, a team of health care providers working together make sure that both you and your baby get the care you need. Your health care provider may recommend that you also see a maternal–fetal medicine subspecialist, a physician who has specialized training in caring for pregnant women with medical problems.

Heart Disease

If you have a history of heart disease, heart murmur, or rheumatic fever, you should talk with your doctor before you try to become pregnant. The risk of problems during pregnancy depends on the type of heart disease you have and how serious it is. For instance, a woman who has congenital heart disease (meaning that it was present at birth) has a higher risk of having a baby with some type of heart defect. Testing to determine whether your baby has the same defect may be needed.

Pregnancy brings about major changes in the circulatory system. The amount of blood volume increases by 40–50%. This increase makes the heart work harder. You should make an appointment with your cardiologist or see a maternal–fetal medicine subspecialist so he or she can provide better details on how your problem may affect your heart and your pregnancy.

It's important to know that some medications that are safe to take before pregnancy should not be used once you become pregnant because they may harm your baby. If you have heart disease and need to take heart medications during your pregnancy, your doctor will prescribe ones that won't harm your baby.

Kidney Problems

Women who only have mild renal (kidney) disease will likely have a successful pregnancy. However, in women with severe kidney disease, becoming pregnant increases the risk of health complications for the mother and baby:

* Hypertension (high blood pressure)
* *Preeclampsia*
* *Preterm* labor
* *Miscarriage*

If you have kidney disease and are thinking about becoming pregnant, it is very important that you contact a maternal–fetal medicine specialist or kidney specialist for preconception care. These specialists will evaluate you and explain any health risks of pregnancy. If you are already pregnant, you likely will be seen by a specialist every 2 weeks.

Women with kidney disease who need dialysis usually are unable to get pregnant or have a healthy pregnancy. The stress of pregnancy for a woman on dialysis can put her and the fetus at greater risk of problems, including miscarriage.

Respiratory System Disorders

The respiratory system consists of the lungs and the airways (the trachea, or windpipe, and the air tubes that branch off it into the lungs). Shortness of breath is common in pregnancy, even in women who do not have a respiratory disorder. As the baby grows, the enlarging uterus compresses the diaphragm, the main muscle of breathing, and elevates it about 4 centimeters above its normal position. The lungs also are compressed. As a result of these changes, a pregnant woman may feel short of breath, especially in the later stages of pregnancy.

For women with certain respiratory disorders, pregnancy can pose additional challenges. Respiratory problems can decrease the amount of oxygen that both the mother and the baby receive. Pregnancy can make some conditions, such as asthma, worse. Managing respiratory conditions requires close cooperation between a woman and her health care provider to ensure both her and her baby's health.

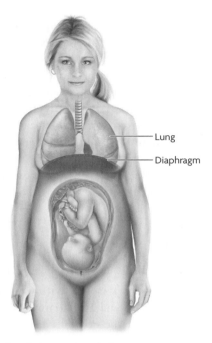

Lung

Diaphragm

Asthma

If you have asthma but keep it well managed, you should be able to have a healthy pregnancy and healthy baby. It is when a woman's asthma is uncontrolled that problems can happen, such as less oxygen getting to the baby.

Respiratory system during pregnancy. During pregnancy, the diaphragm is elevated, compressing the lungs. Shortness of breath is common, especially in the later stages of pregnancy.

Tell your pregnancy health care provider at your first prenatal care visit about your asthma so that the baby's health can be monitored. Although many pregnant women feel uneasy taking medications during pregnancy, if you have asthma, you must continue your medications once your doctor approves them. It's safe to continue using your asthma inhaler during pregnancy.

Some women with asthma may find that their symptoms get worse during pregnancy. It's important to see your allergist or immunologist or maternal–fetal medicine specialist to learn the best way to manage your asthma while you're pregnant and what, if any, other medications you may need to take. You will need to monitor your symptoms throughout pregnancy and may have periodic tests of your lung function to check whether you and your baby are getting enough oxygen.

Pneumonia

Pneumonia is an infection of the lungs caused by bacteria or a virus. It may be more severe if you get it during pregnancy. Pneumonia can cause both you and the baby to get less oxygen.

Some of the symptoms of pneumonia are like those of a cold or the flu, such as a cough and fever. Chest pain is another common symptom. But, many people often do not realize they have this serious condition.

If your doctor thinks you may have pneumonia, he or she may order a chest X-ray to find out for sure. And although this type of X-ray isn't thought to be harmful during pregnancy, tell the X-ray technician that you're pregnant so extra precautions can be taken.

Pneumonia caused by bacteria is treated with antibiotics. If an antibiotic is prescribed, make sure your doctor knows that you are pregnant so the right kind of medication is prescribed. In some cases, a stay in the hospital may be needed until the infection clears up.

Digestive Diseases

If you have a digestive disease that affects how your body digests food, you'll have to work closely with your health care provider throughout your pregnancy. You will have to make sure you and your developing baby are getting enough of the crucial vitamins and nutrients you both need for a healthy pregnancy.

Inflammatory Bowel Disease

Inflammatory bowel disease (IBD) is a condition in which chronic (long-lasting) inflammation occurs in the digestive tract. Researchers believe that the inflammation is the result of a misdirected immune system attack against the normal bacteria found in the digestive system. There are two kinds of IBD: Crohn's disease and ulcerative colitis. Both cause similar symptoms of persistent diarrhea, abdominal pain, fever, and rectal bleeding. Like many *autoimmune disorders*, IBD symptoms may come and go. A person with IBD may experience periods of intense symptoms (flare-ups) followed by periods of mild or no symptoms (remission).

If you have IBD, it probably is difficult for you to get the nutrients you need from the foods you eat. You may not get enough protein, vitamins, or calories in your diet. You also may have intestinal damage. Before you become pregnant, it is very important to see your doctor to discuss your condition and how you will manage it during your pregnancy. It is recommended that pregnancy be attempted only when you are not experiencing a symptom flare-up. You should discuss the medications that you are taking and whether you should continue to use the same drugs while you are pregnant. Consulting with a nutritionist also may be helpful.

Irritable Bowel Syndrome

Irritable bowel syndrome mainly affects women between the ages of 30 years and 50 years. People with this condition seem to have more sensitive colons than usual and can have symptoms such as cramps, gas, and constipation. The symptoms can come and go over time.

Stress, eating large meals, or travel may trigger the symptoms. Certain medicines or foods also can cause symptoms to flare up. When you're pregnant, you will have to become more aware of what triggers your symptoms. This will help make it easier to cope with the body changes that you will experience throughout the 9 months.

Although there is no cure for irritable bowel syndrome, it can be managed to reduce the symptoms. Your doctor or a dietitian can suggest changes in your diet or your doctor may suggest medications to relieve the symptoms.

Celiac Disease

Celiac disease damages the small intestine and interferes with absorption of nutrients from food. If you suffer from this disease, your body cannot digest gluten—a protein found in wheat, rye, oats, and barley.

Gluten is in foods people eat every day, such as pasta, bread, and sauces, and also may be in medicines and vitamins. If celiac disease is not managed, it can cause serious health problems, such as malnutrition, which can lead to anemia, osteoporosis, and miscarriage.

The only way to treat celiac disease is to eat foods that are gluten-free. You will have to work with your doctor and a dietitian during your pregnancy to make sure you have a good gluten-free diet plan that gives you and the baby enough nutrients to stay healthy.

Autoimmune Disorders

In autoimmune disorders, the immune system attacks the body's own tissues. As a result, organs such as the thyroid or other parts of the body can be injured.

Many autoimmune disorders have symptoms that overlap with other illnesses. This makes them hard to detect. Most of these disorders are chronic. Often, they have no cure because the cause isn't always known. Symptoms may go away for a time and then flare up with little warning and for no clear reason.

The effect of an autoimmune disorder on pregnancy depends on the type of disorder and how severe it is. Women who have these disorders need special care during pregnancy.

Lupus

Lupus is an autoimmune disorder that can affect various parts of the body, including the skin, joints, heart, lungs, and kidneys. Today, more than half of women with lupus have completely normal pregnancies. Although some women with lupus are able to have children, the pregnancies are still high risk. Having the disease increases the risk of miscarriage, preterm birth, and fetal growth problems.

If you have lupus, you should be cared for by a maternal–fetal medicine specialist who works closely with your primary doctor. You'll need to see your doctor frequently because many problems that may happen during pregnancy can be prevented, or treated more easily, if found early.

Your doctor also will tell you which of your regular lupus medications are safe to use during pregnancy. Most medications commonly taken for lupus symptoms, such as prednisone and prednisolone, are safe.

Multiple Sclerosis

Multiple sclerosis is a disease that affects the central nervous system. The symptoms of the disease are different for every person but mostly include extreme fatigue, vision problems, loss of balance and muscle control, and stiffness. A person can have relapses or flare-ups when symptoms get worse and also can have periods with no symptoms.

Women with multiple sclerosis are able to have healthy pregnancies. Pregnancy does not make the disease worse, and the baby will grow normally. In fact, some women report that their symptoms get better when they are pregnant. If you have multiple sclerosis, the best therapy is to follow a healthy lifestyle of good nutrition, exercise, rest, and prenatal care.

When you are in labor, the weakness from multiple sclerosis may keep you from pushing hard enough. If this is the case, the doctor may use forceps or vacuum extraction (see Chapter 11, "Operative Delivery, Cesarean Delivery, and Breech Presentation") to help the baby exit the birth canal safely.

Rheumatoid Arthritis

Rheumatoid arthritis is an autoimmune disorder that causes pain and swelling in the joints. It also can cause stiffness in the morning and a general feeling of fatigue and discomfort.

Rheumatoid arthritis can flare up and then lessen for a time, or it can get worse and damage the joints. During pregnancy, rheumatoid arthritis greatly improves for many women.

Rheumatoid arthritis often is treated with antiinflammatory medications, such as aspirin and acetaminophen, which can cause complications in pregnant women. You will have to make sure your doctor tells you which pain relief medications you can use while you are pregnant. There are some drugs that you should avoid during pregnancy, including methotrexate and cyclophosphamide.

Antiphospholipid Syndrome

Antiphospholipid syndrome is a condition caused by high levels of the antiphospholipid antibody. Antibodies are proteins that are made in response to a stimulus. For instance, in some cases, they are helpful in protecting the body against disease. Sometimes antibodies can be harmful.

During pregnancy, the disorder is associated with repeated miscarriage, preeclampsia, and blood clots. However, women with the disease often can be treated successfully during pregnancy to help avoid complications.

Physical Disability

For women who are physically disabled, pregnancy and being a parent pose special challenges. That doesn't mean they can't—or shouldn't—become mothers.

It's a good idea for women with disabilities and their partners to meet with their health care providers before getting pregnant. Preconception care will help reduce the odds of medical problems during pregnancy.

Special care also will be needed after pregnancy begins. Your pregnancy care provider may work closely with the primary care doctor or other specialists. He or she also may suggest occupational or physical therapy to help you better cope with the stresses pregnancy puts on the body.

Before the baby arrives, special equipment may need to be installed or modified at home to help in caring for the baby. Leaving the hospital may require postpartum home care for mother and baby.

Thrombophilias

People with a thrombophilia tend to form blood clots too easily because they either have too much or too little of certain proteins in their blood. About one of every five people in the United States has a thrombophilia.

Most people with a thrombophilia have no symptoms. However, some will develop a thrombosis, a blood clot where it does not belong. Often, blood clots form in veins in the lower leg, causing pain and swelling. This condition is called *deep vein thrombosis.*

Most women with a thrombophilia have healthy pregnancies. The disease, though, does cause some increased risks. Thrombophilias may contribute to pregnancy complications, including miscarriage, placental abruption, or stillbirth.

If you have never been diagnosed with a thrombophilia but have a history of blood clots, let your doctor know at your first prenatal visit so you can be tested. If you do have a thrombophilia, your doctor will let you know if you are at risk for complications. The doctor will decide what treatment may be needed to be sure you have a healthy pregnancy.

Some pregnant women with a thrombophilia are treated with a blood-thinning drug called heparin or low molecular weight heparin. These medications are safe for the baby.

Thyroid Disease

Certain disorders cause the body's thyroid gland to release too much or too little thyroid hormone. Hypothyroidism means the thyroid isn't as active as it should be. Hyperthyroidism means the thyroid is too active. Either condition can harm you or your baby during pregnancy and can increase the risk of high blood pressure, having a low-birth-weight baby, and preterm birth.

If you have a history or symptoms of thyroid disease and are thinking of becoming pregnant or are pregnant already, tell your doctor. Your doctor can monitor your health closely and prescribe medications that will decrease your risk of problems. Your doctor will check the levels of thyroid hormone in your body at regular intervals to be sure they are at healthy levels. The chance of problems during pregnancy is greatest when thyroid disease is not treated or is uncontrolled.

Many medications used to treat thyroid disease are safe during pregnancy. However, radioactive iodine, which is sometimes used to treat hyperthyroidism, should not be taken during pregnancy.

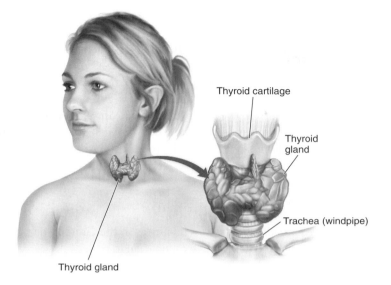

Thyroid gland

Thyroid cartilage

Thyroid gland

Trachea (windpipe)

Thyroid gland

Thyroid gland. The thyroid gland is located in the neck. It releases thyroid hormone. Thyroid hormone plays many roles in the body, including maintaining heart rate and regulating body temperature.

Some women may not have thyroid problems during pregnancy but develop problems after birth. This condition is called postpartum thyroiditis. It often is a short-term problem, and hormone levels quickly return to normal. Sometimes this condition can lead to long-term hypothyroidism, which will require treatment.

Seizure Disorders

Epilepsy and certain other disorders cause seizures (convulsions). A seizure can consist of a few muscle twitches, or it can be a major attack that causes a blackout and loss of bladder or bowel control.

Most women with seizure disorders have healthy babies, but problems can occur. Babies born to mothers with a seizure disorder are two or three times more likely to have a birth defect than babies born to mothers without the condition. Cleft lip, cleft palate, and heart defects are the most common problems, but why these problems occur is not known.

If you have a seizure disorder and get pregnant, do not stop taking your seizure medications without talking to your doctor first. In some cases, seizures may be more harmful than the medication used to control or prevent them.

The amount of medication needed often changes during pregnancy. The doctor will monitor drug levels and adjust the dosage as needed. With good control of drug levels, there should be little change in the number or strength of seizures.

Medications that treat seizure disorders can use up stores of folic acid, a vital nutrient that helps prevent neural tube defects during pregnancy. Taking folic acid supplements will help decrease this risk.

Mental Illness

Millions of women are affected by mental illness in the United States. Some mental illnesses are more common in women than in men:

- Depression
- Bipolar disorder
- Schizophrenia
- Anxiety disorders (panic disorder, obsessive–compulsive disorder, and phobias)
- Personality disorders

Mental illness can affect pregnancy in a number of ways. If you have a mental illness or had one in the past, be sure to tell your doctor about it. The doctor can arrange for counseling or community agencies to provide social or mental health services.

Being pregnant can cause mental illness to worsen. Pregnancy may cause a recurrence of a mental illness. This may be a result of hormonal changes or stress. If a mental illness is not treated, you may do things that could harm your baby. For example, you could have trouble eating well, getting enough rest, or taking care of yourself in other ways. You also may be less likely to get regular prenatal care.

Your pregnancy care provider needs to know about any medications you are taking to control your mental illness. Some medications are safe during pregnancy, but there are some that can harm a growing baby. If you are currently taking a medication, your doctor and mental health care provider can discuss with you whether you should stop taking this medication while you are pregnant, or whether you should continue your medication. This decision is based on several factors, such as severity of your illness, whether the illness has recurred, and whether you currently have symptoms. You and your doctor will need to decide if the benefit of using a drug to control your mental condition outweighs any possible risks from the drug used to treat it. If you decide to discontinue your medication, alternative therapies, such as psychotherapy, may be an option.

Mental health care is vital after the baby is born. Some women have a mental health problem after delivery. Women with mental health problems are 20 times more likely to be admitted to a hospital for a psychiatric illness in the month after giving birth than they are in the 2 years that led up to it. They also are more likely to have *postpartum depression*.

The first weeks after a newborn arrives can be stressful for any new mother. During the early weeks, help and support are important to help you adjust to being a mother.

Part VI
Complications During Pregnancy

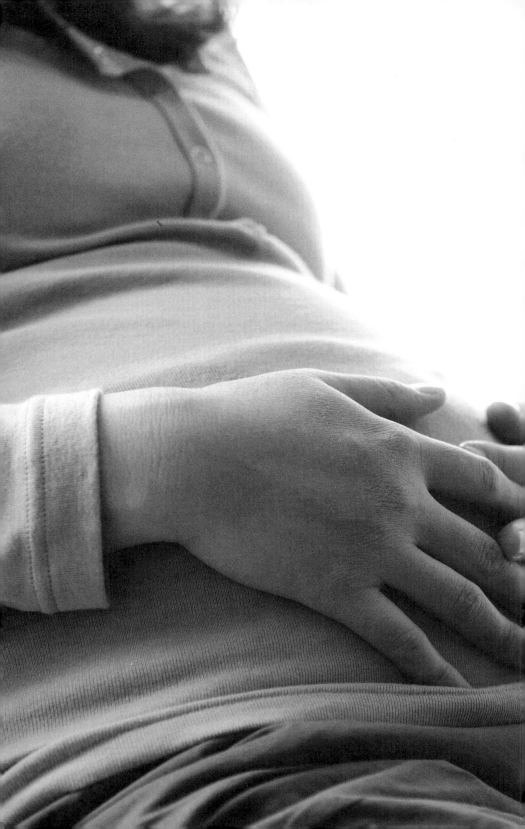

Chapter 21

Early Pregnancy Problems: Miscarriage, Ectopic Pregnancy, and Molar Pregnancy

Miscarriage

A normal pregnancy lasts about 40 weeks. The loss of a pregnancy before 20 weeks is called early pregnancy loss or *miscarriage*. Miscarriages occur in about 15–20% of pregnancies, and most occur in the first 13 weeks of pregnancy. Some miscarriages take place before a woman misses a menstrual period or is even aware that she is pregnant.

Causes

The process of *fertilization*—in which the male *sperm* and the female *egg* join—is complex. Miscarriage can be caused by any one of a number of things before, during, or after this process. The cause of miscarriage often is not known. Most factors that cause a miscarriage are genetic. Sometimes a miscarriage is caused by a woman's health problems.

Genetics

More than half of miscarriages in the first 13 weeks of pregnancy are caused by problems with the *chromosomes* of the *fetus*. Chromosomes are structures inside each of the body's *cells*. Each chromosome carries many *genes*, which determine the traits of a person.

Miscarriages can result from an abnormal number or structure of chromosomes. Most chromosome problems are not inherited (passed on from the parents). They happen by chance and are not likely to occur again in a later pregnancy. In most cases, there is nothing wrong with the woman's or man's health. The chance of these problems increases with the age of the woman.

Your Health

Infections may affect the *uterus* and fetus and, as a result, end the pregnancy. Problems with your hormones also can cause very early miscarriage. If you have a chronic disease, such as *diabetes mellitus*, that is not controlled, you also may have a higher risk for miscarriage.

Sometimes treatment of the illness can improve the chances for a healthy pregnancy. This is even truer if the illness is under control before you become pregnant. Some women with illnesses may need treatment or close watching during pregnancy.

Problems with a woman's uterus or *cervix* also can lead to miscarriage. Problems include an abnormally shaped uterus or an incompetent cervix. An incompetent cervix begins to widen and open too early, usually at 14–26 weeks of pregnancy, without any pain or other signs of labor.

Lifestyle

Smoking cigarettes raises your risk of miscarriage. The same is true for heavy alcohol drinking and using illegal drugs, especially in the early stages of pregnancy.

What Does Not Cause Miscarriage

Most aspects of daily life do not increase the risk of miscarriage. There is no proof that working, exercising, having sex, or having used birth control pills before getting pregnant increases a woman's risk. Morning sickness also does not increase the risk.

Symptoms of Miscarriage

Bleeding is the most common sign of miscarriage. Most women who have vaginal spotting or bleeding during the early months of pregnancy have healthy babies. Some of these women, though, will have a miscarriage. This is why bleeding during early pregnancy is called threatened miscarriage. You should call your health care provider if you have any of these signs and symptoms:

* Spotting or bleeding without pain
* Heavy or persistent bleeding with abdominal pain or cramping

- A gush of fluid from your **vagina**, without pain or bleeding
- Passed fetal tissue

If you bleed while you are pregnant, you and your health care provider will need to be watchful for a few days. In the very early stages, it is hard to tell if the pregnancy is going to miscarry. Your health care provider may order blood tests or perform an **ultrasound** exam.

Sometimes mild cramping of the lower stomach or a low backache may occur along with bleeding. Bleeding may persist, become heavy, or occur along with a pain like menstrual cramps or the breaking of the **amniotic sac**.

If you have heavy bleeding and think you have passed fetal tissue, place it in a clean container and take it to the health care provider for inspection. Your health care provider will want to examine you. If your health care provider thinks a miscarriage has occurred, he or she may do a pelvic exam to see if your cervix has dilated (opened). If the cervix has dilated and fetal tissue is lost, a miscarriage is certain. If the diagnosis of miscarriage is not clear, your health care provider may follow you closely with ultrasound exams or blood tests.

Treatment

If your health care provider does not think that a miscarriage has occurred, you may be asked to rest and avoid having sex. Although these measures have not been shown to prevent miscarriage, they may help reduce bleeding and discomfort.

Often when miscarriage occurs early in pregnancy, tissue remains in the uterus. If there is concern about heavy bleeding or infection, this tissue will be removed by **dilation and curettage (D&C).** With this method, the cervix may be widened if needed. The tissue is then removed from the lining of the uterus. A D&C can be done in a health care provider's office, emergency room, or operating room. It often does not require a hospital stay. Your health care provider also may suggest medication to be used to help pass the tissue that remains in the uterus.

After you've experienced a miscarriage, your menstrual period should return within 4–6 weeks. You can, however, ovulate and become pregnant as soon as 2 weeks after an early miscarriage. If you do not wish to become pregnant again right away, be sure to use birth control. If your blood is Rh negative, you may need a blood product called Rh immunoglobulin (RhIg). This injection prevents you from developing antibodies that could affect a future Rh-positive baby. See Chapter 24, "Blood Type Incompatibility," for more details.

Multiple Miscarriages

If you experience multiple miscarriages, usually more than three in a row, your health care provider will want to do some testing to find the cause. Most of the time, however, a cause is not found. Keep in mind, though, that even without treatment, about 60–70% of women who have had repeated miscarriages go on to have successful pregnancies.

Ectopic Pregnancy

About 2% of pregnancies are ectopic. In a normal pregnancy, a fertilized egg moves through the ***fallopian tube*** and implants in the lining of the uterus, where it starts to grow. When a fertilized egg grows outside of the uterus, it is considered an ***ectopic pregnancy***. About 97% of ectopic pregnancies are in the fallopian tube. Because it is outside of the uterus, an ectopic pregnancy cannot grow to produce a healthy baby, and it can threaten the mother's health. For these reasons, an ectopic pregnancy must be ended either by surgery or with medical treatment.

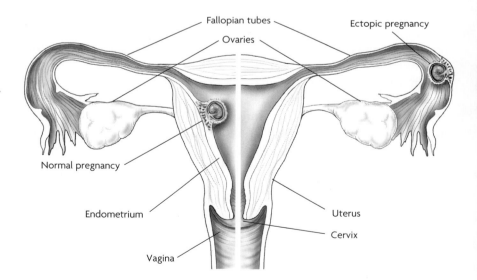

Ectopic pregnancy. In a normal pregnancy (*left*), the fertilized egg or fetus grows in the uterus. In an ectopic pregnancy (*right*), the fertilized egg or fetus grows in the fallopian tube or other abdominal organ.

Risk Factors

Any sexually active woman of childbearing age is at risk for ectopic pregnancy. However, women who have had the following conditions or procedures are at higher risk:

- *Pelvic inflammatory disease*
- Previous ectopic pregnancy
- Pelvic or abdominal surgery
- *Endometriosis*
- Sexually transmitted diseases
- Prior tubal surgery (such as tubal ligation)

Some of these conditions produce scar tissue in the tubes. This may keep a fertilized egg from reaching the uterus.

Other factors that increase a woman's risk of ectopic pregnancy include smoking and the use of *assisted reproductive technology* to become pregnant, such as *in vitro fertilization*.

Symptoms

The symptoms of ectopic pregnancy sometimes include the symptoms of pregnancy, such as tender breasts or an upset stomach. Some women may have no symptoms at all. They may not even know they are pregnant. If ectopic pregnancy can be found early, it can be treated before the tube ruptures. If you have an ectopic pregnancy, you may have any or all of the following symptoms:

- Vaginal bleeding that is not at the time of your normal menstrual period
- Sudden, sharp pain in your abdomen or pelvic area
- Shoulder pain
- Weakness, dizziness, or fainting

These symptoms can occur before you even suspect you are pregnant. If you have these symptoms, call your health care provider.

Diagnosis

If your health care provider thinks you may have an ectopic pregnancy, he or she will do an ultrasound exam or give you a blood test to check your levels of the hormone *human chorionic gonadotropin* (hCG)—the hormone that is produced when a woman is pregnant. This test may be repeated a couple of days later to check the levels of hCG. If your pregnancy is progressing normally, the level of hCG in your blood will increase. If the levels are the same or lower, it may confirm that you have an ectopic pregnancy or are at risk of having a miscarriage.

Tests to find ectopic pregnancy take time. Results may not be clear right away. If your health care provider suspects that you have an ectopic pregnancy that has ruptured, however, it is an emergency. You will need to have surgery right away. If the pregnancy is still in the early stages and the tube is not in danger of rupture, medical treatment may be an option.

Treatment

There are two methods used to treat an ectopic pregnancy: medication and surgery. If your health care provider decides medication is the best choice, you will be given a drug called methotrexate. It will end the pregnancy by stopping the growth of the pregnancy. The ectopic pregnancy is then absorbed by the body.

There are many factors that go into the decision to use methotrexate. It cannot be used for women who are breastfeeding or have certain health problems.

Taking Methotrexate

Methotrexate often is given in either one or two doses. In some cases, it may be given in many doses over several days. After treatment, it takes about 4–6 weeks for the pregnancy to be absorbed.

For this treatment, your health care provider will take a sample of your blood in advance to measure the functions of certain organs as well as the levels of the pregnancy hormone hCG. After receiving the methotrexate, you will have two more blood tests on the fourth and seventh day after taking the medication. The health care provider will check to see if the levels of hCG are decreasing as they should. If levels haven't decreased enough, your health care provider may suggest surgery or another dose of methotrexate to treat the ectopic pregnancy.

After taking methotrexate, you will need to see your health care provider for the next few weeks until hCG is no longer found in your blood.

Surgery

If the pregnancy is small and the fallopian tube is not ruptured, in some cases, the ectopic pregnancy can be removed through a small cut made in the tube during a *laparoscopy*. In this procedure a slender, light-transmitting telescope is inserted through a small opening in your abdomen.

A larger incision in the abdomen may be needed if the pregnancy is large or blood loss is a concern. Some or all of the tube may need to be removed.

It is important that all of the pregnancy is removed from the tube. Blood testing for hCG may be needed for a few weeks after the treatment to check for this.

If you have had surgery and the tubes have been left in place, there is a good chance that you can have a normal pregnancy in the future. Once you have had an ectopic pregnancy, though, you are at higher risk for having another one.

Molar Pregnancy

Molar pregnancy, also called gestational trophoblastic disease, is rare. It results in the growth of abnormal tissue. In the United States, molar pregnancy occurs in 1 of every 1,000–1,200 pregnancies.

Both normal pregnancies and molar pregnancies develop from a fertilized egg. In a molar pregnancy, though, the fertilized egg does not grow as it should. A genetic error causes abnormal cells to grow and form a mass of tissue.

Types of Molar Pregnancy

There are two types of molar pregnancy: complete and partial. The mass in a complete molar pregnancy is made up of all abnormal cells that would have become the *placenta* in a normal pregnancy. There is no fetus. In a partial molar pregnancy, the mass contains the abnormal cells found in a complete molar pregnancy and, often, an abnormal fetus that has severe and fatal defects.

Symptoms and Diagnosis

Most molar pregnancies cause symptoms that signal a problem. The most common symptom is vaginal bleeding during the first trimester. Other signs of molar pregnancy can be found by your health care provider, such as a uterus that is too large for the stage of the pregnancy or cysts on the ovaries.

If your health care provider suspects a molar pregnancy, he or she may do an ultrasound exam or a blood test that measures the level of hCG. If a molar pregnancy is found, a series of tests will be done to check for other medical problems that sometimes occur along with a molar pregnancy.

These problems might include **preeclampsia** and **hyperthyroidism** (overactive thyroid gland). These problems are treated by removing the molar pregnancy.

Treatment

To treat a molar pregnancy, the cervix is dilated, either under **general** or **local anesthesia,** and the tissue is removed by a D&C. About 90% of women whose molar pregnancies are removed require no further treatment. However, they do need careful follow-up. Routine tests for hCG levels continue for about 6 months to 1 year. These tests can determine whether you need further treatment.

After the pregnancy has been removed, abnormal cells may remain. This condition is called persistent gestational trophoblastic disease. It occurs in as many as 10% of women who have a molar pregnancy. It also can occur after a normal pregnancy. One sign of persistent gestational trophoblastic disease is an hCG level that remains high after the molar pregnancy has been removed. Sometimes medication may be needed to remove the abnormal cells that remain.

If you have had a molar pregnancy, your health care provider may advise you to wait 6 months to 1 year before trying to become pregnant again. It is safe to use birth control pills during this time. The chances of having another molar pregnancy are low (about 1%).

Dealing With Grief

For many women, the emotional healing after a pregnancy loss takes a lot longer than healing physically. The feelings of loss can be intense, even if the pregnancy ended very early.

Grief can involve a wide range of feelings. Don't blame yourself for the pregnancy loss. In most cases, it is not likely that it could have been prevented.

Your feelings of grief may differ from those of your partner. You are the one who has felt the physical changes of pregnancy. Your partner also may grieve but may not express feelings in the same way you do. Some partners feel that they need to be strong for both of you. They may be reluctant to share their hurt and disappointment with you. This may create tensions between the two of you when you need each other the most.

If either of you is having trouble handling the feelings that go along with this loss, talk to your health care provider. You also may find it helps to talk with a counselor. Counseling can help both you and your partner if you can't deal with these feelings alone.

Losing a pregnancy often doesn't mean that you can't have more children. Most women who miscarry can have a healthy pregnancy later. You should, however, allow enough time for physical and emotional healing before trying to get pregnant again. Your health care provider can give you some guidance.

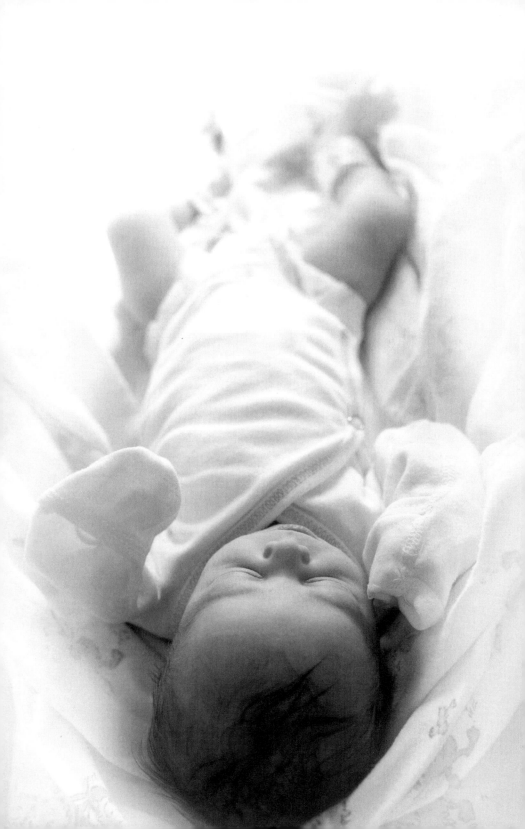

Chapter 22
Birth Defects

Although most babies are born healthy, there is a chance a baby can be born with a birth defect. Some people have risk factors that increase their chances of having a baby with health problems. However, babies with birth defects usually are born to couples who have no known risk factors.

To help ease the concern of parents-to-be, there are tests designed to check the parents' risks for having a baby with certain defects. Some of these tests can be done before pregnancy. The results of these tests, along with genetic counseling, can help potential parents weigh the possible risks and make decisions.

Understanding Birth Defects

A birth defect is a problem that occurs during pregnancy and affects a baby's normal function or appearance. There are more than 4,000 types of birth defects, and they can range from mild to severe. About 1 in 33 babies in the United States is born with a birth defect.

Some birth defects are passed from parent to child. Just as a baby gets hair and eye color from her parents, the baby can inherit certain diseases or conditions. Other birth defects are caused by being exposed to harmful agents during pregnancy. For example, some birth defects can occur if the woman gets certain infections, drinks alcohol, or takes certain medications during pregnancy. In many cases, the reason for a defect isn't known.

It is thought that most birth defects occur in the first 12 weeks of pregnancy, when the organ systems are undergoing intense development. Many birth defects can be seen right after the baby is born, such as clubfoot. Others aren't noticed until later in life. A defect that's present at birth, no matter when it is diagnosed, is called a ***congenital disorder.*** An example is congenital heart disease. Congenital disorders may or may not be inherited.

Genetic Disorders

Genetic disorders may be caused by problems with either genes or chromosomes. A ***gene*** is a small piece of a hereditary material called DNA (short for deoxyribonucleic acid) that controls some aspect of a person's physical makeup. Genes are located on structures called ***chromosomes***, which are found inside each ***cell*** in the body. In humans, most cells have 23 pairs of chromosomes, for a total of 46 chromosomes. Chromosome pairs 1–22 are called autosomes and the 23rd pair are the sex chromosomes. The sex chromosomes are called X and Y.

Sperm and ***egg*** cells have one copy of each of the 23 chromosomes. Joining of an egg and sperm (***fertilization***) results in the creation of a fertilized egg that contains 23 pairs. The egg always has an X chromosome and the sperm can have either an X or a Y chromosome. A combination of XX for the sex chromosomes results in a female and XY results in a male.

Genes come in pairs. Half of a baby's genes come from the mother. The other half come from the father. Some traits, such as blood type, are determined by a single gene pair. Other traits, including skin color, hair color, and height, are the result of many pairs of genes working together.

A gene or a genetic disorder is either dominant or recessive. If one gene in a pair is dominant, the dominant gene overrides the recessive gene. For a recessive trait to show up in the baby, both genes in a pair must be recessive.

Inherited Disorders

An inherited disorder is caused by a gene that is passed from parent to child. These disorders can be dominant, recessive, or X-linked. Table 22-1 lists some inherited disorders.

Dominant Disorders

A dominant disorder is caused by just one gene from either parent. Some dominant disorders are common and not serious. Others are rare but can be life-threatening. If one parent has the gene, each child of the couple has a 50% chance of inheriting the disorder.

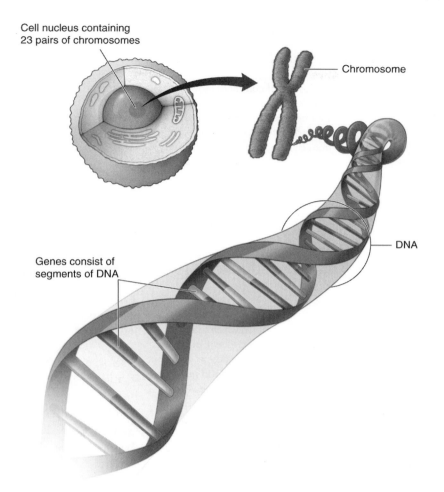

Cell nucleus containing
23 pairs of chromosomes

Chromosome

DNA

Genes consist of
segments of DNA

Chromosomes and genes. Chromosomes are the structures inside cells that carry a person's genes. Each person has 22 pairs of autosomes and one pair of sex chromosomes. A single gene is a segment of a large molecule called DNA.

Recessive Disorders

In recessive disorders, both parents must have the gene in order for it to occur in their child. Everyone carries a few abnormal recessive genes. Most of the time, these genes don't cause a problem because the normal genes override the abnormal ones. A person who has a recessive gene for a certain disorder is a *carrier* for that disorder. Although that person may show no signs of the disorder, the gene can be passed on to his or her children.

Table 22-1 Common Genetic Disorders and Birth Defects

Disorder	What It Means	Who Is At Risk?
Dominant Disorders		
Huntington disease	Causes loss of control of movements and mental function. Symptoms usually start between the ages of 35 years and 50 years, but they can begin any time from childhood to old age.	Those with a family history
Polydactyly	Baby is born with extra fingers or toes	Those with a family history of the disorder, African Americans; commonly occurs without risk factors
Recessive Disorders		
Thalassemia	Causes anemia; there are different types of the disorder and some are more severe than others.	Depends on the type of disorder: Mediterranean (especially Greek or Italian), Middle Eastern, African, or Asian descent
Sickle cell anemia	A blood disorder in which the red blood cells have a crescent, or "sickle," shape rather than the normal doughnut shape. Because of their odd shape, these cells get caught in the blood vessels. This prevents oxygen from reaching organs and tissues, which causes pain.	African Americans
Tay–Sachs disease	A disease in which harmful amounts of a fatty substance called ganglioside GM2 collect in the nerve cells in the brain. It causes severe mental retardation, blindness, and seizures. Symptoms first occur at about 6 months of age.	Ashkenazi Jews; French Canadians
Cystic fibrosis	Causes problems with digestion and breathing. Symptoms appear in child-hood—sometimes right after birth. Some individuals have milder symptoms than others. Over time the problems tend to become worse and harder to treat.	White individuals of Northern European descent
X-Linked Disorders		
Fragile X	The most common cause of inherited mental retardation. People with fragile X syndrome have varying degrees of mental retardation or learning disabilities	Males

Table 22-1 Common Genetic Disorders and Birth Defects, *continued*

Disorder	What It Means	Who Is At Risk?
Fragile X, *continued*	and behavioral and emotional problems. Boys with the disorder have a long, triangular face and ears that stick out. Women can be carriers of the fragile X gene but not have any symptoms.	
Hemophilia	A disorder caused by the lack of a substance in the blood that helps it clot. Affected individuals are at risk for bleeding to death if they are injured.	Males

If both parents are carriers of the same recessive disorder, each of the children has a 25% chance of having the disorder. If one parent has the disorder and the other doesn't (and isn't a carrier), the children will be carriers.

X-Linked Disorders

Disorders that are caused by genes on the X chromosome are called "X-linked" disorders. In most X-linked disorders, the abnormal gene is recessive. When an X-linked disorder is caused by a recessive gene, a woman can carry the gene but usually does not have that disorder. That's because she has two X chromosomes, and the normal gene on the other X chromosome overrides the abnormal gene.

A male baby inherits an X chromosome from his mother and a Y chromosome from his father. If his mother has an X-linked disorder and he inherits an X chromosome with a gene for the disorder, he will have the disorder. His father's Y chromosome does not have a normal gene to override the abnormal gene.

If a woman is a carrier for an X-linked disorder and the father of the baby doesn't have the disorder, there is a 50% chance a son will have the disorder and a daughter will be a carrier. Genetic testing sometimes can show if a woman is a carrier of an X-linked disorder or if the *fetus* is affected.

Chromosomal Disorders

Chromosomal disorders are caused by missing, damaged, or extra chromosomes. These problems usually result from an error that occurs when the egg and sperm are joining. Most children with chromosomal disorders have physical defects or mental defects.

Two examples of chromosomal disorders are **Down syndrome** and **trisomy 18.** In Down syndrome, there is an extra chromosome 21. Children with

Down syndrome have various degrees of mental retardation, abnormal features of the face, and medical problems, such as heart defects. In trisomy 18, there is an extra chromosome 18, which causes severe mental retardation, birth defects, and early death.

Down syndrome is one of the most common chromosomal disorders. It affects about 1 in 800 babies, and in the United States, about 5,500 babies are born with it each year. The risk of Down syndrome increases with the mother's age:

- 1 in 1,250 at age 25 years
- 1 in 1,000 at age 30 years
- 1 in 400 at age 35 years
- 1 in 100 at age 40 years
- 1 in 30 at age 45 years

These statistics can be misleading, though. Although women older than 35 years have been considered most likely to have a baby with Down syndrome, about 80% of babies with Down syndrome are actually born to women who are younger than 35 years, simply because younger women have far more babies.

Environmental Factors

Teratogens are agents that can cause birth defects when a woman is exposed to them during pregnancy. Teratogens can be found in the home, workplace, and environment. They include certain medications, chemicals, and infections. Their effects depend on the amount of the agent a woman is exposed to and when in pregnancy exposure occurs. Some agents have harmful effects only if a woman is exposed to them while certain organ systems are forming.

Medications

Very few medications have been proved to be harmful during pregnancy. The U.S. Food and Drug Administration (FDA) evaluates all of the available information about a drug and determines whether the drug increases the risk of birth defects when taken during pregnancy. Often, the information about a drug is limited. For example, studies of the drug may only have been performed on animals. The FDA considers the source of the information about a drug when determining its risk during pregnancy.

It is important to tell your health care provider about all of the medications you are taking, including over-the-counter medications, vitamin and mineral supplements, and herbal remedies, as soon as you find out you are pregnant. Even better, discuss your medications with your doctor before you become pregnant so they can be adjusted or changed if needed. Do not stop taking prescription medication, however, until you have talked with your health care provider. Although some medications may increase the risk of birth defects, the benefits of continuing to take the medication during pregnancy may outweigh any risk to your baby.

Methyl Mercury

Mercury is an industrial pollutant that builds up to high levels in certain fish species. Mercury can cause defects of the nervous system in a developing fetus. To avoid exposure to high levels of mercury, pregnant women and young children should avoid certain types of fish (see p. 86).

Alcohol

Alcohol abuse during pregnancy is a leading and preventable cause of mental retardation. Alcohol is a known teratogen that is thought to have a dose-related effect on the developing fetus. Drinking alcohol during pregnancy can cause a range of effects, from hyperactivity and poor coordination to various degrees of mental retardation. The most severe alcohol-associated defect is called *fetal alcohol syndrome*, a pattern of major physical, mental, and behavioral problems. Babies with fetal alcohol syndrome may have one or more of the following conditions:

- Problems with joints and limbs
- Small bodies
- Heart defects
- Abnormal facial features
- Behavioral problems
- Mental retardation

All forms of alcohol are equally hazardous. One glass of wine, one beer, and one mixed drink have similar amounts of alcohol. Because it is not known with certainty how much alcohol is safe to drink during pregnancy, you should not drink at all while you are pregnant.

Radiation

We are exposed to low levels of radiation from the earth and the sun every day. Radiation also is used in some medical imaging procedures (such as X-rays). High levels of radiation can cause chromosome damage and changes in genes (called mutations) in a developing fetus. During the first trimester, exposure to 10 rads is required to cause harm to a fetus, and 100 rads are required later in pregnancy. The recommended upper limit of radiation exposure in pregnancy is 5 rads, which is well above the amount of radiation exposure in most X-rays. High-dose radiation for treatment of cancer, however, is not recommended during pregnancy because of the increased risk of miscarriage, birth defects, and fetal death.

Other Chemicals

Pesticides, cleaning solvents, and heavy metals, such as lead, can potentially cause serious problems during pregnancy. Women who work in farming, factories, dry cleaners, electronics, or printing or who have hobbies such as painting or pottery glazing may be exposed to harmful agents. Information about various chemicals can be found at the web sites of the following organizations (see Resources):

• Occupational Safety and Health Administration
• Organization of Teratology Information Specialists
• National Institute for Occupational Safety and Health

Multifactorial Disorders

Multifactorial disorders are disorders that are thought to come from a mix of genetic and environmental factors. The actual cause is unknown. Some of these disorders can be detected during pregnancy. They sometimes can be treated with surgery. Examples of multifactorial disorders are **neural tube defects**, cleft palate, clubfoot, and abdominal and heart defects.

Neural tube defects are caused by the incomplete closure of the coverings over the spinal cord or brain. Examples of neural tube defects are **spina bifida** and **anencephaly.**

Cleft lip or cleft palate is one of the most common birth defects in the United States, and about 6,800 babies are born with it each year. Cleft lip or cleft palate can cause problems with eating, speech, and language. Some affected babies have a small cleft that can be corrected with one surgical procedure, while others have severe clefts and need multiple surgeries.

There are several types of abdominal wall defects. In one type, the muscle and skin that cover the wall of the abdomen are missing and the bowel sticks out through a hole in the abdominal wall (gastroschisis). In another type, abdominal organs protrude into the base of the **umbilical cord** (omphalocele).

Heart defects are another type of multifactorial disorder. In these defects, the chambers or pathways through the heart are not properly developed.

Are You at Risk?

Most babies with birth defects are born to couples with no risk factors. However, the risk of birth defects is higher when certain factors are present:

• Maternal age of 35 years or older when the baby is due

- Family or personal history of birth defects
- Previous child with a birth defect
- Use of certain medicines before and during early pregnancy
- **Diabetes mellitus** before pregnancy

When you have your prepregnancy checkup or start **prenatal care**, your health care provider or a genetic counselor may give you a list of questions to find risk factors. Your answers to these questions will help determine your risk of having a baby with a genetic defect (see box "Risk Factors for Genetic Disorders").

You also may have tests during pregnancy to detect your risk of a problem or to diagnose it. Some tests for birth defects are offered to all pregnant women. Others may be offered if your medical history, family history, or physical exam results raise concerns about your baby's health.

Screening and Diagnostic Testing

A number of tests are available to help parents determine whether they are at risk for having a baby with a certain disorder:

- If you are in a high-risk group, you may be offered carrier testing. The timing of carrier testing varies; some can be done before pregnancy or during pregnancy, whereas some can only be done during pregnancy. You may be at high risk of having a child with a genetic disorder if you or your partner has a family history of that disease. You also are at high risk if you have had a previous child with certain disorders.

- Screening tests show if there is an increased risk that a defect will occur relative to other women. They do not tell you whether the defect is present or not. Certain screening tests are offered to all pregnant women.

- If results of a screening test show an increased risk, you can choose to have diagnostic testing. Diagnostic tests show whether the baby has a specific birth defect.

Carrier Screening

If you are at high risk for having a baby with a genetic disease, genetic counseling (see p. 50) and carrier screening can help you and your partner assess your risk of having a baby with the disorder. In carrier testing, samples of blood or saliva from you are studied in a lab to detect a defective gene for a certain inherited disorder.

Risk Factors for Genetic Disorders

Answer the following questions about risk factors. If you answer yes to any of them, you may be at increased risk for having a baby with a genetic disorder:

___ Will you be age 35 years or older when your baby is due?

___ Will the baby's father be age 50 years or older when your baby is due?

___ If you or the baby's father is of Mediterranean or Asian descent, do either of you or anyone in your families have thalassemia?

___ Is there a family history of neural tube defects?

___ Have you or the baby's father ever had a child with a neural tube defect?

___ Is there a family history of congenital heart defects?

___ Is there a family history of Down syndrome?

___ Have you or the baby's father ever had a child with Down syndrome?

___ If you or the baby's father is of Eastern European Jewish, French Canadian, or Cajun descent, is there a family history of Tay–Sachs disease?

___ If you or your partner is of Eastern European Jewish descent, is there a family history of Canavan disease or any other genetic disorders?

___ If you or your partner is African American, is there a family history of sickle cell disease or sickle cell trait?

___ Is there a family history of hemophilia?

___ Is there a family history of muscular dystrophy?

___ Is there a family history of cystic fibrosis?

___ Is there a family history of Huntington disease?

___ Does anyone in your family or the family of the baby's father have cystic fibrosis?

___ Is anyone in your family or the baby's father's family mentally retarded?

___ If so, was that person tested for fragile X syndrome?

___ Do you, the baby's father, anyone in your families, or any of your children have any other genetic diseases, chromosomal disorders, or birth defects?

___ Do you have a metabolic disorder such as diabetes mellitus or phenylketonuria?

___ Do you have a history of pregnancy issues (miscarriage or stillbirth)?

Carrier testing is available for some, but not all, inherited birth defects. Carrier testing detects if a person is a carrier of a genetic defect. All pregnant women should be informed about carrier screening for cystic fibrosis. Carrier screening for other disorders can be done if your family history, ethnic background, or other factors increase your risk of being a carrier. For example, individuals of Eastern European (Ashkenazi) Jewish ancestry may be offered carrier screening for Tay–Sachs disease, Canavan disease, cystic fibrosis, and familial dysautonomia and may want to have tests for other diseases, including mucolipidosis IV, Niemann-Pick disease type A, Fanconi anemia group C, Bloom syndrome, and Gaucher disease.

Results

If your test result is negative, no further testing is needed. If your test result is positive, the next step is to test the baby's father. If results of both tests are positive, a genetic counselor or your health care provider will help you understand your risks of having a child with the disorder, as well as your options. Further testing may be available to show if the baby has the disorder or is a carrier. Once you know your carrier status, your test does not need to be repeated in subsequent pregnancies. If you are found to be a carrier, you may wish to consider telling your family members, as they may be at risk as well.

Timing

Carrier screening can be done either before pregnancy or during the early weeks of your pregnancy. If the screening is done before you are pregnant, you can use the results to decide if you want to get pregnant. If it's done after you are pregnant, for some disorders, the baby can then be tested for the defect.

Screening Tests

Screening tests for birth defects are offered to all pregnant women, even when there are no symptoms or known risk factors, to help ease prospective parents' concerns that their developing baby may have a problem. Screening tests for birth defects consist of blood tests and an **ultrasound** exam. The ultrasound exam usually is given between 18 weeks and 20 weeks of pregnancy and includes a check of the baby's anatomy for abnormalities, and thus serves as a screening test for low-risk women. Some of the common problems found through screening tests include neural tube defects, heart defects, and Down syndrome. In fact, every pregnant woman may be offered a screening test for Down syndrome, regardless of her age.

Results

A screening test result could be positive (showing there is a risk of a problem) even though the baby is healthy. Keep in mind, though, that screening tests won't tell if your child has Down syndrome or another condition. They only give the odds of your baby having a problem. The test results may help you decide whether to undergo further testing.

Timing

Screening tests for birth defects are done at different times during your pregnancy. Some are carried out in the first trimester and some are done during the second trimester. Results of screening tests also can be combined. Table 22-2 provides a comparison of the different types of screening tests that are available and their detection rates:

- *First-trimester screening*—First-trimester screening includes a blood test that measures the levels of two proteins in your blood and a special ultrasound exam called a **nuchal translucency screening** test. Together, these two tests are known as first-trimester combined screening and are done between weeks 10 and 14. The blood test measures two proteins that are made by your placenta during pregnancy: **human chorionic gonadotropin (hCG)** and pregnancy-associated plasma protein A. A woman who is carrying a baby with Down syndrome is more likely to have higher levels of these two proteins in her blood than normal. The nuchal translucency screening test measures the clear (translucent) space in the back of your baby's neck. Babies with chromosomal abnormalities tend to build up more fluid at the back of their neck, making the clear space larger.

- *Second-trimester screening*—Second-trimester screening involves a blood test that is done between 15 weeks and 20 weeks of pregnancy. The test has many different names, such as the quadruple screen, quad screen, multiple marker screen, and maternal serum screen. The test measures the levels of these four substances in your blood, which can tell whether the baby may have a chromosomal problem (see p. 355):

Table 22-2 Down Syndrome Screening Tests and Detection Rates

Screening Test	Detection Rate
First Trimester	
NT screening	64–70%
NT screening plus blood tests for PAPP-A and hCG levels	82–87%
Second Trimester	
Triple screen	69%
Quadruple screen	81%
First Trimester Plus Second Trimester	
Integrated (NT screening, PAPP-A blood test, quadruple screening)	94–96%
Integrated (PAPP-A plus quadruple screening)	85–88%
Contingent sequential	88–94%

Abbreviations: hCG, human chorionic gonadotropin; PAPP-A, pregnancy-associated plasma protein A; NT, nuchal translucency

Adapted from Screening for fetal chromosomal abnormalities. ACOG Practice Bulletin No. 77. American College of Obstetricians and Gynecologists. Obstet Gynecol 2007;109:217–27.

1. ***Alpha-fetoprotein***—a protein made by the baby's liver
2. hCG
3. Estriol—a pregnancy-related hormone
4. Inhibin A—a pregnancy-related protein

• *Combined screening*—The results of first-trimester and second-trimester screening tests can be combined in a number of ways to increase their ability to detect Down syndrome. With this type of testing, the final result may not be available until all the tests are completed. When tests are used together and depending on the tests used, 85–96% of Down syndrome cases can be detected:

—In integrated screening, results of the first-trimester and second-trimester tests are analyzed together. Integrated screening is highly accurate and has the lowest false-positive rate of all of the testing strategies.

—In sequential screening, results of the first-trimester screening tests are used to determine further testing. If results show that you are at high risk, you can opt to have a diagnostic test. If results show you are at low or intermediate risk, you can go on to have second-trimester screening.

Diagnostic Tests

If a screening test or other factors raise concerns about the baby, further tests will be offered to diagnose certain birth defects. In the past, women at increased risk of having a baby with a birth defect—for instance, maternal age older than 35 years—were offered diagnostic testing first, rather than having screening tests. Currently, both screening tests and diagnostic tests may be offered as a first choice to all women before 20 weeks of pregnancy. It is up to you to decide if you want any testing at all and, if so, whether to undergo screening or diagnostic testing. However, some diagnostic tests carry risks, including an increased risk of pregnancy loss. It is important to understand all of the risks if you choose this option.

Detailed Ultrasound Exam

A detailed ultrasound exam may be done if there is an abnormal result from a screening test. This type of exam allows a more extensive view of the baby's organs and features. A detailed ultrasound exam generally can be done after 18 weeks of pregnancy. Even a detailed ultrasound, however, cannot detect all birth defects. Detailed ultrasound testing is best used to detect structural abnormalities, such as abdominal wall defects.

Amniocentesis

Most often, ***amniocentesis*** is performed at 15–20 weeks of pregnancy. To perform the procedure, a doctor guides a thin needle through the abdomen and uterus. A small sample of amniotic fluid is withdrawn and sent to a lab.

In the lab, cells that have been shed from the baby are grown in a special culture. This can take up to 3 weeks. Next, the chromosomes in these cells are studied under a microscope. This shows if there is an extra chromosome (as in Down syndrome). It also can show if there are other chromosomal defects and certain other birth defects, such as cystic fibrosis. How-

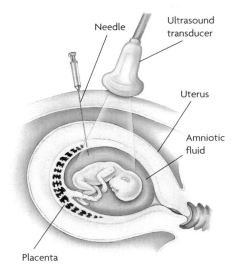

Amniocentesis. In this procedure, a small sample of amniotic fluid is removed with a needle to be studied.

ever, these other tests must be specifically requested. Testing the levels of alpha-fetoprotein in the ***amniotic fluid*** can help determine if the fetus has a neural tube defect.

Complications from amniocentesis include cramping, vaginal bleeding, and leakage of amniotic fluid, which occur in 1–2% of women having this procedure. There is a slight chance (about 0.5%) of miscarriage as a result of amniocentesis (although a recent study found the risk to be as low as 0.06%).

Chorionic Villus Sampling

Chorionic villus sampling (CVS) detects the same chromosomal problems that amniocentesis does. It can be performed earlier than amniocentesis—often at 10–12 weeks of pregnancy.

To do CVS, a doctor guides either a small tube through the ***vagina*** and ***cervix*** or a thin needle through the abdomen and uterine wall. The doctor then takes a small sample of ***chorionic villi*** from the placenta. Chorionic villi (the plural of villus) are tiny, finger-like projections of placental tissue. Villi come from the same fertilized egg as the fetus. This means they have the same genetic makeup.

The sample is sent to a lab, where it is grown in a culture. This can take up to 2 weeks. Chromosomes from the villi then are studied under a microscope to check for chromosomal or other defects.

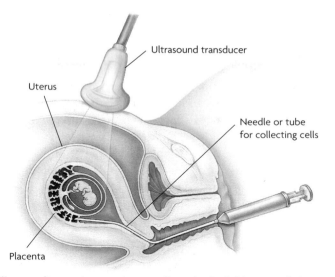

Chorionic villus sampling. In this procedure, a small sample of cells (chorionic villus) is removed from the placenta for study.

The risk of miscarriage as a result of CVS is about 1%. If it is performed earlier than 10 weeks, the risks associated with the procedure, including the risk of a limb abnormality, are increased. For this reason, CVS should not be performed before 10 weeks of pregnancy.

Cordocentesis

Cordocentesis (also called *fetal blood sampling*) is used to test for chromosomal defects and other abnormalities. At 18 weeks of pregnancy or later, blood is taken from a *vein* in the umbilical cord. This test usually is done when the results of amniocentesis, chorionic villus sampling, or ultrasound are unclear. As with amniocentesis, possible side effects from this procedure are cramping and bleeding. The miscarriage rate after cordocentesis is about 1–2%.

Preimplantation Genetic Diagnosis

For couples undergoing *in vitro fertilization* to become pregnant, a test can be done on the *embryo* to check for certain problems. This test is called *preimplantation genetic diagnosis*. With this procedure, embryos that are found to be affected by a disorder are not implanted in the mother's uterus. Preimplantation genetic diagnosis has been used for diagnosis of some chromosomal disorders; genetic disorders, such as cystic fibrosis; X-linked recessive conditions; and other inherited problems.

Genetic Counseling

How do you make decisions about what tests to have? Genetic counseling can help a couple assess the risk of having a baby with a genetic disorder, decide whether to be tested, and consider their options. A genetic counselor has special training in genetics. He or she can offer expert advice on types of genetic disorders and how they affect babies born with them.

The genetic counselor will take a detailed medical, genetic, and family history. If a family member has a problem, the counselor may ask to see that person's medical records. He or she also may refer the woman or her partner for physical exams, blood tests, or prenatal tests. Using all the information gathered, the counselor will try to figure out the baby's risk of having a problem. The counselor then will explain and discuss the options.

Options

When you receive the results of your test, you will need to process the information and decide what to do. Your health care provider or genetic counselor can help guide you through your options.

If You or Your Partner Is a Carrier

If you learn that you or your partner is a carrier for a disease before you become pregnant, the test results can help you both decide whether to try to conceive a child. You may want to explore other options for starting a family, such as adopting a child or using donor sperm or a donor egg to get pregnant. You also may want to inform siblings and other family members who may want to have children in the future.

If you are already pregnant and testing shows there is a high chance the baby will be born with a genetic disorder, you may want to have diagnostic testing, if it is available, to see whether the baby will be born with the disorder.

If Your Baby Has a Disorder

If diagnostic testing shows that your baby has a disorder, you have two options. You may choose to continue the pregnancy. Or, you may end the pregnancy. There is no right choice in these cases. Your health, values, beliefs, and situation all play a role in the decision.

If you decide to continue with the pregnancy, you can use the rest of your pregnancy preparing for the birth of a child with special needs. Learn all you can about the condition and what it will mean for your baby's health. You may want to find a pediatrician who specializes in caring for babies with the disorder. Your health care provider or staff may be able to help you find this special care. You also can seek out support groups for you and your partner. Ask whether the hospital where you are planning to deliver has pediatric doctors who can provide the best possible care for your infant. If it doesn't, consider requesting a transfer of care to deliver at such a facility.

Remember that educating yourself about your child's condition is crucial. You may find it helpful to visit the March of Dimes Foundation's web site and find the local chapter in your area (see Resources).

Prevention

Some birth defects can be prevented or the risk of having a baby with a certain disorder can be decreased by taking certain steps. Many involve making certain lifestyle changes before and during pregnancy. For example, getting the recommended amount of folic acid before and during pregnancy has been shown to decrease the risk of neural tube defects (see Chapter 1, Months 1 and 2 [Weeks 1–8], p. 23). There are other steps you can take as well:

- Seeing your doctor to evaluate your risks (pp. 36–37)
- Taking care of medical conditions before becoming pregnant (p. 319)
- Avoiding harmful agents during pregnancy (pp. 348–350)
- Limiting your intake of fish that contain high levels of mercury (p. 86)
- Maintaining a healthy weight (pp. 24–25)
- Avoiding alcohol, smoking, and illegal drugs (pp. 29–31)
- Preventing infections (pp. 379–381)

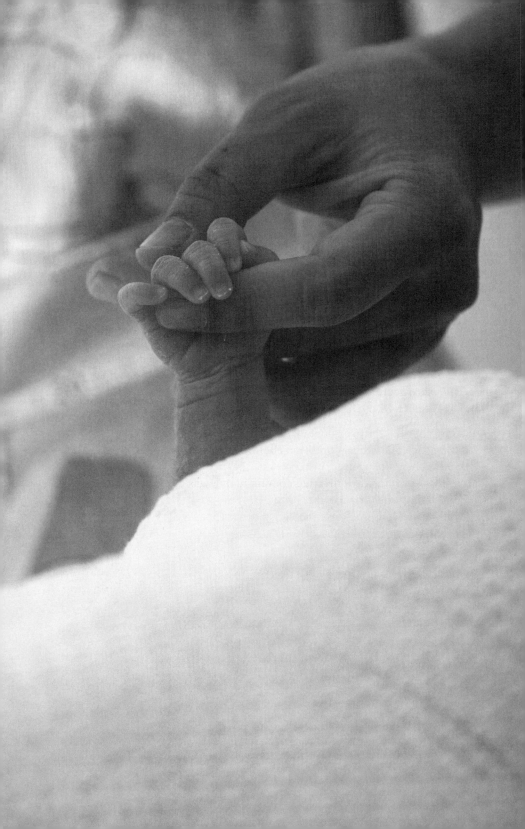

Chapter 23
Preterm Labor, Preterm Birth, and Premature Rupture of Membranes

Pregnancy usually lasts about 40 weeks. Labor or birth that happens too early—before 37 weeks of pregnancy—is called *preterm*. Another problem that may occur is preterm *premature rupture of membranes*—when the *amniotic sac* that cushions the baby breaks before 37 weeks of pregnancy.

Preterm Labor and Preterm Birth

When a baby is born between 32 weeks and 37 weeks of pregnancy, she is preterm (premature) and is not fully grown. Babies born before 32 weeks of pregnancy are called "early preterm." The earlier a baby is born, the less likely she is to survive. Those who do survive may have serious, life-long health problems. About 12% of babies are born prematurely in the United States each year.

The *Eunice Kennedy Shriver* National Institutes of Child Health and Human Development (NICHD) studies the outcomes of early preterm births in 16 hospitals. Between 1998 and 2002, the studies found that babies born before the 23rd week of pregnancy were not likely to survive. About one half of the babies born at the 25th week survived. By the 26th week of pregnancy, the survival chances increased to 76%. But most of the babies who survived had serious health problems 18–22 months later, including respiratory problems, bleeding in the brain, infection, cerebral palsy, and developmental delays. Many of these medical conditions may be lifelong.

Birth weight and sex are important factors in your baby's chances of survival and risk of health problems. Survival rates and outcomes also differ from hospital to hospital.

How Birth Weight and Sex Affect a Baby's Survival Chances and Risk of Health Problems

Doctors consider these factors when making treatment decisions:

- Babies born weighing between 501 and 750 grams (1.10–1.65 pounds) have a 55% chance of survival. Of the babies who survive, 65% have serious health problems.

- Babies born weighing between 751 and 1,000 grams (1.66–2.20 pounds) have an 88% chance of survival. Of the babies who survive, 43% have serious health problems.

- Babies born weighing between 1,001 and 1,250 grams (2.21–2.76 pounds) have a 94% chance of survival. Of the babies who survive, 22% have serious health problems.

- Babies born weighing between 1,251 and 1,500 grams (2.76–3.31 pounds) have a 96% chance of survival. Of the babies who survive, 11% have serious health problems.

- Girls who are born at the 25th week of pregnancy and weigh about 700 grams (1½ pounds) may have a higher chance of survival than boys born at the same age and weight.

- For twins, the chances for survival are less than for single births at the same age and weight.

Risk Factors

Preterm labor can happen to anyone, without warning. There are some factors, however, that can increase your risk of preterm labor:

- Having preterm labor or birth in your past pregnancies
- Having twins
- Certain infections
- Bleeding in mid-pregnancy
- *Placenta previa*
- High blood pressure
- Having a chronic illness
- Too much fluid in the amniotic sac
- Birth defects in the baby

What to Watch For

Preterm birth can result if labor starts before the end of the 37th week. If preterm labor is found early, attempts may be made to postpone birth to give your baby extra time to grow and mature. Even a few more days in the womb may mean a healthier baby. Be aware of these signs that you may be going into preterm labor and call your doctor or nurse right away:

- Change in your vaginal discharge (it becomes watery, mucus-like, or bloody)
- Pressure in your pelvis or lower abdomen
- Constant, low backache
- Mild abdominal cramps
- Regular contractions, often painless
- Your water breaks

Sometimes the signs that preterm labor may be starting are fairly easy to detect. For instance, you can monitor yourself to see if you are having contractions. Lie down on your side and gently feel the entire surface of your lower abdomen with your fingertips. Feel for a firm tightening over the surface of your **uterus**. Often this tightening is not painful. If you feel these contractions, keep track of them for an hour. Note when each one starts and ends. If you have contractions that occur four times every 20 minutes or if you have contractions eight times an hour that last for more than an hour, call your health care provider right away.

Diagnosis

The only way for your health care provider to be sure that you are truly in preterm labor is to check your **cervix**. In labor, the cervix shortens and thins out (effacement) and opens up (**dilation**) so the baby can enter the birth canal. To see if your cervix has dilated, your health care provider will check your cervix by performing a **pelvic exam**. Fetal monitoring also can be done to check the heartbeat of the baby and contractions of the uterus. **Ultrasound** may be used to estimate the size and **gestational age** of the baby.

There are two tests that can help determine if you are at high risk for preterm birth: 1) ultrasound exam to assess the length of the cervix, and 2) a test that measures the amount of fetal fibronectin in the vaginal discharge. Fetal fibronectin is a substance that "glues" the amniotic sac to the uterine wall. Towards the end of pregnancy, this glue starts to break down and can be detected in the vaginal discharge. These two tests can be used together or singly. They may be most useful in identifying women who are least likely to deliver. If results of the tests are negative—if cervical length and fetal fibronectin amounts are normal, preterm birth is unlikely. The fetal fibronectin test often is given to women who have symptoms of preterm labor.

Managing Preterm Birth

If you are at risk for preterm birth, you may be referred to a subspecialist in maternal–fetal medicine, an obstetrician who specializes in treating problems affecting a pregnant woman and her baby. Medications sometimes can be given to women at risk for preterm birth to help the baby's lungs mature (**corticosteroids**) or help prolong pregnancy (**tocolytics** and **progesterone**). During labor, a woman may receive **antibiotics** to prevent early-onset infection of her baby with Group B streptococci (see p. 381). You may be transported to a hospital with special facilities for treating preterm infants (neonatal intensive care unit). Once the baby is born, she may receive other medications and breathing support, if necessary.

Corticosteroids

Corticosteroids are drugs that help speed up the development of your baby's lungs and some other organs. Giving the mother one course of this medication can greatly increase the chances of a baby's survival. The babies whose mothers received this treatment also are much less likely to have trouble breathing.

Progesterone

Progesterone may be given to help prevent preterm birth if you have had a previous preterm birth. It sometimes is given to women who have been found to have a very short cervix but no symptoms of preterm labor. More research is being done to find out whether progesterone can prevent preterm birth in women with other risk factors.

Tocolytics

Tocolytics are drugs that stop or slow labor. Sometimes tocolytics are given to allow corticosteroids to help the baby's lungs mature. Also, delaying labor can allow time for you to be transferred to a hospital with a high-level neonatal intensive care unit that is better equipped and has specially trained doctors and nurses who are experienced in caring for preterm infants. If you are given tocolytics, you may have side effects of a rapid pulse, chest pain, dizziness, and headache.

Neonatal Intensive Care Units

Preterm infants who are delivered at hospitals with high-level neonatal intensive care units have a better chance of survival. High-level neonatal intensive care units provide specialized care for infants with serious health problems. These units are better equipped and have doctors and nurses with advanced training and experience in caring for preterm infants. You and the baby usually will be cared for by a team of health care providers. The team may include a neonatologist, a doctor who specializes in treating problems in newborns.

You may be moved to such a hospital for delivery if you go into labor very early. It is safer to give birth to a preterm baby at these hospitals than to transport the baby after birth.

Surfactant Replacement Therapy

If your baby is born preterm, she may be given surfactant replacement therapy. Surfactant is a liquid substance in the body that very preterm babies don't have enough of. When surfactant is given to the baby it can stop the lungs from collapsing and help the baby breathe. Although this treatment often works well, it usually is given only in hospitals where the staff is experienced in caring for very preterm infants born with breathing problems.

Resuscitation and Breathing Support

If the birth cannot be delayed and the baby is born early, doctors have to take quick action to help the baby breathe on its own because the lungs may not be mature enough and able to work well. If the baby is not breathing on her own, she may be put on a ventilator (or respirator) that breathes for her.

The decisions to try to revive a baby who is not breathing when it is born, as well as how long to continue having the baby on a ventilator, are complex. Many factors are considered, including gestational age, the baby's birth weight, and the baby's condition at birth. Sometimes, a condition such as an infection may become apparent after the baby is born, which can worsen the prognosis for a baby on breathing support. Your health care team will discuss with you the realistic chances that your baby will survive and help you make decisions.

Premature Rupture of Membranes

When the sac that holds the *amniotic fluid* ruptures and your water breaks, it usually is followed by other signs of labor. If these membranes rupture at or around the time of a woman's due date, but labor does not begin soon afterward, it is called premature rupture of membranes ("term PROM" or just "PROM"). When the membranes rupture before 37 weeks, it is called preterm premature rupture of membranes (or "preterm PROM").

Term PROM happens in about 8% of pregnancies. It is caused by the normal weakening of the amniotic sac as birth approaches, as well as by the force of uterine contractions. In about 95% of cases, labor begins within 28 hours. The risks of PROM include infection of the uterus and **umbilical cord** problems. The likelihood of these complications occurring increases the longer labor is delayed.

Because it occurs before 37 weeks of pregnancy, preterm PROM may lead to serious problems for the baby related to prematurity. Other complications that can occur are infection (of you or the baby or both of you) and **placenta** and umbilical cord problems. There is a 1–2% risk of fetal death as a result of preterm PROM.

There are several risk factors for preterm PROM, although many cases occur in the absence of any risk factors. The risk factors associated with PROM include infection, a low body mass index (less than 19), bleeding during the second or third trimesters, smoking, and dietary deficiencies. A significant risk factor is having had preterm PROM in a previous pregnancy. The risk for recurrence is between 16% and 32%.

Diagnosis

The main symptom of PROM is leakage of fluid from your **vagina**. Call your health care provider if you have any fluid leakage. Your health care provider will want to determine whether your membranes have ruptured. Sometimes you may have a discharge for other reasons, including **urine** leakage, cervical mucus, vaginal bleeding, or a vaginal infection. You probably will have a physical exam and maybe lab tests to confirm if there is amniotic fluid in the vagina.

Management

Once the diagnosis of PROM is confirmed, one of the first things that your health care provider will do is determine your baby's gestational age. If you have any conditions that put your or your baby's life in danger, such as **placental abruption** or infection of the uterus, your baby will be delivered right away, regardless of her gestational age. But if you do not have any of these conditions, the gestational age of your baby is an important factor in determining how your condition will be managed.

If you have term PROM and your baby is in the correct position for delivery, you probably will have your labor induced using *oxytocin*. If the baby is not in the correct position (*breech presentation*), you will have a *cesarean delivery*. In either case, you also will receive antibiotics for group B streptococci based on your prior test results or risk factors if you have not been tested.

If you have preterm PROM that occurs between 23 weeks and 33 weeks of pregnancy, your health care provider may try to delay birth until the baby is more developed. You most likely will need to stay in the hospital so that you can be monitored closely. You may receive antibiotics to prevent infection and corticosteroids to help the baby's lungs mature. Tocolytics also may be given. Strict bed rest may be prescribed, and you will be told not to have sex. These measures may stop the leakage of amniotic fluid. In about 10% of women with preterm PROM, the amniotic fluid level returns to normal.

If you have preterm PROM before 24 completed weeks of pregnancy, your health care provider will explain the risks of having a very preterm baby and the potential risks and benefits of trying to delay labor. If you do go into labor, your baby may be born with severe health problems.

Caring for a Preterm Baby

Once the baby is born, your baby's doctor will have a better idea of the baby's health and whether any other problems exist. If your baby is healthy enough to overcome the challenges of being born preterm, she will still require special care. There are pediatricians who specialize in the care of preterm babies (called neonatologists) and children. Some clinics focus on follow-up care for preterm babies. Make sure you find a doctor you like and trust. The doctor will closely watch how your baby grows and check to see if any other problems develop during childhood.

You also can find information for parents about caring for preterm babies. It is a good idea to become as informed as you can so you can give your baby the best care. As your child reaches school age, you also may need to find a special school or teachers to help with any learning problems. For more information about preterm birth and caring for a preterm child, contact the March of Dimes or the *Eunice Kennedy Shriver* National Institute of Child Health and Human Development (see Resources).

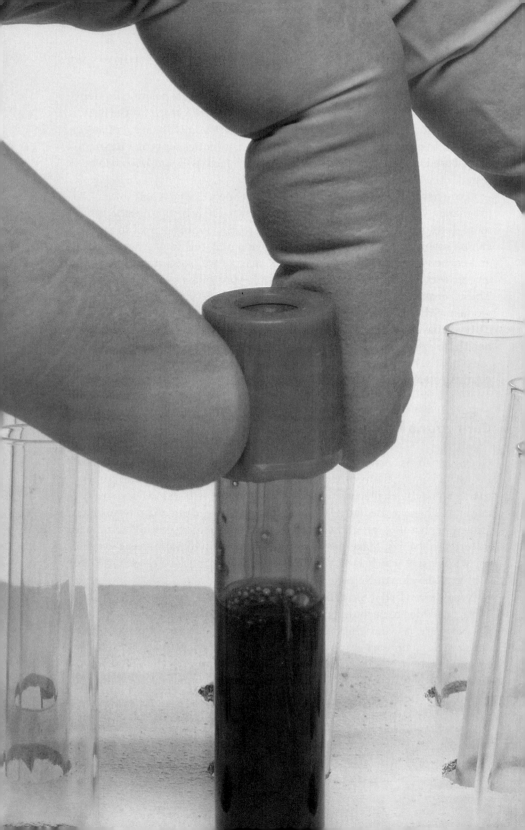

Chapter 24
Blood Type
Incompatibility

A s part of your prenatal care, you will have blood tests to find out your blood type and determine your Rhesus (or Rh) factor. Knowing your blood type and Rh status is important because complications can occur if you are a certain blood type and your baby is another type. Experts call this problem blood type incompatibility. In the past, these problems were a major cause of newborn sickness and even death. Now, however, early testing and treatment can prevent these complications.

Blood Types and Rh Factor

Your blood type is A, B, AB, or O. Blood types are determined by the types of *antigens*—tiny proteins—on your blood *cells*. Type A blood has only A antigens, type B has only B antigens, type AB has both A and B antigens, and type O has neither A nor B antigens.

Your prenatal blood tests also determine your Rh factor. The Rh factor is a type of antigen sometimes found on the surface of red blood cells. If your blood does contain the protein, you are Rh positive. If it does not have the protein, you are Rh negative.

Most people (about 85%) are Rh positive. Your Rh status does not affect your health at all except during pregnancy. And then, it only may cause concern when your Rh status does not match your baby's status.

Rh Incompatibility

Some women are Rh negative and carry a baby who is Rh positive—which can happen if the father is Rh positive. This may cause a problem called Rh factor incompatibility.

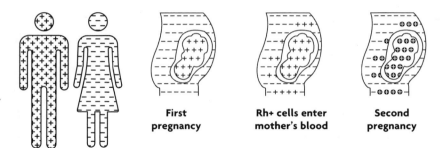

First pregnancy — **Rh+ cells enter mother's blood** — **Second pregnancy**

| - Rh-negative |
| + Rh-positive |
| ⊕ Antibodies |

Rh incompablity. Rh incompatibility occurs when a baby is Rh positive and the mother has developed Rh antibodies during a previous pregnancy. First pregnancy: An Rh-negative woman has an Rh-positive baby. Cells from the Rh-positive baby enter the mother's bloodstream. She may make antibodies that attack Rh-positive cells. Second pregnancy: If she becomes pregnant again with an Rh-positive baby, the Rh antibodies will attach to the baby's blood cells.

How It Affects Your Baby

If a small amount of the baby's blood mixes with your blood, it may cause your body to make *antibodies* to attack the Rh-positive factor in the baby's blood. This mixing can occur during labor and delivery as well as during some procedures, such as *amniocentesis* and *chorionic villus sampling* (tests that are done to diagnose birth defects and other problems early in pregnancy). It also may occur spontaneously with no apparent cause. If your body has made these antibodies, you are said to be sensitized. Sensitization usually does not cause problems until you become pregnant again. During a subsequent pregnancy, these antibodies can destroy the red blood cells in your baby's blood if he is Rh positive. This condition is called hemolytic disease of the newborn, a condition that can cause *anemia*. If it is not treated, it can cause mild or even severe damage to your baby. It can cause death in very rare cases.

Treatment

If you are Rh negative, you will be tested at 28 weeks of pregnancy to see if you have made Rh antibodies. This test is called the indirect Coombs test. If the test result shows that you are not producing Rh antibodies, your doctor will give you an injection (shot) of *Rh immunoglobulin (RhIg)* to prevent harm to the next child. These shots prevent antibodies to the Rh antigens from forming. They are safe for pregnant women. The only side effects may be soreness from the injection or a slight fever.

In addition to the RhIg shot at 28 weeks, you will receive another injection within 72 hours after the birth (if the baby is Rh positive). The effects of RhIg last for about 12 weeks. For this reason, anti-RhIg also is given any time blood from the baby and the mother might mix, such as a miscarriage or before certain procedures, such as amniocentesis. It also may be given if you have had an abdominal injury (because of the risk that some of the baby's blood has entered your bloodstream as a result of the injury), bleeding during pregnancy, or if your baby needs to be turned in the **uterus** to prevent a **breech presentation**. You don't need RhIg if it is known (and can be confirmed) that the father is Rh negative. Two Rh-negative parents can only have an Rh-negative baby, and there is no risk of the mother making antibodies.

If, however, blood tests show that you are producing Rh antibodies, RhIg is not going to be beneficial. In this case, you will have regular blood tests during pregnancy to check the level of antibodies. If they become high, further tests may be done to check the health of the baby. The baby may be anemic and need a blood transfusion. After 18 weeks of pregnancy, a transfusion can be given while the baby is still in the uterus. If the baby is old enough, early birth may be an option. The baby most likely will be cared for in a special-care nursery.

ABO Incompatibility

Although it occurs very rarely, some pregnant women's blood types are incompatible with their babies' blood types. When this happens, it is usually when the mother is type O and her baby is type A, B, or AB. This is known as ABO incompatibility.

How It Affects Your Baby

Newborns born with ABO incompatibility can have mild hemolytic disease and high levels of bilirubin in the blood. Bilirubin is a substance that forms when old red blood cells break down. **Jaundice** (yellowish skin) is a sign of high levels of bilirubin. Too much of the substance can be harmful, especially to the baby's nervous system, and can cause developmental problems.

Treatment

If your baby has jaundice caused by hemolytic disease, the doctor will check the level of bilirubin in his blood. If it's high, special treatment, such as the use of special lights, will bring the level down. If this treatment does not decrease the bilirubin level, if the level is very high to begin with, or if the infant is showing signs of bilirubin toxicity, a blood transfusion may be needed.

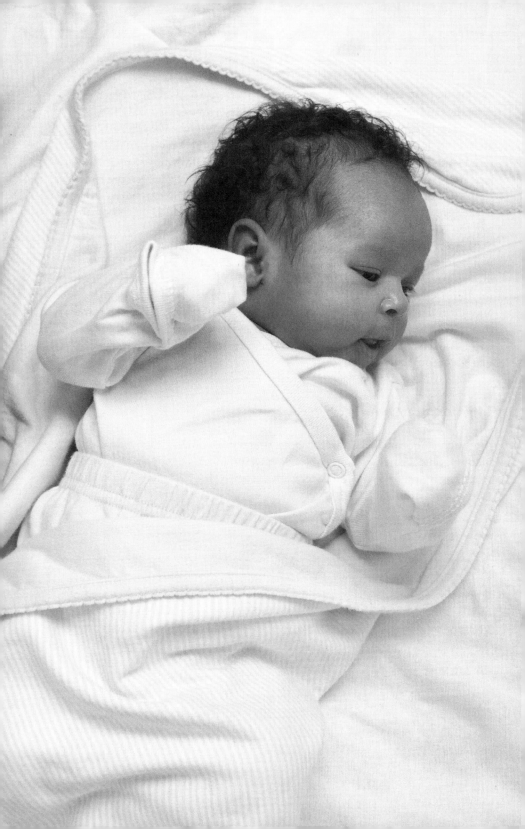

Chapter 25
Placental Problems

I n a normal pregnancy, the ***placenta*** is attached high on the uterine wall away from the ***cervix***. It remains attached until shortly after the baby is born, when it detaches from the wall of the ***uterus***. The placenta is important to provide the baby with nutrients and oxygen. Certain problems with the placenta can occur during pregnancy. They can cause serious complications if they are not identified early. You should be aware of the signs and symptoms of these problems and alert your health care provider immediately if you think you are experiencing them.

Placenta Previa

Placenta previa is a condition in which the placenta lies low in the uterus and covers part (called partial placenta previa) or all (called complete placenta previa) of the cervix. Because it's covering the cervix, the placenta blocks the baby's exit from the uterus. Also, the placenta is attached to the uterus with blood vessels. When the cervix begins to thin and opens in preparation for labor, bleeding can occur before or during delivery. Bleeding may be excessive and pose a danger to the mother and baby.

Placenta previa occurs in 1 in 200 pregnant women. Although the reasons why placenta previa happens in some women are unknown, it is more common in women with the following conditions:

* Have had more than one child
* Have had a ***cesarean delivery***
* Have had surgery on the uterus
* Are carrying twins or triplets

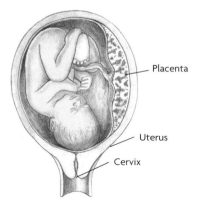

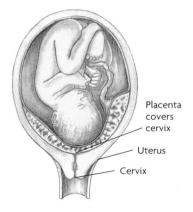

Normal position of placenta. The placenta normally attaches high on the uterine wall, away from the cervix.

Placenta previa. In this condition, the placenta lies low in the uterus and either partly or completely blocks the cervix.

Warning Signs

Painless vaginal bleeding is the main sign of placenta previa. The bleeding usually occurs near the end of the second trimester or the start of the third trimester (from about weeks 20–32). Placenta previa is a serious condition that needs to be treated quickly, so call your health care provider right away if you have any bleeding in your third trimester.

Some women learn that they have placenta previa early in pregnancy during an *ultrasound* examination, before any bleeding occurs. Women with early-diagnosed placenta previa will be checked closely with ultrasound exams throughout their pregnancy. In most (90%) of cases, placenta previa resolves on its own, and labor and delivery can proceed normally.

Treatment

You will receive initial treatment that depends on the stage of your pregnancy. Your health care provider will decide which treatment is best depending on your condition and how far along you are in your pregnancy. Early in pregnancy, you will be told to restrict your activities (including no sex). Later in pregnancy, placenta previa usually requires hospitalization and intravenous fluids. Your baby then will be monitored to check his condition. Occasionally a blood transfusion may be necessary. Ultrasound will be used to check the position of the placenta within the uterus.

Placenta previa may be severe enough to require that the baby be delivered early. Women with this condition usually will need to have a cesarean delivery. Sometimes, the bleeding stops on its own, and the pregnancy is allowed to continue. If this happens and you are less than 34 weeks along, it may be possible to monitor your condition on an outpatient basis (you don't have to stay in the hospital), but you will need to see your health care provider frequently and call immediately if you have any vaginal bleeding. You may receive drugs called *corticosteroids* to help the baby's lungs develop. At 36–37 weeks, a test may be done to see if the baby's lungs have matured. If they have, you may have a cesarean delivery at this time.

Placental Abruption

Placental abruption occurs when the placenta detaches from the wall of the uterus before or during birth. This often causes vaginal bleeding and severe pain in the abdomen. Placental abruption is a potentially dangerous problem for both the mother and baby. The baby may get less oxygen than he needs to survive, and the mother can lose a large amount of blood. Prompt treatment is needed.

Only 1% of pregnant women have this problem, and it usually occurs in the last 12 weeks before birth. Placental abruption happens more often in women who have high blood pressure, who smoke, or who use cocaine or amphetamines during pregnancy. It also is more common in women with the following conditions:

- Have already had children
- Are older than 35 years
- Have had placental abruption before
- Have sickle cell disease

Warning Signs

The most common warning signs are vaginal bleeding and abdominal or back pain. Some women do not have a lot of bleeding with placental abruption because the blood becomes trapped inside the uterus by the placenta.

Treatment

Just as with placenta previa, the treatment for placental abruption depends on your condition and how far along you are in your pregnancy. Ultrasound

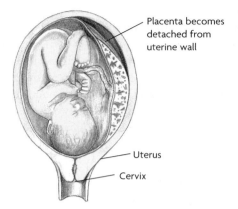

Placenta becomes detached from uterine wall

Uterus

Cervix

Placental abruption. The placenta becomes detached from the uterine wall.

examination may be done, but sometimes it's not possible to identify placental abruption with ultrasound. If you have lost a lot of blood, you may need a blood transfusion and intravenous fluids. After your condition is stabilized, your health care provider will monitor your baby to make sure he is safe. You may have to stay in the hospital so doctors can watch your condition closely.

If the abruption is small, and you are near your due date, labor may be induced, or you may have a cesarean delivery if there are other problems. Sometimes bleeding stops on its own. In this case, you will be monitored closely to make sure the abruption does not get worse. If your due date is still far off (you're between 24 weeks and 34 weeks), you may receive drugs called **tocolytics** to help stop labor and corticosteroids to help the baby's lungs mature. After 34 weeks of pregnancy, the baby usually is delivered. Although there is a risk of the baby having health problems related to prematurity, it often is safer to deliver the baby in some cases.

Placenta Accreta

Placenta accreta is a condition in which the blood vessels of the placenta grow too deeply into the uterine wall. It can cause severe, life-threatening blood loss during delivery. A major risk factor for this condition is a previous cesarean delivery. The risk increases with the number of prior cesarean deliveries. Placenta accreta may cause bleeding during the third trimester, and it also commonly occurs with placenta previa. Placenta accreta often is not diagnosed until after the baby is delivered, although occasionally it may be diagnosed with ultrasound or with a procedure called magnetic resonance imaging (MRI) during pregnancy. Sometimes a *hysterectomy* is needed following a vaginal or cesarean delivery if a woman has placenta accreta, although every effort is made to preserve the uterus. However, there may be no other option but to remove the uterus if the bleeding becomes life threatening when the placenta partially separates from the uterus.

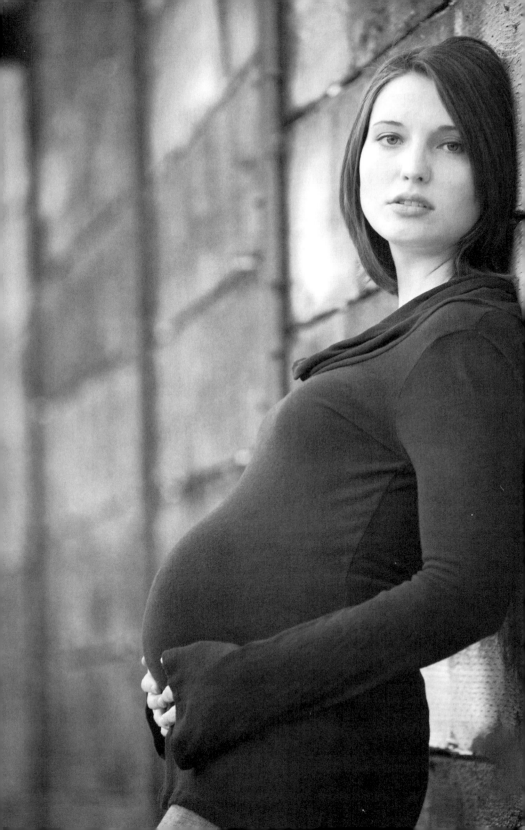

Chapter 26
Infections

C ertain infections can pose risks to you and your unborn baby. Many of the tests and exams given during prenatal care visits are directed at detecting these infections. If an infection is diagnosed, it's important to get prompt treatment. But by far the best way to reduce your risk of problems caused by infections is prevention.

Infections are diseases caused by bacteria, viruses, or parasites that invade the body and then spread. Infections also can be caused by the bacteria that normally live on the skin and in the body's digestive, respiratory, and reproductive systems. If the balance of these bacteria is disrupted, for example, by an injury that allows skin bacteria to get into the body, it can cause some bacteria to grow out of control. If the growth is not stopped, an infection can result.

The body's immune system consists of a variety of **cells** and tissues that detect the presence of foreign invaders, sound an alarm, and unleash defenses to fight off the infection. A key part of the **immune system** is **antibodies**. These special proteins are formed in the blood in response to an infection. They "tag" foreign cells for destruction by other parts of the immune system.

For some infections, blood tests can show whether antibodies have formed in your body. If they have, it means you have been exposed to that infection. In many cases, once the body makes antibodies to a disease, the person becomes immune to the disease and will not get it in the future.

An infection may not cause any symptoms or the symptoms may not occur right away. The earlier an infection is found and treated, the less likely it is for long-term health problems to develop.

Some infections can be prevented with vaccines. However, some vaccines are not safe to get during pregnancy. If you think you have been exposed to an

Vaccines

Vaccines help prevent diseases caused by infection. Like all medicines, a vaccine should be used during pregnancy only when it is needed and safe. It is best for you to have all your vaccinations before you become pregnant. If a vaccination is needed during pregnancy, waiting until your fourth month is best.

Avoid being exposed to measles, rubella, mumps, and chickenpox during pregnancy. You should be vaccinated against measles, rubella, and mumps at least 1 month before you become pregnant. You also should be vaccinated against chickenpox at least 1 month before becoming pregnant. Vaccination is safe for both you and your baby while you are breastfeeding. Pregnant women should be vaccinated against influenza if they will be pregnant during the flu season (October through March).

The following vaccines are not usually given to pregnant women, but the benefits may outweigh the risks if you are likely to come in contact with the infections:

- Hepatitis A virus
- *Hepatitis B virus*
- Pneumonia caused by pneumococcus
- Rabies
- Polio
- Tetanus–diphtheria–pertussis booster or the tetanus booster depending on the need for tetanus or diphtheria protection during pregnancy

The following vaccines should be avoided during pregnancy:

- Lyme disease
- Measles
- Mumps
- Rubella
- Varicella (chickenpox)

infection, tell your health care provider right away. Sometimes steps can be taken to avoid problems and decrease any risk to your baby.

The best way to protect yourself against infections is to take steps to prevent them:

- Know which childhood diseases you have had, and make sure your vaccines are up-to-date before you become pregnant.
- Know the symptoms of infections so you can alert your health care provider right away if they occur.
- Do not engage in behavior that increases the risk of infections.

- Use good hygiene, including washing your hands often.
- Avoid contact with people who are sick.

Group B Streptococci

About 10–30% of pregnant women carry a bacterium known as Group B streptococcus (GBS). In women, GBS most often is found in the **vagina** and rectum. Both men and women can have GBS, and usually the bacteria live in the body without causing any harm—you won't have any symptoms.

Although GBS is fairly common in pregnancy, very few babies actually become sick with GBS infection. If GBS bacteria are passed from a woman to her baby, the baby may become infected. This is rare and happens to only 1–2% of babies. Babies who do become infected may have early or late infections:

- *Early infections*—A baby typically gets sick within the first 6 hours after birth or up to the first 7 days. These infections can cause severe problems, such as inflammation of the brain (meningitis), pneumonia, and fever. About 5% of babies with early infections die even with immediate treatment.

- *Late infections*—A baby gets sick within a week to a few months after birth. About half of late infections are passed from the mother to the baby during birth. The rest are from other sources of infection, such as contact with people who have GBS. Late infections are serious and can cause meningitis.

Because women infected with GBS do not show any symptoms, all pregnant women are screened for GBS as part of their **prenatal care** visits. Testing usually is done between week 35 and week 37 of pregnancy and is done by taking a culture from the vagina and rectal area. The culture is then tested for the GBS bacteria. If the results show GBS is present, **antibiotics** are given to you once you go into labor to help prevent the baby from being infected.

Some women do not need to be tested for GBS. If you have had a previous child who had a GBS infection, you won't be tested, but you will receive antibiotics during labor. If you have GBS bacteria in your **urine** at any point during your pregnancy, you also will not be tested and you also will receive antibiotics during labor.

Urinary Tract Infections

Urinary tract infections—infections of the **bladder**, **kidney**, or **urethra**—are common in pregnancy. Severe infections can cause problems for both you and the baby, so it is important to treat the infections early. Because some urinary tract infections may not cause any symptoms, you will be tested at your first prenatal visit. If an infection is found, it can be treated easily with antibiotics.

When an infection of the bladder does cause symptoms, you may feel a burning pain when you urinate. Bladder infections also can cause an increased urge to urinate, blood in the urine, and abdominal pain.

If a bladder infection is not treated or is not cured by treatment it may result in a kidney infection. It is important to finish any medications prescribed for a bladder infection, even after your symptoms go away. A kidney infection can cause symptoms such as chills, fever, back pain, rapid heart rate, and nausea or vomiting. Contact your health care provider right way if you have any of these symptoms so that you can be treated with antibiotics. If left untreated, a kidney infection can lead to premature labor or severe infection.

Tuberculosis

Tuberculosis (TB) is a disease caused by bacteria that are carried through the air and are passed on to others when an infected person coughs or sneezes. Tuberculosis infection usually occurs in the lungs.

If your health care provider determines you have risk factors for TB, such as moving from a country that has a high rate of TB infection, you should be tested with a Mantoux test with purified protein derivative during pregnancy. If the test results are positive, you will need a chest X-ray to confirm the result.

Tuberculosis can be either active or latent. Active TB can cause symptoms such as fever, weight loss, night sweats, a cough, chest pain, and fatigue. Active TB usually shows up on a chest X-ray.

Latent TB, however, usually does not cause any symptoms and will not show up on a chest X-ray. Most people who are infected with TB have latent TB. Their bodies are able to stop the bacteria from growing. The bacteria become inactive but remain alive in the body and can become active later.

In most pregnant women, treatment of latent TB should be delayed until 2 or 3 months after delivery. If TB is latent but threatens to become active, treatment should start right away. There are many drugs used to treat latent TB, and you will have to take medication for 2–9 months. It is important to finish the treatment. It is safe to breastfeed if you are still being treated after the baby is born.

If you have active TB, you will need treatment with several medications for at least 9 months. Most of the drugs used to treat TB are safe to use during pregnancy. The baby also may be given treatment for TB after birth to pre-

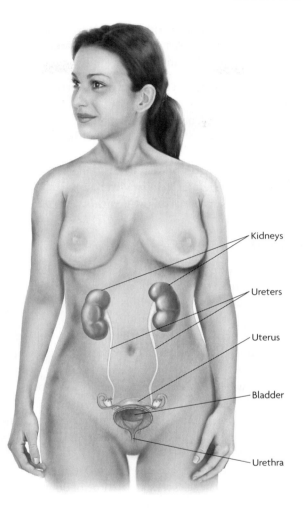

Kidneys

Ureters

Uterus

Bladder

Urethra

Female urinary tract. If not treated, an infection of the bladder can spread to the kidneys.

vent infection. After birth, you and the baby may need to be kept apart for some time until you are no longer contagious.

Sexually Transmitted Diseases

Sexually transmitted diseases (STDs) are infections that are spread by sexual contact. They can be caused by bacteria, viruses, or parasites. STDs can cause severe damage to your body if they are not diagnosed and treated.

Some STDs can be harmful during pregnancy. Pregnant women receive screening for some STDs as part of their routine prenatal care. It also is important to protect yourself against STDs by following these guidelines:

- Limit your sexual partners. The more sexual partners you have, the higher your risk of getting STDs.
- Know your partner. Ask about your partner's sexual history. Ask whether he or she has had STDs. Even if your partner has no symptoms, he or she still may be infected.
- Use a condom. Both male and female condoms are sold over-the-counter in drug stores. They help protect against STDs.
- Avoid contact with any sores on the *genitals.*

Genital Herpes

Genital herpes is an infection that can cause painful sores and blisters on or around the sex organs as well as on the mouth, eyes, and fingers. Other symptoms include swollen glands, fever, chills, muscle aches, fatigue, and nausea. Sometimes, however, there are no symptoms.

The infection is spread by direct contact with a person who has active sores. In some cases, the virus can be passed to others even when the sores have healed. Although the sores heal, the virus stays in your body until some event triggers a new bout, and a new outbreak of sores occurs. For most people, these outbreaks are not as painful or severe as the initial outbreak.

There is no cure for genital herpes. Antiviral medications are available that may prevent some outbreaks or decrease their length or severity. These medications must be taken every day.

In rare cases, newborns can become infected with the herpes virus during birth if the mother has herpes sores at the time of delivery. Newborn herpes infection can cause damage to the nervous system, blindness, mental retardation, or death. The risk is increased when a woman gets herpes for the first time late in pregnancy.

If you have ever had genital herpes or have had sex with someone who has, tell your health care provider. For women with a history of herpes, antiviral medication may be recommended during the last 4 weeks of your pregnancy. This treatment has been shown to reduce the recurrence of herpes at delivery. If you have had herpes in the past but have no herpes sores at the time of delivery, the baby can be born vaginally. If there are signs of active infection when you are in labor, you may need to have your baby by cesarean delivery to decrease the chance the baby will be infected.

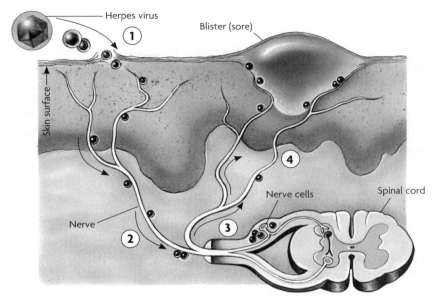

Herpes virus

Blister (sore)

Skin surface

Nerve cells

Spinal cord

Nerve

How herpes reappears after you are infected. When you are first infected, the herpes virus passes through your skin (1). It travels along nerves (2) and settles at nerve cells near your spine (3). If something triggers the virus, it travels back along the nerves (4) to the surface of the skin, and a new outbreak occurs.

If your sexual partner has herpes, you need to take extra steps to avoid becoming infected during pregnancy. Your health care provider may recommend antiviral medication for you or your partner. You should use condoms during sex (although condoms are only 50% effective in reducing transmission of the herpes virus). In the last 6–8 weeks of pregnancy, you should not have sexual contact if your partner has an outbreak (if your partner has oral herpes, oral–genital contact should be avoided).

Gonorrhea and Chlamydia

Both *gonorrhea* and *chlamydia* are caused by bacteria. Women 25 years and younger are at greater risk for both of these infections, although they can occur at any age. These infections can occur in the mouth, reproductive organs, and rectum. In women, the most common place these infections occur is the *cervix.* From the cervix, the bacteria can spread into the *uterus* and *fallopian tubes* and cause *pelvic inflammatory disease (PID).* PID is a serious infection that can damage the fallopian tubes, which can lead to infertility. Scarring in the fallopian tubes as a result of the damage caused by PID also increases the risk of *ectopic pregnancy.*

Pregnant women who are infected with chlamydia or gonorrhea have an increased risk of miscarriage, **premature rupture of membranes,** and **preterm** birth. The infection can be passed from mother to baby. Babies born to infected mothers may have conjunctivitis (an infection of the eyes) or birth defects. Chlamydia may cause pneumonia in an infected infant. To prevent conjunctivitis, the eyes of all newborns are treated at birth whether or not the mother is infected or not.

Women with chlamydia or gonorrhea often have only mild symptoms or no symptoms at all. Symptoms may include the following:

• A discharge from a woman's vagina or a man's penis
• Painful or frequent urination
• Pain in the pelvis or abdomen
• Burning or itching in the vaginal area
• Redness or swelling of the **vulva**
• Bleeding between periods
• Sore throat with or without fever
• Swollen or enlarged lymph nodes

All pregnant women are tested for chlamydia early in pregnancy, and women with certain risk factors are screened later in pregnancy as well. Women at increased risk for gonorrhea or who have symptoms are tested for this infection early in pregnancy and may be tested again in the third trimester. Both infections can be treated with antibiotics during pregnancy.

Human Immunodeficiency Virus

Human immunodeficiency virus (HIV) is spread through contact with body fluids—mainly blood or semen—from an infected person. The most common ways that HIV is passed to others are by sexual contact and by sharing needles used to inject drugs.

Once in the body, HIV destroys cells that are part of the immune system—the body's natural defense against disease. This leaves the body open to infections that can cause death. When a person with HIV gets one of these infections or has a very low level of these immune-system cells, he or she is said to have **acquired immunodeficiency syndrome (AIDS).**

Once infected with HIV, there is no cure. An infected person will have the virus for the rest of his or her life. In most cases, a person who has been infected with HIV doesn't get sick right away because it can take 5 years or more for some people to get symptoms. Sometimes people infected with

HIV have a brief illness like the flu. Later symptoms can include weight loss, fatigue, swollen lymph nodes, night sweats, fever, diarrhea, and cough.

HIV can be passed from mother to baby during pregnancy, at the time of vaginal delivery, or during breastfeeding. In the United States, an estimated 120,000 to 160,000 women are living with HIV, and many do not know it. About 80% of these women are of childbearing age. For this reason, all pregnant women are tested for HIV as part of routine prenatal testing. If a pregnant woman finds out she is infected, she can start treatment. By starting treatment during pregnancy, the risk of the baby getting infected is greatly reduced. For best results, the medication for HIV should be taken during pregnancy, labor, and delivery. Some women may benefit from cesarean delivery. The baby will also be given the medication during the first 6 weeks of life. A woman infected with HIV should not breastfeed her baby.

Human Papillomavirus

Human papillomavirus (HPV) is a very common virus that can be passed from person to person. There are more than 100 types of HPV, and some are spread through sexual contact.

Like many other STDs, there often are no signs of HPV infection. However, a few types of HPV cause warts on your genitals and other parts of your body. Warts can be treated with medication applied to the area or you can have surgery to remove them. The type of treatment depends on where the warts are located.

Some types of HPV can cause cancer of the cervix. Human papillomavirus also may be linked to cancer of the anus, vulva, and vagina. Genital warts usually are not linked with cancer.

There is no cure for HPV, so it is best to try to prevent it. The Pap test is used to find changes in the cells of the cervix that could lead to cancer. Most women should have Pap tests on a regular basis. Using condoms with your sexual partner may reduce your risk of infection. There are also vaccines that protect against some types of HPV. You should not be given the HPV vaccine during pregnancy, but it is safe to get while breastfeeding.

Syphilis

Syphilis is caused by organisms called spirochetes. Syphilis occurs in stages. It is more easily spread in some stages than in others. If not treated, syphilis can cause heart and brain damage, blindness, paralysis, and death. If found early and treated, syphilis may cause less damage.

Syphilis can be passed from a pregnant woman's bloodstream to her baby. It may cause miscarriage, stillbirth, or premature rupture of membranes. Infants born with syphilis may have birth defects. Treating an infected infant after birth often prevents more damage from occurring, but it cannot reverse any harm already done.

Syphilis can be hard to detect in women. The sore that marks the site of infection—called a *chancre*—is painless. It may be in the vagina where it cannot be seen. A chancre appears only in the early stage of syphilis. Later symptoms are a rash, sluggishness, or slight fever.

In the very early stages of syphilis, a blood test may or may not find the disease. If a chancre is present, syphilis can be diagnosed by scraping tissue from the chancre. The chancre will go away even without treatment, but the infection remains. After the chancre goes away, the only sure way to diagnose syphilis is by a blood test.

All women are tested for syphilis early in pregnancy. Treatment during the first 3–4 months of pregnancy most likely will prevent any long-term damage.

Trichomoniasis

Trichomoniasis is caused by the microscopic parasite *Trichomonas vaginalis*. Women who have trichomoniasis are at an increased risk of infection with other STDs. Trichomoniasis can increase the risk of certain pregnancy problems, such as premature rupture of membranes and preterm birth.

Signs of trichomoniasis may include a yellow-gray or green vaginal discharge. The discharge may have a fishy odor. There may be burning, irritation, redness, and swelling of the vulva. Sometimes there is pain during urination. Often, a woman has mild or no symptoms. Trichomoniasis can be treated during pregnancy with medication.

Bacterial Vaginosis

An imbalance of the bacteria growing in the vagina can cause the infection *bacterial vaginosis*. It is the most common cause of a vaginal discharge that has a fishy odor. Bacterial vaginosis is not an STD. Some studies suggest that women who have the infection during pregnancy are at greater risk for *preterm* birth or *premature rupture of membranes*. Other studies do not show this association.

Bacterial vaginosis may cause a thin grayish or white discharge. The odor may be worse after intercourse. Itching around the vagina also may occur. However, 50% of women with bacterial vaginosis do not have any symptoms.

If during pregnancy bacterial vaginosis is diagnosed in a woman with symptoms, it is treated with medication.

Listeriosis

Listeriosis is a serious infection caused by eating food contaminated with the bacterium *Listeria monocytogenes*. Pregnant women are about 20 times more likely than other healthy adults to get listeriosis, and about one third of listeriosis cases happen during pregnancy.

If you get infected during pregnancy you may have symptoms similar to the flu. The infection is very serious, however, and can lead to miscarriage or stillbirth, premature delivery, or infection of the baby.

To lower your risk of getting listeriosis, take these precautions:

- Thoroughly cook raw food from animal sources, such as beef, pork, or poultry.
- Do not eat hot dogs, luncheon meats, bologna, or other deli meats unless they are reheated until steaming hot.
- Wash raw vegetables thoroughly before eating.
- Keep uncooked meats separate from vegetables and from cooked foods and ready-to-eat foods.
- Avoid unpasteurized (raw) milk or foods made from unpasteurized milk.
- Wash hands, knives, and cutting boards after handling uncooked foods.

Hepatitis

Hepatitis is a viral infection that affects the liver. The four common kinds of hepatitis infection are hepatitis A virus, **hepatitis B virus**, hepatitis C virus, and hepatitis D virus. Hepatitis A virus cannot be passed to others, and hepatitis D virus is rare. Hepatitis B virus is of the greatest concern during pregnancy because it is most likely to be passed to the baby.

Hepatitis B virus can be passed between people through infected body fluids, such as blood, semen, vaginal fluids, and saliva. The following activities put a person at increased risk for hepatitis B virus infection:

- Injecting drugs and sharing needles
- Having multiple sexual partners
- Working in a health-related job that exposes you to blood or blood products
- Living with someone infected with hepatitis B virus
- Receiving blood products (for example, for a clotting disorder)

Some people infected with hepatitis B virus have chronic hepatitis. Chronic hepatitis can be life threatening and cause **cirrhosis** (hardening) of the liver and liver cancer. Most people who get hepatitis can't pass it on to anyone else after the disease has run its course.

Some people with hepatitis B virus may not feel sick or show any signs of the disease. They are **carriers** of the infection. They keep the virus in their bodies all their lives and can pass it to other people.

All pregnant women should be given a blood test for the hepatitis B virus. The infection can be hard to find without testing because its symptoms—nausea and vomiting—often occur in pregnancy anyway. If you might be infected, your health care provider may give you **hepatitis B immune globulin**. It contains antibodies to the virus. It can make the illness less severe. Rest, a healthy diet, and liquids also may be prescribed.

A woman who is a carrier can pass the hepatitis B virus to her baby at birth. Whether the baby will get the virus depends on when the mother was infected. If it was early in pregnancy, the chances are less than 10% that the baby will get the virus. If it was late in pregnancy, there is up to a 90% chance the baby will be infected. Hepatitis may be severe in babies and can be life threatening. Even babies who appear well may be at risk for serious health problems.

Infected newborns have a high risk (up to 90%) of becoming chronic hepatitis B carriers. If they become carriers, as adults they have a 25% risk of dying of cirrhosis or liver cancer.

There is a vaccine to prevent hepatitis B virus infection. Any teen or adult with a high risk of getting the hepatitis B virus should be vaccinated. All infants should get the vaccine too. The vaccine is given in three doses. The first two doses are given 1 month apart, and the third is given 6 months later.

Babies born to infected mothers also will receive hepatitis B immune globulin soon after birth. With this treatment, the chance of the baby getting the infection is only 1 in 20. If the baby is given the vaccine, it is safe to breastfeed.

Rubella

Rubella (also known as German measles) is a virus that causes fever, swollen lymph glands, joint pain, and a rash. Rubella is very rare in the United States because most people are vaccinated against it as children.

If you were never vaccinated in your childhood, it is possible for you to become infected as an adult and during pregnancy. If this happens, rubella can be dangerous. The infection can cause miscarriage or birth defects.

Testing for rubella is done as part of early *prenatal care*. If you are not immune, you will not be given the rubella vaccine during pregnancy. You can be vaccinated, though, after you give birth to protect you in the future.

Cytomegalovirus

Cytomegalovirus (CMV) is the most common virus transmitted during pregnancy. Women at highest risk for CMV are health care and lab workers, mothers of young children in child care, and child care providers.

Cytomegalovirus is hard to detect because it rarely causes symptoms. When it does, however, the symptoms include fever, sore throat, and fatigue. Infected women can pass it to their babies during pregnancy, birth, or by breastfeeding. However, healthy full-term babies born to women infected with CMV have protective antibodies, and they can be breastfed without any problems.

When a woman has CMV for the first time during pregnancy, there is a greater risk of her passing it to her baby during birth. It can cause serious problems including *jaundice* (yellow skin), neurologic problems, and hearing loss.

If you are at high risk for CMV, talk with your health care provider about being tested. If you are diagnosed with the infection, *amniocentesis* may be recommended to check for the infection in the baby. The baby will be monitored closely by *ultrasound* as well.

Toxoplasmosis

Toxoplasmosis is an infection caused by a parasite that usually is passed to people through undercooked contaminated meat or from animals. Toxoplasmosis may cause no symptoms. When symptoms do appear, they are like flu symptoms, such as fatigue and muscle aches. If you were infected before you were pregnant, you won't pass toxoplasmosis on to your baby. You can, however pass it on to your baby if you are infected for the first time while you are pregnant.

Although you may not have symptoms, there is a possibility of serious problems for the baby, such as diseases of the nervous system and eyes. If you are infected during pregnancy, medication is available. You and your baby should be closely monitored during your pregnancy and after your baby is born.

Cats that go outside and hunt wild prey play a role in the spread of toxoplasmosis. They become infected by eating infected rodents, birds, or other small animals. The parasite then is passed in the cat's feces. You don't have to get rid of your cat while you are pregnant, but you need to take some precautions:

- Only eat meat that has been thoroughly cooked.

- Wash cutting boards, counters, utensils, and hands with hot soapy water after contact with raw meat, poultry, seafood, or unwashed fruits or vegetables.

- Wear gloves when gardening and during any contact with soil or sand because it might be contaminated with cat feces.

- Wash hands thoroughly after gardening or contact with soil or sand.

- If you own a cat that goes outdoors, avoid changing cat litter if possible. If no one else can do it, wear disposable gloves and wash your hands thoroughly with soap and water afterwards. Change the litter daily. (Clean litter is not dangerous. It's only used cat litter that can transmit the infection.)

- Do not adopt or handle stray cats, especially kittens. Do not get a new cat while you're pregnant.

Parvovirus

Parvovirus is a contagious infection also known as "fifth disease." It's common among school children, and if you had it during your childhood, you aren't likely to get it again.

Parvovirus can cause cold-like symptoms, followed by a rash on the cheeks, arms, and legs. It also often causes pain and swelling in the joints that can last from days to weeks.

If you think you have been exposed to parvovirus or are having any of the symptoms, see your health care provider so that you can have a blood test to confirm whether you have been infected. Parvovirus rarely causes problems for pregnant women. In a few cases, there may be a chance of **anemia** in the baby. If you are diagnosed with parvovirus, your health care provider will monitor you and the baby to make sure you both stay in good condition.

Influenza

Influenza (the flu) is a contagious infection of the respiratory system. It is caused by a virus. Major symptoms are fever, headache, fatigue, muscle aches, coughing, congestion, runny nose, and sore throat. Pregnancy can increase the risk for complications from the flu, such as pneumonia.

All women who are pregnant during the flu season (October through March) should be vaccinated against the flu. Protection from the vaccine usually begins 1–2 weeks after getting your flu shot. The protection lasts 6 months or longer. A flu shot is considered safe at any stage of pregnancy. However, the nasal flu mist vaccine is not approved for use in pregnant women.

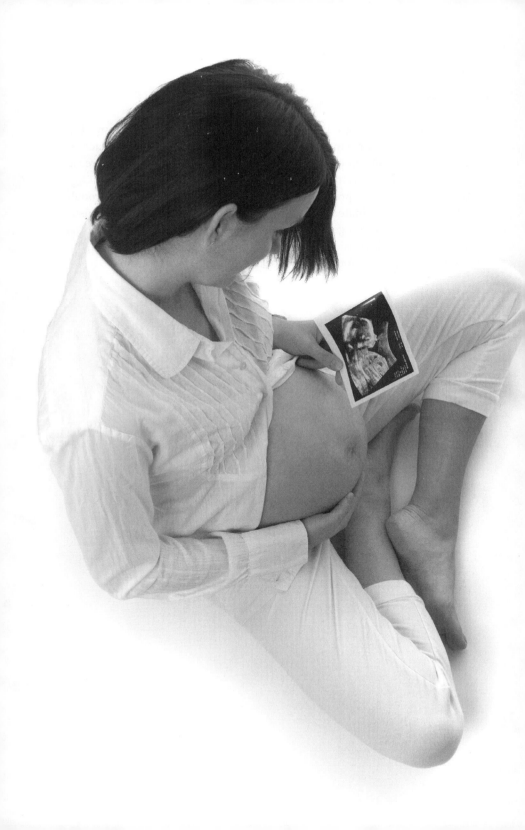

Chapter 27
Growth Problems

In some pregnancies, the unborn baby does not grow and develop normally. Babies can be too small or too large, both of which can cause complications for the baby and the mother. Your health care provider will monitor you throughout your pregnancy for both of these conditions.

Intrauterine Growth Restriction

When a developing baby is smaller than expected, it can be because the baby is smaller than average or it can be because the baby is having trouble growing. The term "intrauterine growth restriction" (IUGR) is used to describe babies who are developing in the *uterus* and whose estimated weight appears to be less than expected. The term "small for gestational age" (SGA) is used to describe babies who are born at a weight that is below normal. Babies are considered to be SGA when they are born smaller than 9 out of 10 babies at the same gestational age.

About 25% of stillborn babies will have IUGR. Up to half of babies affected by IUGR have complications such as heart rate abnormalities during labor and delivery. There also may be long-term consequences, such as behavioral and developmental problems, for some babies who are born too small. The risk of having long-term complications depends on the cause of IUGR and its severity. Some babies will have no long-term complications, whereas others will be severely affected. For example, if SGA is the result of a problem with the *placenta* but the baby is otherwise normal, the baby probably will "catch up" in weight by the age of 2 years.

Risk Factors

The mother's health can be one of the main risk factors for IUGR. Having chronic health problems such as the following conditions put you at more at risk:

- High blood pressure
- *Kidney* disease
- *Lupus*
- *Diabetes mellitus*
- Certain heart diseases
- Severe *anemia*

The use of certain drugs to treat some medical conditions, such as hypertension, also can lead to IUGR. Certain pregnancy conditions can increase the risk of IUGR, including multiple pregnancies and placental problems. Certain infections, such as cytomegalovirus, increase the risk of IUGR. Conditions that affect the baby, such as some genetic disorders, may cause IUGR.

Intrauterine growth restriction also is caused by having poor nutrition and unhealthy lifestyle habits during pregnancy. Smoking, alcohol use, and use of illegal drugs are known risk factors for IUGR. A pregnant woman who smokes is three and one half times more likely to have an SGA baby than nonsmokers. It's not known for certain how much alcohol it takes to affect the baby's weight, but it appears that the more a woman drinks, the greater the risk of having a smaller than normal baby. Illegal drugs, such as heroin and cocaine, greatly increase the risk of having an SGA baby. In fact, up to 50% of women who abuse heroin during pregnancy and up to 30% of women who abuse cocaine have babies affected by SGA.

Diagnosis

There are several ways that IUGR is found during pregnancy. Many of the exams that you have during *prenatal care* visits are designed to find this problem as early as possible:

- *Fundal height measurement*—Beginning at about month 5 of your pregnancy, your health care provider will measure the fundal height—the distance from your pubic bone to the top of your uterus. This measurement allows your health care provider to assess your baby's size and growth rate (see pages 96–97).

- *Ultrasound exam*—Between week 18 and week 22, you may have an **ultrasound** examination. During this exam, measurements are taken of the baby that are used to estimate his weight.

The drawback of these methods is that they are not very accurate. About 50% of cases of IUGR are not detected during pregnancy.

If your health care provider suspects that you have IUGR as a result of these methods, or if you have risk factors for IUGR, you will have more frequent ultrasound exams—about every 3–6 weeks to track the growth of your baby throughout your pregnancy. Other exams that also may be done on a regular basis are Doppler velocimetry (a special ultrasound exam that measures the blood flow in the baby's umbilical artery), nonstress test, contraction stress test, and biophysical profile. These tests are discussed in Chapter 28, "Testing to Monitor Fetal Health."

Management

An effort will be made to determine the cause of your baby's IUGR. If a medical condition is thought to be the cause, for example, your health care provider will make sure that you are getting the optimal treatment. If a genetic disorder is suspected, you may have tests to find out the type of disorder. But even if the cause is found, there is little that can be done during pregnancy to reverse IUGR. Stopping smoking, however, has been shown to be helpful. Women who stop smoking before 16 weeks of pregnancy have infants with birth weights similar to those of babies of women who never smoked. Even stopping as late as the seventh month can have a positive effect on the baby's weight.

Prevention

You can improve your chances of having a normal-weight baby by following healthy eating habits and making sure you're getting all the proper nutrients recommended by your health care provider and in the month-to-month sections of this book. What's even more crucial is giving up any lifestyle habits you may have that could be harmful. Do not drink alcohol or smoke while you are pregnant. If you are using illegal drugs, such as heroin or cocaine, get counseling right away to help you stop.

Taking steps to prevent having a baby that is smaller than normal is important. Talk with your doctor honestly if you are having trouble giving up unhealthy habits so he or she can get you the help you need.

Macrosomia

Macrosomia is the term that describes a baby that has grown very large—one that weighs more than about 4,000–4,500 grams at birth (between 8 pounds,

13 ounces and 9 pounds, 14 ounces). Several risk factors are associated with macrosomia, including pregestational and gestational *diabetes mellitus*, a prior history of macrosomia, being overweight before pregnancy, excessive weight gain during pregnancy, having had more than one child, and having a male baby.

Diabetes can lead to macrosomia if your blood sugar level is high throughout pregnancy. The baby receives too much sugar and can grow too large. Because macrosomia can cause problems during delivery, it is important to manage your diabetes and follow your health care provider's advice closely (see Chapter 19, "Diabetes Mellitus," for more discussion on diabetes during pregnancy).

Diagnosis

Like SGA, it is difficult to diagnose macrosomia. It is only diagnosed with certainty after the baby is born. Measuring fundal height and feeling the abdomen, as well as ultrasound exams, may be used to help diagnose macrosomia.

Complications

Macrosomia can cause complications for both mother and baby. The most common are problems with labor and delivery. Women who have large babies are more likely to have *cesarean deliveries*. The baby can be affected by a difficult delivery—large babies are at greater risk for low *Apgar scores* (see Chapter 12, "The Postpartum Period") and are more likely to need specialized care in a neonatal intensive care unit.

Shoulder dystocia is a problem during labor and delivery and occurs when the baby's shoulders are too big (wide) to fit through the mother's birth canal. Although shoulder dystocia also can occur during delivery of normal-sized babies, it happens more often in cases of macrosomia. It cannot be predicted before labor. It can lead to injury of the baby, including fracture of the collarbone and damage to the brachial plexus. The brachial plexus is a collection of nerves near the shoulder. These nerves can become compressed or stretched, and this compression can lead to a condition called Erb-Duchenne palsy. This condition often resolves on its own by 1 year of age. Brachial plexus injury is rare, and it also can occur in babies of normal size, during cesarean deliveries, and in the absence of shoulder dystocia.

When a baby's shoulders are having difficulty passing through the birth canal, the health care provider can try to change your position to open the pelvis wider. There are also a number of techniques that can be used to ease delivery of the baby's shoulders and prevent injury.

Suspected macrosomia in itself is not always an indication for cesarean delivery, because predicting macrosomia before birth is so inaccurate, and because cesarean deliveries carry more risks for mothers than vaginal deliveries. Damage to the baby can still occur even when a cesarean delivery is performed. Cesarean delivery is indicated, however, if the baby is estimated to weigh more than 5,000 grams (about 11 pounds) in women without diabetes mellitus and more than 4,500 grams in women with diabetes mellitus.

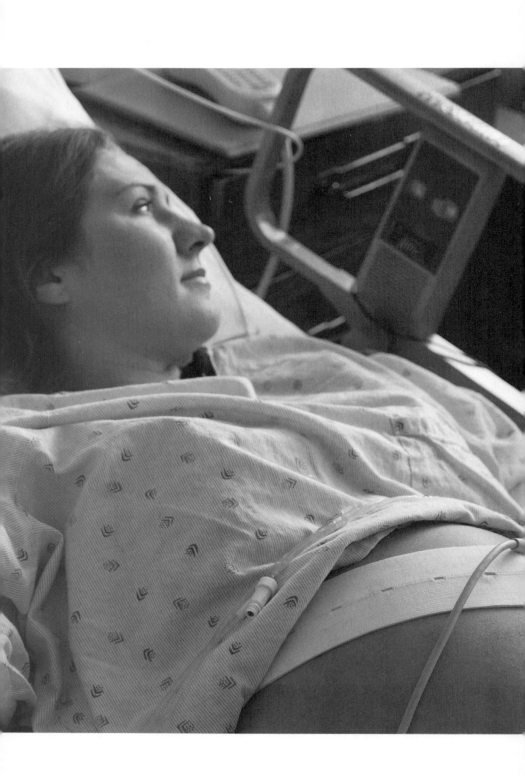

Chapter 28
Testing to Monitor Fetal Health

There are many different techniques that are available to check the well-being of your baby throughout your pregnancy. These tests may be done to confirm other test results or to provide your doctor with additional information. The results of these tests will help assure you and your doctor that your pregnancy is going well or tell you whether you may need special care.

The need for and the type of tests that are done depend on the stage of your pregnancy, any risk factors, and the results of routine tests. Some maternal conditions that may require more frequent testing include the following:

- Blood disorders
- Thyroid disease
- Heart disease
- *Lupus*
- *Kidney disease*
- *Diabetes mellitus*
- High blood pressure

Some pregnancy-related conditions that may signal a need for more frequent testing include the following:

- High blood pressure from pregnancy
- Decreased fetal movement
- Too much or too little *amniotic fluid*
- Fetal growth problems
- *Postterm pregnancy*
- *Rh sensitization*

- Prior fetal death
- *Multiple pregnancy,* if there are complications

No test is perfect. Keep in mind that tests cannot always find a problem, or the results may show that there is a problem when one does not exist.

When Tests Are Done

In most cases, special testing is started between 32 and 34 weeks of the pregnancy. If your baby has growth problems or you have more than one condition, you might be tested as early as 26 weeks. Your health care provider decides when to begin testing based on the following factors:

- Whether the baby can survive if delivered early
- How serious the mother's condition is
- The risk of *stillbirth*

Types of Special Tests

The tests used to monitor fetal health include fetal movement counts, ultrasound, Doppler ultrasound, nonstress test, biophysical profile, and contraction stress test. Some of these tests may be repeated regularly until delivery as long as the pregnancy is still at risk. Some tests are done weekly. In certain high-risk cases, they may be done twice weekly.

Fetal Movement Counts

Fetal movement counting (also called "kick counts") is a test that you can do at home. Your health care provider will tell you how often to do it and when to notify him or her.

One way to do kick counts is to note how long it takes your baby to make 10 movements. If it takes fewer than 2 hours, the result is "reassuring" (which means that all is going well at the time). Once you have felt 10 movements, you can stop counting that day. This test is repeated daily. Another way to do kick counts is to note fetal movements for 1 hour 3 times a week. You should feel at least as many movements as you have usually felt before.

Whichever method you use, be sure that you are counting fetal movements. Don't count the baby's hiccups, for instance. Also, when doing your kick counts, choose a time when the baby is most active, such as after you have had a meal.

If you do not feel enough movement, your health care provider may do other tests to check the baby. These tests include the nonstress test and amniotic fluid assessment, biophysical profile, modified biophysical profile, or contraction stress test.

Ultrasound

An **ultrasound** creates pictures or sounds of the baby from sound waves. It does not cause any harm to you or the baby. An ultrasound provides useful information about your pregnancy:

* The baby's age
* Estimated weight of your baby
* Position of the **placenta**
* The baby's position, movement, breathing, and heart rate
* Amount of amniotic fluid in your uterus
* Whether you are carrying multiples

Ultrasound also is used along with other tests to screen for birth defects in early pregnancy. If you have bleeding or pelvic pain, ultrasound may be done to find the cause.

When performed by a trained technician for medical reasons, ultrasound is safe during pregnancy. Ultrasonography without a medical reason—such as to find out the sex of the baby or to create a "keepsake" photo—is not recommended. It may even violate state or local laws or regulations. Ultrasonography is a medical tool that should be used only when there is a valid medial reason.

Your health care provider or a technician will perform the ultrasound exam using a device called a transducer. There are two types of transducers: one that is moved over the abdomen (**transabdominal ultrasound**) and one that is inserted into the **vagina** (**transvaginal ultrasound**).

For a transabdominal ultrasound exam, you will lie on your back on the table with your abdomen exposed. A gel will be used on your abdomen to improve the contact between the transducer and the skin surface. The transducer then is moved over your abdomen and records sound waves as they bounce off parts of your baby. These sound waves create images that are shown on a viewing screen. For a transvaginal ultrasound, a vaginal transducer is inserted in the vagina to help view the pelvic organs and the baby and delivers images the same way. Both types of ultrasound exams are shown on page 54.

If the baby is not growing well, ultrasound exams may be done every 2–4 weeks. If results are "nonreassuring" (which means that more information

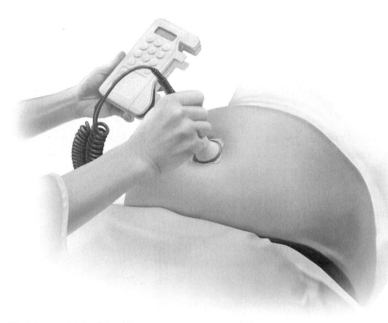

Listening to the fetal heartbeat. During this test, a small, handheld device is pressed against your abdomen to detect your baby's heartbeat.

is needed to make sure all is going well), other tests may be done. These include Doppler velocimetry, amniotic fluid assessment, or biophysical profile.

Doppler Velocimetry

Sometimes a special ultrasound test called Doppler velocimetry is used to check the blood flow in the baby's **umbilical cord**. It uses a type of ultrasound that allows the health care provider to both see and hear the waveform produced by ultrasound. This test may be performed if the baby is not growing normally or with other tests to detect fetal **anemia**.

Listening to the Fetal Heartbeat

The baby's heartbeat can be heard using a Doppler ultrasound device. Doppler ultrasound changes sound waves into signals that can be heard. A small, handheld device is pressed against your abdomen to detect your baby's heartbeat. With the Doppler device, the fetal heartbeat can be detected as early as 12 weeks of gestation.

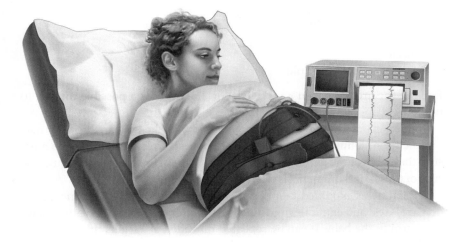

Electronic fetal monitoring. During these tests, you may wear a belt that has a Doppler ultrasound device.

Nonstress Test

The **nonstress test** measures the baby's heart rate in response to the baby's own movements—when the baby moves, the heart beats faster. These changes in your baby's heart rate are signs of good health.

The nonstress test can be performed in your health care provider's office or in a hospital or other health care facility. During the nonstress test, you lie on your back. A belt with Doppler ultrasound transducers is placed around your abdomen. You will be told to push a button each time you feel the baby move. This causes a mark to be made on a paper that is recording the fetal heart rate. (The nonstress test also can be done with a device that senses the baby's movement.) It takes 10–40 minutes to complete the test.

If the baby does not move for a while during the nonstress test, your baby may be asleep. A device like a buzzer may be used to produce sound and vibration to wake the baby and cause movement. This test is called vibroacoustic stimulation. The doctor also may suggest you have something to eat or drink to make the baby more active.

Biophysical Profile

The **biophysical profile** assesses the baby's well-being in these five areas during a 30-minute period:

1. Fetal heart rate (the nonstress test will be done again if results of the previous test were not reassuring)

2. Breathing movements
3. Body movements
4. Muscle tone
5. Amount of amniotic fluid

Each of the areas is given a score of 0 or 2 points, for a possible total of 10 points. A score of 8 or 10 is normal.

In measuring the amount of amniotic fluid, your health care provider may use the term "amniotic fluid index." For this test, ultrasound is used to measure the depth of the amniotic fluid in four different areas of your uterus. The sum of these measurements is the amniotic fluid index.

Sometimes a modified biophysical profile is performed. This includes a nonstress test and amniotic fluid index. The biophysical profile does not cause any harm to the baby. It can be repeated if needed at various times to check the baby's well-being. The score will help decide whether you need special care or whether your baby should be delivered sooner than planned.

Contraction Stress Test

The contraction stress test measures how the baby's heart rate reacts when the **uterus** contracts. To stimulate contractions, your health care provider will give you a drug called **oxytocin** or you may be asked to rub your nipples to make your uterus contract mildly. The baby's heart rate is recorded at the same time the contractions of the uterus are measured. The contraction stress test often is used if the nonstress test shows no change in the baby's heart rate when she moves. However, most health care providers now prefer the easier biophysical profile.

During a contraction, the blood flow to the **placenta** normally decreases for a brief time. This decrease in blood flow also briefly decreases the flow of oxygen to the baby. A healthy baby is not affected by this brief decrease in oxygen, and the baby's heart rate remains normal (the test result is negative). If the baby's heart rate decreases during a contraction (the test result is positive), it may indicate a problem. Several tests usually are performed if the results of a contraction stress test are positive.

Test Results

Results of these tests can help your health care provider detect any problems and treat them as needed. Results can confirm other test results or show the need for more testing. Keep in mind, however, that tests cannot always find a problem, or the results may indicate a problem when there isn't one.

Even if your test results are reassuring, tests may need to be repeated regularly to make sure the baby continues to do well for the rest of the pregnancy. If your results are nonreassuring, repeat tests can show your health care provider if results were accurate. Additional care for your baby may be necessary.

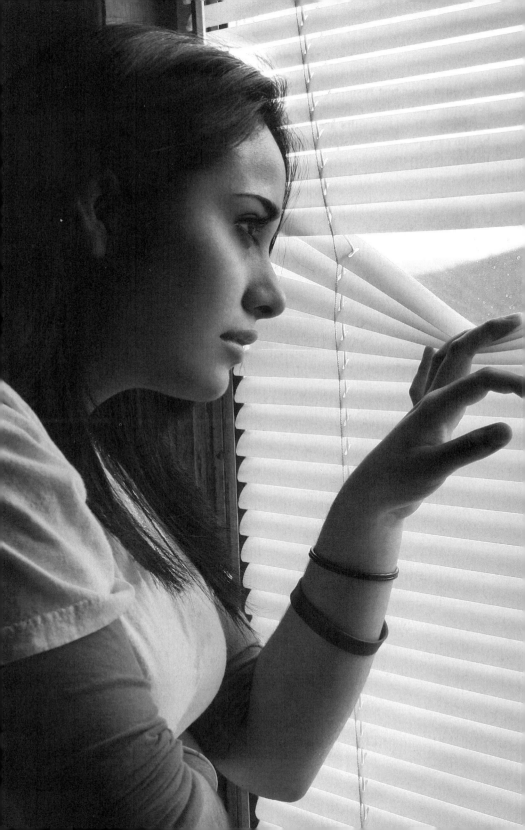

Chapter 29

Stillbirth

When a baby dies after 20 weeks of pregnancy, it is called a ***stillbirth***. The loss of a baby is tragic, and you will be faced with intense feelings of sadness and shock. It may help to understand what may have gone wrong, but you may never get an answer to this question. Most important, it will help to grieve however long you need and to have the support of your partner and loved ones during this difficult time.

What Went Wrong?

Perhaps the most difficult question for your health care provider to answer is what happened. Unfortunately, the reasons for many stillbirths are unknown. The death may have been caused by a birth defect. There also may be complications during labor and delivery that can cause a baby's death. These include problems with the ***placenta***, the ***umbilical cord***, infection, lack of oxygen, or maternal disease.

If there are concerns about your baby, ***ultrasound*** will be used to see if the baby is alive. If your baby dies in the ***uterus***, your health care provider will talk with you about the best options for delivery. Often, the best thing may be to induce labor. This decision depends on your health and the stage of your pregnancy. Your health care provider may recommend ***amniocentesis***, which may be able to provide information about the cause of the baby's death, such as infection or a genetic problem.

After the baby's birth, your health care provider may ask to do an autopsy—an exam of your baby's organs—to help find the cause of death. The placenta also may be examined to look for problems. Although the health care provider may not be able to tell the exact reason why your baby died, an autopsy may help answer questions about what happened.

Grieving

Grief is a normal, natural response to the loss of your baby. Mourn your loss for as long as you need. It's best to go through the complete grieving period to help you cope and move ahead. Remember that each parent grieves in a different way. It is important to talk with your partner or other person whom you trust about what you are feeling.

The Stages of Grief

Grieving includes a wide range of feelings. Just as each pregnancy is unique, ways to react to a pregnancy loss also are unique. The process you follow will be affected by your experiences with death, the culture you were raised in, your role in the family, and what you think others expect of you.

The death of a baby is a profoundly painful event. Your grief may last for years. The grieving process involves certain stages that can overlap and repeat. Each person who goes through the grieving process will heal in his or her own way. However, the process often seems to follow a common pattern in many people and consists of shock, numbness, and disbelief; searching and yearning; anger or rage; depression and loneliness; and acceptance.

Shock, Numbness, and Disbelief
When faced with news of their baby's death, parents often think that it is not really happening or that it can't be true. You may deny that the loss has occurred. You may have trouble grasping the news or feel nothing at all. Even though you and your partner may be together physically, you may each feel a very private sense of being alone or empty.

Searching and Yearning
These feelings tend to overlap with your initial shock and get stronger over time. You may start looking for a reason for your baby's death—who or what caused him or her to die. It is common during this stage to feel very guilty. You may think that somehow you brought about your baby's death and blame yourself for things you did or did not do. You may have dreams about the baby and yearn for what might have been.

Coping With the Pain

Grieving your loss will take time. There are a few things that may make dealing with the pain a little easier:

- *Saying good-bye*—Right after your baby is born, it is often helpful to hold your baby to say good-bye. The hospital staff may take pictures of your baby or give you keepsakes, such as the baby's cap, a handprint or footprint, an identification bracelet, or a crib card from your baby. If these things are not offered to you, ask for them.

- *Express yourself*—Talk about your feelings with your partner, family, and friends. It often helps to write down your thoughts in a journal or in letters to the baby and others.

- *Reach out*—Tell your family and friends what they can do to help you and your partner whether it's cooking a meal, doing house chores, running errands, or just spending time with you.

- *Take care of yourself*—Eat healthy, try to get enough sleep every night, and stay physically active. Avoid using alcohol or drugs to cope with the grief.

- *Choose a name*—Naming the baby helps give him or her an identity. A name allows you, your friends, and your family to refer to a specific child, not just "the baby you lost." You may want to use the name you first chose or pick another one.

- *Plan a funeral or memorial service*—For many parents, it's a great comfort to have family and friends acknowledge the life and death of their baby and to express their sorrow at a special service. You may wish to contact a funeral home for burial or cremation.

Anger or Rage

"What did I do to deserve this?" and "How could this happen to me?" are common questions after losing a baby. In this stage of grief you may direct your anger at your partner, the doctors or health care providers, the hospital staff, or even other women whose babies were born healthy. If you or your partner feel angry toward each other, it may be hard for you to comfort each other. It's good to accept your anger, express it, and try to get it out of your system. Anger becomes unhealthy if you turn it inward and direct it toward yourself.

Depression and Loneliness

In this stage, the reality sinks in that you have lost your baby. You may feel tired, sad, and helpless. You may have trouble getting back into your normal routine. The support from friends and family that you received during the early weeks of your loss may be gone, even though you still need comfort and kindness. Slowly you will start to get back on your feet and work through your loss.

Acceptance
In this final stage of grieving, you come to terms with what has happened. Your baby's death no longer rules your thoughts. You start to have renewed energy. Although you will never forget your baby, you begin to think of him or her less often and with less pain. You pick up your normal daily routine and social life. You laugh with friends and make plans for the future. You may feel ready to start planning your next pregnancy.

Anniversary days of your due date or the baby's birthday may be sad times. You need to plan your next pregnancy when you are physically and emotionally ready for another pregnancy (see "Another Pregnancy" on page 413).

As you come to terms with your baby's death, you may feel guilty about moving through the worst of your grief. However, it's okay to accept what has happened. A normal part of life is to start to plan for the future. Moving on does not mean that you will forget your baby; it just means that you are healing and are ready to accept what life has to offer.

You and Your Partner

Your relationship with your partner may be affected by the stress of the loss of your child. You may have trouble getting your thoughts and feelings across to each other. One or both of you may feel hostile toward the other. You may find it hard to have sex again or do other things together that you used to enjoy. This is normal. Try to be patient with each other. Let your partner know what your needs are and what you are feeling. Take time to be tender, caring, and close. Make an extra effort to be open and honest.

Throughout the grieving process, your partner may not respond in the same way as you do. Your partner may feel differently from you and may be able to move on before you are ready. Your partner may not want to talk about the loss when you are. Each person should be allowed to grieve in his or her own way. Try to understand and respond to your partner's needs as well as your own.

Seeking Support

Surround yourself with your partner, family, and friends for support during the coming months. Know you are not alone. A number of people have the knowledge and skills to help you. Ask your health care provider to direct you to support systems in your community. These can include childbirth educators, self-help groups, social workers, and clergy. Take time to find one that suits you best (see Resources).

Many grieving parents find it helpful to get involved with groups of parents who have gone through the same loss. Members of such support groups respect your feelings, understand your stresses and fears, and have a good sense of the kindness you need.

Professional counseling also can help to relieve your pain, guilt, and depression. Talking with a trained counselor can help you understand and accept what has happened. You may wish to get counseling for yourself only, for you and your partner, or for your entire family.

Another Pregnancy

Before thinking about getting pregnant again, allow time for you and your partner to work through your feelings. After losing a baby, some couples feel a need to have another baby right away. They think it will fill the empty feeling or take away the pain. A new baby cannot replace the baby that was lost. If you have another baby too soon after your loss, you may find it hard to think of the new child as a separate and special person.

Should you choose to have another pregnancy, keep in mind that the chances of losing another baby are very small in most cases. Even so, you may be anxious and worried during your next pregnancy. Talk with your health care provider about the baby's death. Find out the chances that it could happen again and what you can do to reduce these risks. Your doctor or care provider may suggest certain tests before or during your pregnancy to find problems as early as possible.

The Future

The pain of losing your baby will never vanish completely, but it will not always be the main focus in your life and thoughts. At some point you will be able to talk and think about the baby more easily and with less pain. One day you'll find yourself doing more of the things you used to do, such as enjoy favorite activities, renew friendships, and look forward to the future.

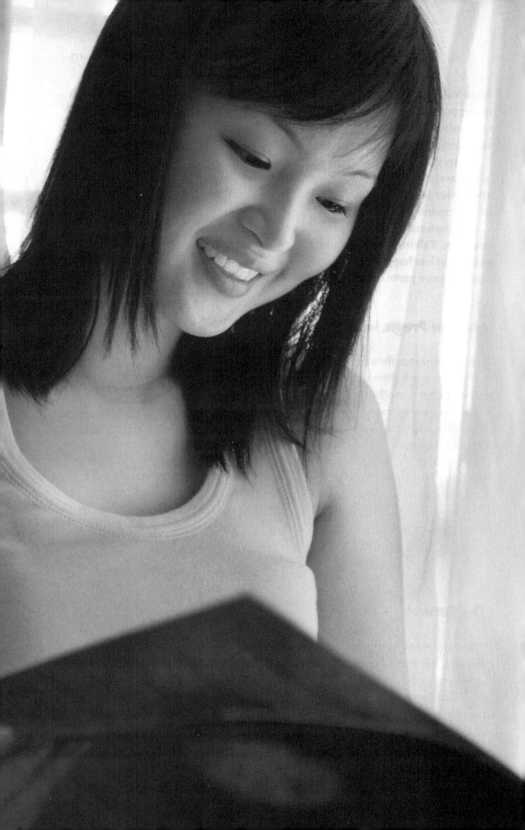

Glossary

Acquired Immunodeficiency Syndrome (AIDS): A group of signs and symptoms, usually of severe infections, occurring in a person whose immune system has been damaged by infection with human immunodeficiency virus (HIV).

Alpha-fetoprotein (AFP): A protein produced by a growing fetus; it is present in amniotic fluid and, in smaller amounts, in the mother's blood.

Amniocentesis: A procedure in which a needle is used to withdraw and test a small amount of amniotic fluid and cells from the sac surrounding the fetus.

Amniotic Fluid: Water in the sac surrounding the fetus in the mother's uterus.

Amniotic Sac: Fluid-filled sac in the mother's uterus in which the fetus develops.

Analgesic: A drug that relieves pain without causing loss of consciousness.

Anemia: Abnormally low levels of blood or red blood cells in the bloodstream. Most cases are caused by iron deficiency, or lack of iron.

Anencephaly: A type of neural tube defect that occurs when the fetus's head and brain do not develop normally.

Anesthesia: Relief of pain by loss of sensation.

Anesthetic: A drug used to relieve pain.

Anesthesiologist: A doctor who is an expert in pain relief.

Anorexia Nervosa: An eating disorder in which distorted body image leads a person to diet excessively.

Antibiotics: Drugs that treat infections.

Antibody: A protein in the blood produced in reaction to foreign substances.

Antidepressants: Medications used to treat depression.

Antigen: A substance, such as an organism causing infection or a protein found on the surface of blood cells, that can induce an immune response and cause the production of an antibody.

Apgar Score: A measurement of a baby's response to birth and life on its own, taken 1 and 5 minutes after birth.

Areola: The darker skin around the nipple.

Assisted Reproductive Technologies: A group of infertility treatments in which an egg is fertilized by a sperm outside of the body; the fertilized egg is then transferred to the uterus.

Autoimmune Disorder: A condition in which the body attacks its own tissues.

Bacterial Vaginosis: A type of vaginal infection caused by the overgrowth of a number of organisms that are normally found in the vagina.

Biophysical Profile: An assessment by ultrasound of fetal breathing, fetal body movement, fetal muscle tone, and the amount of amniotic fluid. May include fetal heart rate. Sometimes the profile includes only the nonstress test and an estimate of the amniotic fluid.

Bladder: A muscular organ in which urine is stored.

Braxton Hicks Contractions: False labor pains.

Breech Presentation: A situation in which a fetus's buttocks or feet would be born first.

Bulimia: An eating disorder in which a person binges on food and then forces vomiting or abuses laxatives.

Calcium: A mineral stored in bone that gives it hardness.

Calorie: A unit of heat used to express the fuel or energy value of food.

Carrier: [genetics] A person who shows no signs of a particular disorder but could pass the gene on to his or her children.

Carrier: [infections]: A person who is infected with the organism of a disease without showing symptoms and who can transmit the disease to others.

Catheter: A tube used to drain fluid or urine from the body.

Cell: The smallest unit of a structure in the body; the building blocks for all parts of the body.

Cephalopelvic Disproportion: A condition in which a baby is too large to pass safely through the mother's pelvis during delivery.

Cervix: The opening of the uterus at the top of the vagina.

Cesarean Delivery: Delivery of a baby through incisions made in the mother's abdomen and uterus.

Chancre: A sore appearing at the place of infection.

Chlamydia: A sexually transmitted disease caused by bacteria that can lead to pelvic inflammatory disease and infertility.

Chloasma: The darkening of areas of skin on the face during pregnancy.

Chorionic Villi: Microscopic, finger-like projections that make up the placenta.

Chorionic Villus Sampling (CVS): A procedure in which a small sample of cells is taken from the placenta and tested.

Chromosomes: Structures that are located inside each cell in the body and contain the genes that determine a person's physical makeup.

Cirrhosis: A disease caused by loss of liver cells, which are replaced by scar tissue that impairs liver function.

Colostrum: A fluid secreted in the breasts at the beginning of milk production.

Congenital Disorder: A condition that is present in a baby when it is born.

Contraction Stress Test: A test in which mild contractions of the mother's uterus are induced and the fetus's heart rate in response to the contractions is recorded using an electronic fetal monitor.

Corticosteroids: Hormones given to mature fetal lungs, for arthritis, or other medical conditions.

Crowning: The phase in Stage 2 of childbirth when a large part of the baby's scalp is visible at the vaginal opening.

Deep Vein Thrombosis: A condition in which a blood clot forms in veins in the leg or other areas of the body.

Depression: Feelings of sadness for periods of at least 2 weeks.

Diabetes Mellitus: A condition in which the levels of sugar in the blood are too high.

Digestive System: A system in the body made up of the stomach, bowels, liver, gallbladder, and pancreas. This system breaks down food and removes waste from the body.

Dilation: Widening of the opening of the cervix.

Dilation and Curettage (D&C): A procedure in which the cervix is opened and tissue is gently scraped or suctioned from the inside of the uterus.

Discordant: A large difference in the size of fetuses in a multiple pregnancy.

Down Syndrome: A genetic disorder in which mental retardation, abnormal features of the face and body, and medical problems such as heart defects occur.

Eclampsia: Seizures occurring in pregnancy and linked to high blood pressure.

Ectopic Pregnancy: A pregnancy in which the fertilized egg begins to grow in a place other than inside the uterus, usually in one of the fallopian tubes.

Edema: Swelling caused by fluid retention.

Egg: The female reproductive cell produced in and released from the ovaries; also called the ovum.

Electronic Fetal Monitoring: A method in which electronic instruments are used to record the heartbeat of the fetus and contractions of the mother's uterus.

Embryo: The developing fertilized egg from the time it implants in the uterus up to 8 completed weeks of pregnancy.

Endometriosis: A condition in which tissue similar to that normally lining the uterus is found outside of the uterus, usually on the ovaries, fallopian tubes, and other pelvic structures.

Endometrium: The lining of the uterus.

Epidural Block: A type of anesthesia given through a tube placed in the space at the base of the spine.

Episiotomy: A surgical incision made into the perineum (the region between the vagina and the anus) to widen the vaginal opening for delivery.

Estrogen: A female hormone produced in the ovaries.

External Cephalic Version: A technique, performed late in pregnancy, in which the doctor manually attempts to move a breech baby into the head-down position.

Fallopian Tubes: Tubes through which an egg travels from the ovary to the uterus.

Fertilization: Joining of the egg and sperm.

Fetal Alcohol Syndrome: A pattern of physical, mental, and behavioral problems in the baby that are thought to be due to alcohol abuse by the mother during pregnancy.

Fetal Blood Sampling: A procedure in which a sample of blood is taken from the umbilical cord and tested.

Fetal Monitoring: A procedure in which instruments are used to record the heartbeat of the fetus and contractions of the mother's uterus during labor.

Fetus: The developing offspring in the uterus from the ninth week of pregnancy until the end of pregnancy.

Fibroids: Benign growths that form in the muscle of the uterus.

Folic Acid: A vitamin that has been shown to reduce the risk of certain birth defects when taken in sufficient amounts before and during pregnancy.

Follicle-Stimulating Hormone (FSH): A hormone produced by the pituitary gland that helps an egg to mature.

Forceps: Special instruments placed around the baby's head to help guide it out of the birth canal during delivery.

Foreskin: A layer of skin covering the end of the penis.

Fraternal Twins: Twins that have developed from two fertilized eggs that are not genetically identical.

Gene: A DNA "blueprint" that codes for specific traits, such as hair and eye color.

General Anesthesia: The use of drugs that produce a sleep-like state to prevent pain during surgery.

Genital Herpes: A sexually transmitted disease caused by a virus that produces painful, highly infectious sores on or around the sex organs.

Genitals: The sexual or reproductive organs.

Gestational Age: The number of weeks that have elapsed between the first day of the last normal menstrual period and the date of delivery.

Gestational Diabetes Mellitus: Diabetes that arises during pregnancy.

Glucose: A sugar that is present in the blood and is the body's main source of fuel.

Gonadotropin-releasing Hormone (GnRH) Agonists: Medical therapy used to block the effects of certain hormones.

Gonorrhea: A sexually transmitted disease that may lead to pelvic inflammatory disease, infertility, and arthritis.

Hepatitis: Inflammation of the liver.

Hepatitis B Immune Globulin: A substance given to provide temporary protection against infection with hepatitis B virus.

Hepatitis B Virus (HBV): A virus that attacks and damages the liver, causing inflammation.

Hormones: Substances produced by the body to control the functions of various organs.

Human Chorionic Gonadotropin (hCG): A hormone produced during pregnancy; its detection is the basis for most pregnancy tests.

Human Immunodeficiency Virus (HIV): A virus that attacks certain cells of the body's immune system and causes acquired immunodeficiency syndrome (AIDS).

Human Papillomavirus (HPV): The name for a group of related viruses, some of which cause genital warts and are linked to cervical changes and cervical cancer.

Hydramnios: A condition in which there is an excess amount of amniotic fluid in the sac surrounding the fetus.

Hyperemesis Gravidarum: Severe nausea and vomiting during pregnancy that can lead to loss of weight and body fluids.

Hyperthyroidism: A condition in which the thyroid gland makes too much thyroid hormone.

Hypothyroidism: A condition in which the thyroid gland makes too little thyroid hormone.

Hysterectomy: Removal of the uterus.

Hysterosalpingography: A special X-ray procedure in which a small amount of fluid is placed into the uterus and fallopian tubes to detect abnormal changes in their size and shape or to determine whether the tubes are blocked.

Hysteroscopy: A procedure in which a slender, light-transmitting device, the hysteroscope, is inserted into the uterus through the cervix to view the inside of the uterus or perform surgery.

Identical Twins: Twins that have developed from a single fertilized egg that are usually genetically identical.

Immune System: The body's natural defense system against foreign substances and invading organisms, such as bacteria that cause disease.

Incontinence: Inability to control bodily functions such as urination.

Intrauterine Device (IUD): A small device that is inserted and left inside the uterus to prevent pregnancy.

Insulin: A hormone that lowers the levels of glucose (sugar) in the blood.

In Vitro Fertilization: A procedure in which an egg is removed from a woman's ovary, fertilized in a dish in a laboratory with the man's sperm, and then reintroduced into the woman's uterus to achieve a pregnancy.

Jaundice: A buildup of bilirubin that causes a yellowish appearance.

Kegel Exercises: Pelvic muscle exercises that assist in bladder and bowel control.

Kick Count: A record kept during late pregnancy of the number of times a fetus moves over a certain period.

Kidney: One of two organs that cleanse the blood, removing liquid wastes.

Labia: Folds of skin on either side of the opening of the vagina.

Lactation: Production of breast milk.

Lactose Intolerant: Being unable to digest dairy products.

Laminaria: Slender rods (natural and synthetic) inserted into the opening of the cervix to widen it.

Lanugo: The fine hair on the body of the fetus.

Laparoscopy: A surgical procedure in which a slender, light-transmitting instrument, the laparoscope, is inserted into the pelvic cavity through small incisions. The laparoscope is used to view the pelvic organs. Other instruments can be used to perform surgery.

Laxative: A product that is used to empty the bowels.

Linea Nigra: A line running from the navel to pubic hair that darkens during pregnancy.

Listeriosis: A type of food-borne illness caused by bacteria found in unpasteurized milk, hot dogs, luncheon meats, and smoked seafood.

Local Anesthesia: The use of drugs that prevent pain in a part of the body.

Lochia: Vaginal discharge that occurs after delivery.

Low Birth Weight: Weighing less than 5 ½ pounds at birth.

Lupus: An autoimmune disorder that causes changes in the joints, skin, kidneys, lungs, heart, or brain.

Luteinizing Hormone (LH): A hormone produced by the pituitary glands that helps an egg to mature and be released.

Macrosomia: A condition in which a fetus grows very large.

Masturbation: Self-stimulation of the genitals, usually resulting in orgasm.

Meconium: A greenish substance that builds up in the bowels of a growing fetus.

Menstruation: The monthly discharge of blood and tissue from the uterus that occurs in the absence of pregnancy.

Metabolism: The physical and chemical processes in the body that maintain life.

Miscarriage: Early pregnancy loss.

Molar Pregnancy: Growth of abnormal placental tissue in the uterus. Also called gestational trophoblastic disease (GTD).

Multiple Pregnancy: A pregnancy in which there are two or more fetuses.

Neural Tube Defect (NTD): A birth defect that results from incomplete development of the brain, spinal cord, or their coverings.

Nonstress Test: A test in which changes in the fetal heart rate are recorded, using an electronic fetal monitor.

Nuchal Translucency Screening: A test in which the size of a collection of fluid at the back of the fetal neck is measured by ultrasound to screen for certain birth defects, such as Down syndrome, trisomy 18, or heart defects.

Obesity: A condition characterized by excessive body fat.

Obstetrician–Gynecologist: A physician with special skills, training, and education in women's health.

Oral Contraceptives: Birth control pills containing hormones that prevent ovulation and thus pregnancy.

Orgasm: The climax of sexual excitement.

Osteoporosis: A condition in which the bones become so fragile that they break more easily.

Ovaries: Two glands, located on either side of the uterus, that contain the eggs released at ovulation and that produce hormones.

Ovulation: The release of an egg from one of the ovaries.

Oxytocin: A hormone used to help bring on contractions of the uterus.

Pap Test: A test in which cells are taken from the cervix and vagina and examined under a microscope.

Pelvic Exam: A manual examination of a woman's reproductive organs.

Pelvic Inflammatory Disease: An infection of the uterus, fallopian tubes, and nearby pelvic structures.

Penis: An external male sex organ.

Perineum: The area between the vagina and the rectum.

Pica: The urge to eat nonfood items.

Placenta: Tissue that provides nourishment to and takes waste away from the fetus.

Placental Abruption: A condition in which the placenta has begun to separate from the inner wall of the uterus before the baby is born.

Placenta Previa: A condition in which the placenta lies very low in the uterus, so that the opening of the uterus is partially or completely covered.

Polycystic Ovary Syndrome (PCOS): A condition characterized by two of the following three criteria: the presence of multiple cysts on the ovaries as seen by ultrasonography, irregular menstrual periods, and increased androgen levels. This syndrome may cause infertility and may increase the risk of diabetes and heart disease.

Postpartum Depression: Intense feelings of sadness, anxiety, or despair after childbirth that interfere with a new mother's ability to function and that do not go away after 2 weeks.

Postterm Pregnancy: A pregnancy that extends beyond 42 weeks.

Preeclampsia: A condition of pregnancy in which there is high blood pressure and protein in the urine.

Preimplantation Genetic Diagnosis: A type of genetic testing that can be done during *in vitro fertilization.* Tests are performed on the fertilized egg before it implants in the uterus.

Premature Rupture of Membranes: A condition in which the membranes that hold the amniotic fluid rupture before labor.

Prenatal Care: A program of care for a pregnant woman before the birth of her baby.

Preterm: Born before 37 weeks of pregnancy.

Progesterone: A female hormone that is produced in the ovaries and that prepares the lining of the uterus for pregnancy.

Progestin: A synthetic form of progesterone that is similar to the hormone produced naturally by the body.

Prostaglandins: Chemicals that are made by the body that have many effects, including causing the muscle of the uterus to contract, usually causing cramps.

Quickening: The mother's first feeling of movement of the fetus.

Rectum: The final segment of the digestive system.

Regional Anesthesia: The use of drugs to block sensation in certain areas of the body.

Respiratory Distress Syndrome (RDS): A condition of some babies in which the lungs are not mature and causes breathing difficulties.

Rh Immunoglobulin (RhIg): A substance given to prevent an Rh-negative person's antibody response to Rh-positive blood cells.

Screening Test: A test that looks for possible signs of disease in people who do not have symptoms.

Scrotum: The external genital sac in the male that contains the testes.

Sexual Intercourse: The act of the penis of the male entering the vagina of the female (also called "having sex" or "making love").

Sexually Transmitted Disease (STD): A disease that is spread by sexual contact, including chlamydial infection, gonorrhea, human papillomavirus infection, herpes, syphilis, and infection with human immunodeficiency virus (HIV, the cause of acquired immunodeficiency syndrome [AIDS]).

Sperm: A male cell that is produced in the testes and can fertilize a female egg cell.

Spermicides: Chemicals (creams, gels, foams) that inactivate sperm.

Spina Bifida: A neural tube defect that results from incomplete closure of the fetal spine.

Spinal Block: A form of anesthesia where medication is administered into the spinal fluid to lessen labor pain or provide anesthesia for a cesarean delivery.

Spleen: An organ located in the abdomen that stores blood, traps organisms for destruction by the immune system, and creates cells that dispose of old, worn-out red blood cells.

Sterilization: A permanent method of birth control.

Stillbirth: Delivery of a baby that shows no sign of life.

Sudden Infant Death Syndrome (SIDS): The unexpected death of an infant and in which the cause is unknown.

Surfactant: A substance produced by cells in the respiratory system that contributes to the elasticity of the lungs and keeps them from collapsing.

Syphilis: A sexually transmitted disease that is caused by an organism called *Treponema pallidum;* it may cause major health problems or death in its later stages.

Teratogens: Agents that can cause birth defects when a woman is exposed to them during pregnancy.

Testes: Two male organs that produce the sperm and male sex hormones.

Testosterone: A hormone that regulates male sex characteristics, such as a deep voice and beard. In men, it also regulates sperm production.

Tocolytic: A drug that slows contractions of the uterus.

Toxoplasmosis: An infection caused by *Toxoplasma gondii,* an organism that may be found in raw and rare meat, garden soil, and cat feces and can be harmful to the fetus.

Transabdominal Ultrasound: A type of ultrasound in which a transducer is moved across the abdomen.

Transducer: A device that emits sound waves and translates the echoes into electrical signals.

Transvaginal Ultrasound: A type of ultrasound in which a transducer specially designed to be placed in the vagina is used.

Transverse Incision: An incision used for cesarean delivery, made horizontally across the lower, thinner area of the uterus.

Trichomoniasis: A type of vaginal infection caused by a one-celled organism that is usually transmitted through sex.

Trimester: Any of the three 3-month periods into which pregnancy is divided.

Trisomy 18: A chromosomal disorder in which an individual has an extra 18th chromosome.

Tubal Ligation: Surgical sterilization procedure in which the fallopian tubes are blocked in order to prevent an egg from reaching the uterus.

Twin–Twin Transfusion Syndrome (TTS): A condition of identical twin fetuses when the blood passes from one twin to the other through a shared placenta.

Ultrasonography, Ultrasound: A test in which sound waves are used to examine internal structures. During pregnancy, it can be used to examine the fetus.

Umbilical Cord: A cord-like structure containing blood vessels that connects the fetus to the placenta.

Urethra: A short, narrow tube that conveys urine from the bladder out of the body.

Urine: A liquid that is excreted by the body and is made up of wastes, water, and salt removed from the blood.

Uterus: A muscular organ located in the female pelvis that contains and nourishes the developing fetus during pregnancy.

Vacuum Extraction: The use of a special instrument attached to the baby's head to help guide it out of the birth canal during delivery.

Vagina: A tube-like structure surrounded by muscles leading from the uterus to the outside of the body.

Vas Deferens: A small tube that carries sperm from a male testis to the prostate gland.

Vasectomy: A method of male sterilization in which a portion of the vas deferens is removed.

Veins: Blood vessels that carry blood from various parts of the body back to the heart.

Vernix: The greasy, whitish coating of a newborn.

Vertex Presentation: A normal position assumed by a fetus in which the head is positioned down ready to be born first.

Vulva: The external female genital area.

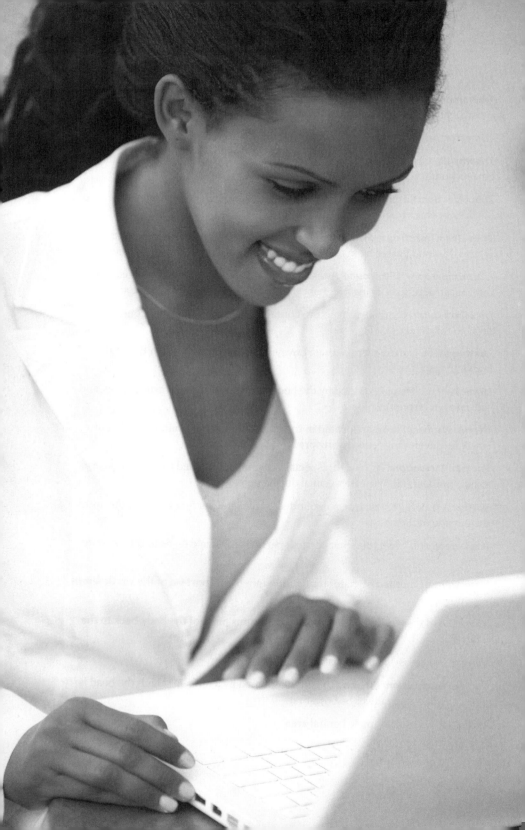

Resources

Birth Defects

March of Dimes
1275 Mamaroneck Avenue
White Plains, NY 10605-5201
(914) 997-4488
www.marchofdimes.com

Provides materials in English and Spanish on genetic conditions, birth defects, recommended newborn screening tests, and bereavement materials for pregnancy loss.

National Center on Birth Defects and Developmental Disabilities
1600 Clifton Road, MS E-86
Atlanta, GA 30333
(800) 232-4636
E-mail: cdcinfo@cdc.gov
www.cdc.gov/ncbddd

Provides information on birth defects, developmental disabilities, and hereditary blood disorders.

Breastfeeding

American Academy of Pediatrics (AAP)
141 Northwest Point Boulevard
Elk Grove Village, IL 60007
(847) 434-4000
Fax: (847) 434-8000
E-mail: lactation@aap.org
www.aap.org

Provides written materials about breastfeeding.

International Lactation Consultant Association (ILCA)
2501 Aerial Center Parkway, Suite 103
Morrisville, NC 27560
(919) 861-5577 or (888) ILCA-IS-U
Fax: (919) 459-2075
E-mail: info@ilca.org
www.ilca.org
Provides a directory of lactation consultants.

La Leche League International (LLLI)
PO Box 4079
Schaumburg, IL 60168-4079
(800) 525-3243 or (847) 519-7730
Fax: (847) 969-0460
E-mail: LLLI@LLLI.org
www.llli.org
Provides information and support on breastfeeding and referrals to local support groups.

National Women's Health Information Center Breastfeeding Helpline
(800) 994-9662
www.womenshealth.gov/breastfeeding/
Provides telephone support from breastfeeding information specialists and written materials in English, Spanish, and Chinese.

Childbirth Education and Assistance

American Academy of Husband-Coached Childbirth (The Bradley Method)
PO Box 5224
Sherman Oaks, CA 91413-5224
(800) 422-4784 or (818) 788-6662
www.bradleybirth.com
Provides information on natural childbirth and referrals to childbirth educators.

Association of Labor Assistants & Childbirth Educators (ALACE)
PO Box 390436
Cambridge, MA 02139
(877) 334-4207
E-mail: info@alace.org
www.alace.org
Provides referrals to childbirth educators and doulas.

Doulas of North America (DONA)
PO Box 626
Jasper, IN 47547
(888) 788-3662
Fax: (812) 634-1491
E-mail: doula@dona.org
www.dona.org
Provides referrals to birth doulas and postpartum doulas.

Hypnobirthing
5640 E. Bell Road #1073
Scottsdale, AZ 85254
(602) 788-6198
Fax: (602)466-2841
E-mail: hypnobirthing@hypnobirthing.com
www.hypnobirthing.com
Explains the HypnoBirthing® method; offers information about classes, books, articles, testimonials, and practitioner training.

International Cesarean Awareness Network (ICAN)
PO Box 98
Savage, MN 55378
(800) 686-4226
E-mail: info@ican-online.org
www.ican-online.org
Provides information about cesarean delivery and recovery.

International Childbirth Education Association (ICEA)
1500 Sunday Drive, Suite 102
Raleigh, NC 27607
(800) 624-4934 or (919) 863-9487
Fax: (919) 787-4916
E-mail: info@icea.org
www.icea.org
Offers lists of certified childbirth educators and doulas.

Lamaze International
2025 M Street NW, Suite 800
Washington, DC 20036-3309
(800) 368-4404 or (202) 367-1128
Fax: (202) 267-2128
E-mail: info@lamaze.org
www.lamaze.org
Provides information about pregnancy and childbirth and referrals to Lamaze-trained childbirth educators.

Cord Blood Donation

National Marrow Donor Program
3001 Broadway Street NE, Suite 100
Minneapolis, MN 55413-1753
(800) 627-7692
E-mail: patientinfo@nmdp.org
www.marrow.org

Provides information about storing and donating cord blood.

Domestic Violence

National Domestic Violence Hotline
PO Box 161810
Austin, TX 78716
(800) 799-7233 (voice) or (800) 787-3224 (TTY)
www.ndvh.org

Offers materials about abuse and domestic violence and has referrals to shelters and other community resources.

Environmental Exposure to Toxins

Motherisk
c/o the Hospital for Sick Children
555 University Avenue
Toronto, Ontario, Canada M5G 1X8
(416) 813-1500
E-mail: momrisk@sickkids.ca
www.motherisk.org

Answers questions about potential reproductive risks from exposure to drugs, chemicals, radiation, and infections during pregnancy and breastfeeding; will answer inquiries from Canada or the United States.

Organization of Teratology Information Specialists
University of Arizona
Drachman Hall
PO Box 210202
1295 N. Martin, Room B308
Tucson, AZ 85721-0202
(520) 626-3547
E-mail: contatus@otispregnancy.org
www.otispregnancy.org

Provides facts sheets about specific hazards and links to specialists who provide free information to patients and medical practitioners.

Teratology Society
1821 Michael Faraday Drive, Suite 300
Reston, VA 20190
(703) 438-3104
Fax: (703) 438-3113
E-mail: tshq@teratology.org
www.teratology.org

Supports research and provides information about substances that contribute to or cause birth defects.

Food Safety

U.S. Environmental Protection Agency
1200 Pennsylvania Avenue, NW
Washington, DC 20460
(202) 272-0167
www.epa.gov

Federal agency that conducts research, provides assessments, and educates the public about human health and environmental issues.

General

American College of Obstetricians and Gynecologists
PO Box 96920
Washington, DC 20090-6920
(202) 638-5577
E-mail: resources@acog.org
www.acog.org

Membership society of over 52,000 members that promotes excellence in women's health care through advocacy and education.

American College of Nurse-Midwives
8403 Colesville Road, Suite 1550
Silver Spring, MD 20910
(240) 485-1800
Fax: (240) 485-1818
E-mail: info@acnm.org
www.acnm.org

Membership society for certified nurse–midwives.

American Medical Association
311 S. Wacker Drive, Suite 5800
Chicago, IL 60606
(800) AMA-1150 or (312) 542-9000
Fax: (312) 542-9001
www.ama-assn.org
Membership society for physicians.

***Eunice Kennedy Shriver* National Institute of Child Health and Human Development (NICHD)**
PO Box 3006
Rockville, MD 20847
(800) 370-2943
Fax: (866) 760-5947
E-mail: NICHDInformationResourceCenter@mail.nih.gov
www.nichd.nih.gov
Provides information and education on pregnancy, infertility, preterm birth, birth defects, contraception, and sexually transmitted diseases.

National Healthy Mothers, Healthy Babies Coalition
200 N. Beauregard Street, 6th Floor
Alexandria, VA 22311
(703) 837-4792
Fax: (703) 684-5968
E-mail: info@hmhb.org
www.hmhb.org
Provides resources and education about healthy pregnancy and prenatal care.

National Women's Health Information Center
Office on Women's Health
Department of Health and Human Services
200 Independence Avenue, SW, Room 712E
Washington, DC 20201-0004
(800) 994-9662 or (202) 690-7650
Fax: (202) 205-2631
www.4woman.gov
Offers information and resources in Spanish and English about pregnancy, contraception, and diseases affecting women.

High-Risk Pregnancy

Confinement Line
c/o Childbirth Education Association
PO Box 1609
Springfield, VA 22151
(703) 941-7183

Provides telephone support and a newsletter for women confined to bed during pregnancy.

Sidelines National Support Network
PO Box 1808
Laguna Beach, CA 92652
(888) 447-4754
Fax: (949) 497-5598
E-mail: sidelines@sidelines.org
www.sidelines.org

Offers emotional support and resources for women with high-risk pregnancies.

Infertility

RESOLVE: The National Infertility Association
1760 Old Meadow Road, Suite 500
McLean, VA 22102
(703) 556-7172
Fax: (703) 506-3266
www.resolve.org

Provides information about fertility treatments and resources for infertile couples.

Loss and Grieving

CLIMB: Center for Loss in Multiple Birth, Inc.
PO Box 91377
Anchorage AK 99509
(907) 222-5321
E-mail: climb@pobox.alaska.net
www.climb-support.org

Offers support for families that have lost twins or high-order multiples during pregnancy and through infancy and childhood.

The Compassionate Friends
PO Box 3696
Oak Brook, IL 60522
(877) 969-0010 or (630) 990-0010
Fax: (630) 990-0246
E-mail: nationaloffice@compassionatefriends.org
www.compassionatefriends.org

Offers support for families experiencing grief following the death of a child of any age.

First Candle/ SIDS Alliance
1314 Bedford Avenue, Suite 210
Baltimore, MD 21208
(800) 221-7437
E-mail: info@firstcandle.org
www.sidsalliance.org

Supports research and education about sudden infant death syndrome; counseling service available at all times.

International Stillbirth Alliance
1314 Bedford Avenue, Suite 210
Baltimore, MD 21208
(800) 221-7437
E-mail: info@stillbirthalliance.org
www.stillbirthalliance.org

Supports stillbirth research, education, and awareness.

SHARE: Pregnancy and Infant Loss Support, Inc.
The National SHARE Office
402 Jackson Street
St. Charles, MO 63301
(636) 947-6164 or (800) 821-6819
Fax: (636) 947-7486
www.nationalshare.org

Offers support for families who have lost a baby through miscarriage, stillbirth, or newborn death.

Multiple Pregnancies

Mothers of Supertwins (MOST)
PO Box 306
East Islip, NY 11730-0306
(631) 859-1110
Fax: (631) 859-3580
E-mail: Info@MOSTonline.org
www.mostonline.org

Provides education, resources, and support during pregnancy, infancy, and childhood for families with triplets or higher numbers of babies.

National Organization of Mothers of Twins Clubs
2000 Mallory Lane, Suite 130-600
Franklin, TN 37067-8231
(248) 231-4880
E-mail: info@nomotc.org
www.nomotc.org

Provides support and practical advice for women expecting or rearing multiples.

Triplet Connection
PO Box 429
Spring City, UT 84662
(435) 851-1105
Fax: (435) 462-7466
E-mail: tc@tripletconnection.org
www.tripletconnection.org

Provides information and support for families preparing for or rearing multiples.

Nutrition

American Dietetic Association
120 South Riverside Plaza, Suite 2000
Chicago, IL 60606-6995
(800) 877-1600
E-mail: knowledge@eatright.org
www.eatright.org

Offers documents and information about nutrition during pregnancy and breastfeeding and provides referrals to nutrition professionals.

Special Supplemental Nutrition Program for Women, Infants, and Children (WIC Program)
Supplemental Food Programs Division
Food and Nutrition Science
U.S. Department of Agriculture
3101 Park Center Drive, Room 520
Alexandria, VA 22302
(703) 305-2746
Fax: (703) 305-2196
E-mail: wichq-web@fns.usda.gov
www.fns.usda.gov/wic
Provides supplemental foods, nutrition education, and health care referrals for low-income pregnant, postpartum, and breastfeeding women and for infants and children up to 5 years of age.

U.S. Department of Agriculture (My Pyramid Plan for Moms)
USDA Center for Nutrition Policy and Promotion
3101 Park Center Drive, Room 1034
Alexandria, VA 22302-1594
(888) 779-7264
E-mail: support@cnpp.usda.gov
www.mypyramid.gov/mypyramidmoms
Provides an interactive program for designing a personalized pregnancy diet.

Smoking and Substance Abuse

Alcoholics Anonymous
PO Box 459
New York, NY 10163
(212) 870-3400
www.aa.org
Nonprofit, self-supporting, international group that helps alcoholics achieve sobriety.

American Cancer Society
2200 Lake Boulevard NE
Atlanta, GA 30319
(800) ACS-2345
www.cancer.org
Offers tips for quitting smoking and staying quit.

Narcotics Anonymous
PO Box 9999
Van Nuys, CA 91409
(818) 773-9999
Fax: (818) 700-0700
E-mail: customer_service@na.org
www.na.org

Nonprofit group that helps drug addicts abstain from drugs.

National Clearinghouse for Alcohol and Drug Information
SAMHSA's Health Information Network
PO Box 2345
Rockville, MD 20847-2345
(800) 729-6686
Fax: (301) 443-5447
www.ncadi.samhsa.gov

Offers materials for prevention and intervention in alcohol and drug abuse and provides a directory of alcoholism and drug abuse treatment and prevention services nationwide.

National Organization on Fetal Alcohol Syndrome
900 17th Street, NW, Suite 910
Washington, DC 20006
(800) 666-6327 or (202) 785-4585
Fax: (202) 466-6456
E-mail: info@nofas.org
www.nofas.org

Offers education and information about fetal alcohol syndrome and provides a directory to drug and alcohol abuse treatment programs nationwide.

Quitnet
www.quitnet.org

Supplies an online support group for people quitting smoking.

Substance Abuse and Mental Health Services Administration
SAMHSA's Health Information Network
PO Box 2345
Rockville, MD 20847-2345
(877) 726-4727
Fax: (240) 221-4292
www.samhsa.gov/shin

Offers a locator service for mental health and substance abuse programs and providers.

Specific Concerns

DES Action
PO Box 7296
Jupiter, FL 33468
(800) 337-9288
E-mail: info@desaction.org
www.desaction.org

Provides materials in English and Spanish and support for people exposed to diethylstilbestrol (DES) in utero.

Group B Strep Association
PO Box 16515
Chapel Hill, NC 27516
E-mail: bstrep@mindspring.com
www.groupbstrep.org

Provides information in Spanish and English and referrals to promote testing and treatment of GBS.

Motherisk Hotline
c/o the Hospital for Sick Children
555 University Avenue
Toronto, Ontario, Canada M5G 1X8
(800) 436-8477
E-mail: momrisk@sickkids.ca
www.motherisk.org

Provides a hotline for questions about nausea and vomiting in pregnancy.

Tax Credit

U.S. Internal Revenue Service
(800) 829-1040
www.irs.gov

Travel Tips

International Travelers Hotline
(Operated by Centers for Disease Control and Prevention)
1600 Clifton Road
Atlanta, GA 30333
(888) 232-3228
www.cdc.gov

Provides safety tips about travel in and up-to-date vaccination facts for many countries.

The International Association for Medical Assistance to Travelers
1623 Military Road #279
Niagara Falls, NY 14304-1745
(716) 754-4883
www.iamat.org
Offers health information for travelers; maintains a database of physicians worldwide.

Workplace

Equal Employment Opportunity Commission (EEOC)
131 M Street NE
Washington, DC 20507
(202) 663-4900 or (800) 669-4000
E-mail: info@eeoc.gov
www.eeoc.gov
Agency of the United States government that enforces federal employment discrimination laws.

National Institute for Occupational Safety and Health (NIOSH)
Centers for Disease Control and Prevention
1600 Clifton Road
Atlanta, GA 30333
E-mail: cdcinfo@cdc.gov
www.cdc.gov/niosh/homepage.html
Identifies workplace hazards and suggests ways to limit the dangers; will inspect workplaces for hazards on request.

Occupational Safety and Health Administration (OSHA)
200 Constitution Avenue NW
Washington, DC 20010
(800) 321-6742
(877) 889-5627 (TTY)
www.osha.gov
Prevents work-related injuries, illnesses, and deaths by enforcing laws designed to protect workers' health and safety.

U.S. Department of Labor
200 Constitution Avenue NW
Washington, DC 20210
(866) 487-2365
www.dol.gov
(Family Medical Leave Act Information: www.dol.gov/dol/topic/benefits-leave/fmla.htm)
Administers various federal labor laws.

To calculate your body mass index, find your height in inches in the left column. Then look across the line to find your weight in pounds. The number at the top of that column is your body mass index (BMI).

Body Mass Index Table

	NORMAL						OVERWEIGHT					OBESE					
BMI	19	20	21	22	23	24	25	26	27	28	29	30	31	32	33	34	35
HEIGHT (Inches)	BODY WEIGHT (Pounds)																
58	91	96	100	105	110	115	119	124	129	134	138	143	148	153	158	162	167
59	94	99	104	109	114	119	124	128	133	138	143	148	153	158	163	168	173
60	97	102	107	112	118	123	128	133	138	143	148	153	158	163	168	174	179
61	100	106	111	116	122	127	132	137	143	148	153	158	164	169	174	180	185
62	104	109	115	120	126	131	136	142	147	153	158	164	169	175	180	186	191
63	107	113	118	124	130	135	141	146	152	158	163	169	175	180	186	191	197
64	110	116	122	128	134	140	145	151	157	163	169	174	180	186	192	197	204
65	114	120	126	132	138	144	150	156	162	168	174	180	186	192	198	204	210
66	118	124	130	136	142	148	155	161	167	173	179	186	192	198	204	210	216
67	121	127	134	140	146	153	159	166	172	178	185	191	198	204	211	217	223
68	125	131	138	144	151	158	164	171	177	184	190	197	203	210	216	223	230
69	128	135	142	149	155	162	169	176	182	189	196	203	209	216	223	230	236
70	132	139	146	153	160	167	174	181	188	195	202	209	216	222	229	236	243
71	136	143	150	157	165	172	179	186	193	200	208	215	222	229	236	243	250
72	140	147	154	162	169	177	184	191	199	206	213	221	228	235	242	250	258
73	144	151	159	166	174	182	189	197	204	212	219	227	235	242	250	257	265
74	148	155	163	171	179	186	194	202	210	218	225	233	241	249	256	264	272
75	152	160	168	176	184	192	200	208	216	224	232	240	248	256	264	272	279
76	156	164	172	180	189	197	205	213	221	230	238	246	254	263	271	279	287

Source: National Heart, Lung, and Blood Institute. Clinical guidelines on the identification, evaluation, and treatment of overweight and obesity in adults. U.S. Department of Health and Human Services, 1998 June: 139

Appendix A
Body Mass Index Chart

				EXTREME OBESITY														
36	37	38	39	40	41	42	43	44	45	46	47	48	49	50	51	52	53	54
172	177	181	186	191	196	201	205	210	215	220	224	229	234	239	244	248	253	258
178	183	188	193	198	203	208	212	217	222	227	232	237	242	247	252	257	262	267
184	189	194	199	204	209	215	220	225	230	235	240	245	250	255	261	266	271	276
190	195	201	206	211	217	222	227	232	238	243	248	254	259	264	269	275	280	285
196	202	207	213	218	224	229	235	240	246	251	256	262	267	273	278	284	289	295
203	208	214	220	225	231	237	242	248	254	259	265	270	278	282	287	293	299	304
209	215	221	227	232	238	244	250	256	262	267	273	279	285	291	296	302	308	314
216	222	228	234	240	246	252	258	264	270	276	282	288	294	300	306	312	318	324
223	229	235	241	247	253	260	266	272	278	284	291	297	303	309	315	322	328	334
230	236	242	249	255	261	268	274	280	287	293	299	306	312	319	325	331	338	344
236	243	249	256	262	269	276	282	289	295	302	308	315	322	328	335	341	348	354
243	250	257	263	270	277	284	291	297	304	311	318	324	331	338	345	351	358	365
250	257	264	271	278	285	292	299	306	313	320	327	334	341	348	355	362	369	376
257	265	272	279	286	293	301	308	315	322	329	338	343	351	358	365	372	379	386
265	272	279	287	294	302	309	316	324	331	338	346	353	361	368	375	383	390	397
272	280	288	295	302	310	318	325	333	340	348	355	363	371	378	386	393	401	408
280	287	295	303	311	319	326	334	342	350	358	365	373	381	389	396	404	412	420
287	295	303	311	319	327	335	343	351	359	367	375	383	391	399	407	415	423	431
295	304	312	320	328	336	344	353	361	369	377	385	394	402	410	418	426	435	443

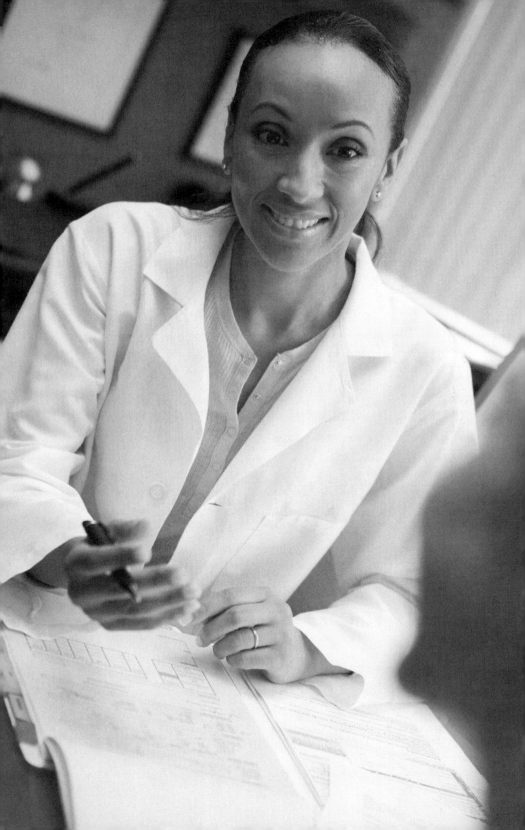

Appendix B
Health Questions for
Your First Prenatal Care Visit

Before your first prenatal care visit, make sure that you know the answers to these questions. You can fill out the form if you'd like, but be aware that your health care provider may have his or her own form for you to complete.

What was the date of your last menstrual period? _____

Was it a normal period in terms of length and amount? _____

What symptoms have you had since your last menstrual period? _____

Past Pregnancies

Total number of pregnancies:

Number of pregnancies that were:

Full term _____

Premature _____

Miscarriages _____

Induced abortions _____

Ectopic pregnancies _____

Multiple births _____

Number of living children _____

Fill in the following information for each of your past live births:

Date of Birth	Gestational Age at Birth (Weeks)	Length of Labor (Hours)	Birth Weight	Sex	Type of Delivery	Anesthesia	Place of Delivery	Complications, Including Preterm Labor

Your Medical History

Please check off whether you have or have had any of the following conditions:

Diabetes mellitus _____

High blood pressure (hypertension) _____

Heart disease_____

Autoimmune disease (lupus, multiple sclerosis, inflammatory bowel disease)_____

Kidney disease or urinary tract infection_____

Neurologic disease or epilepsy_____

Psychiatric disorder_____

Depression, including postpartum depression_____

Hepatitis or liver disease_____

Varicose veins or blood clots in the legs_____

Thyroid disease_____

Trauma or violence_____

Lung disease, such as asthma_____

Rh sensitization_____

Seasonal allergies_____

Drug reactions or allergies_____

Breast disease_____

Surgery_____

Gynecologic disorders_____

Abnormal Pap test result_____

Infertility_____

Assisted reproductive technology treatment_____

Uterine abnormalities_____

Lifestyle Issues

Smoking

Did you smoke before pregnancy? ❏ **Y** ❏ **N**   If yes, how much?_____

Do you currently smoke now? ❏ **Y** ❏ **N**   If yes, how much?_____

Alcohol

Did you drink alcohol before pregnancy? ❏ **Y** ❏ **N**   If yes, how much?_____

Do you drink alcohol now? ❏ **Y** ❏ **N**   If yes, how much?_____

Illegal Drugs

Did you use illegal drugs before pregnancy? ❏ **Y** ❏ **N**   If yes, what type and how much?

_____

Do you use illegal drugs now? ❏ **Y** ❏ **N**   If yes, what type and how much?

_____

Your Home Life

Do you feel safe in your current living situation? ❏ **Y** ❏ **N**

Do you feel safe with your current partner? ❏ **Y** ❏ **N**   If you answered "No" to either of these questions, please exercise caution and do not leave this form where your partner may see it. Both you and your baby may be at risk in this situation. It is important that you protect yourself and your baby by finding a safe place.

Genetic Background

Please indicate whether you, your baby's father, or anyone in either family has had any of the following conditions:

Condition	Y	N
Thalassemia (Italian, Greek, Mediterranean, or Asian background)		
Neural tube defect (spina bifida, meningomyelocele, anencephaly)		
Congenital heart defect		
Down syndrome		
Tay–Sachs disease (Ashkenazi Jewish, Cajun, French Canadian)		
Canavan disease (Ashkenazi Jewish)		
Familial dysautonomia (Ashkenazi Jewish)		

Have you or your baby's father had a child with a birth defect not listed above? ❏ **Y** ❏ **N**
If yes, what type?_____

Are you age 35 years or older? ❏ **Y** ❏ **N**

Do you have a metabolic disorder, such as type 1 diabetes mellitus or phenylketonuria?
❏ **Y** ❏ **N**

446 • APPENDIX B

Please list all medications you have taken since your last menstrual period (include supplements, vitamins, herbs, and over-the-counter drugs). Please include the strength and dosage.

Drug	Strength (eg, milligrams)	Dosage

Infection History

Do you live with someone with tuberculosis or have you been exposed to tuberculosis?
❏ Y ❏ N

Do you or your sexual partner have oral or genital herpes? ❏ Y ❏ N

Have you had a rash or viral illness since your last menstrual period? ❏ Y ❏ N

Do you have hepatitis B virus or hepatitis C virus? ❏ Y ❏ N

Have you ever had the following childhood diseases or have you been vaccinated against them?

Chickenpox	❏ Y	❏ N	❏ vaccine
Measles	❏ Y	❏ N	❏ vaccine
Mumps	❏ Y	❏ N	❏ vaccine
Rubella	❏ Y	❏ N	❏ vaccine

Have you had parvovirus? ❏ Y ❏ N

Have you ever had a sexually transmitted disease, such as gonorrhea, chlamydia, human immunodeficiency virus (HIV) infection, syphilis, or human papillomavirus infection?
❏ Y ❏ N

Please circle all that apply.

Your Questions

Please list any questions that you would like to ask your pregnancy health care provider.

_____

_____

_____

_____

_____

_____

_____

_____

_____

_____

_____

_____

_____

_____

_____

_____

_____

_____

_____

_____

_____

_____

_____

_____

Adapted from The American College of Obstetricians and Gynecologists. ACOG Antepartum Record. Version 6. ACOG: Washington, DC; 2007.

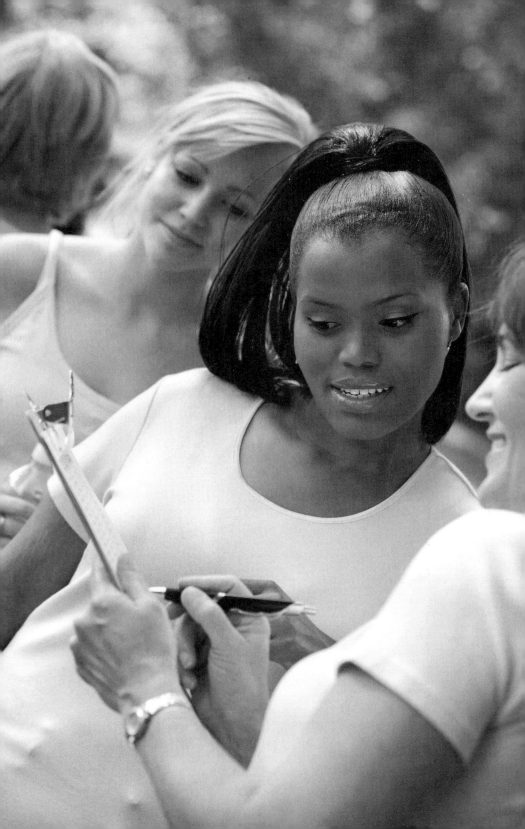

Index

Information in figures, tables, and boxes is denoted by *f, t,* and *b,* respectively

Sciatica, 119
Screening
for birth defects, 351–357
carrier, 351–353
genetic, 90
nuchal translucency, 354
Searching, in grief, 410
Seasickness, 94
Seat belts, 93*b*, 164*b*
Seizure disorders, 327–328
Selenium, dietary reference intake for, 243*t*
Settings, birth, 72
Sex, of baby, 89–90
Sex
Braxton Hicks contractions and, 121
concerns with, 111–112
feelings about, 110–111
postpartum, 226
premature rupture of membranes and, 151
at term, 175
Sexually transmitted diseases (STDs)
definition of, 383
risks of, 58
testing for, 53, 57
Shark, 86
Shellfish, 86
Shock, in grief, 410
Shoulder lifts, 222*b*
Sickle cell disease
definition of, 346*t*
folic acid and, 23
genetic counseling for, 50
risk factors for, 346*t*
Skiing, 108
Skin
acne and, 44
changes in third month, 52
in chloasma, 52
itchy, 141
stretch marks on, 52
Sleep
difficulty, 156
and newborn, 212
positions for, 95
in third month, 43
Sleeping, trouble with, 156

Smells
appetite and, 22
morning sickness and, 21
Smoking
complications with, 29
miscarriage and, 334
nicotine replacement therapy for, 30
postpartum, 225
quitting, 29–30
toxins in, 29
Snacks
healthy, 87
morning sickness and, 21
at work, 36
Snoring, 171
Soda, 38–39
Sodium, 105
Spacing between pregnancies, 282*b*
Sperm, in fertilization, 13
Spermicides, 228*f*, 231
Spina bifida
folic acid and, 23
as multifactorial disorder, 350
Spines, ischial, 186, 187*f*
Sponge, 228*f*, 232
Sports, to avoid, 108
Spotting, 177
State Children's Health Insurance Program, 75
Station, 186–188, 187*f*
STDs. *See* Sexually transmitted diseases
Sterilization, as birth control, 133, 228*f*, 234–236
Sterilization, of bottle, 274
Stevia, 46
Stillbirth
autopsy in, 409–410
causes of, 409–410
coping with, 411*b*
definition of, 409
depression and, 411–412
diabetes and, 312
future pregnancies after, 413
grief and, 410–412
support after, 412–413
Storage
of breast milk, 271
of cord blood, 128

U

Ultrasound
  detailed, 355
  Doppler velocimetry, 404
  early, 39
  in first trimester, 53
  information in, 403
  keepsake, 114
  mechanism of, 53
  in preterm labor, 363
  in second trimester, 97
  three-dimensional, 114
  transabdominal, 53, 54f, 403
  transducer, 53
  transvaginal, 53, 54f, 403
Umbilical cord, 14, 15f
  banking of blood from, 125, 128–129
  cesarean and, 201
  cutting, 193
  in postterm pregnancy, 178
Underweight, 254t
Upper body bend, 157
Urethra, infections of, 76
Urinary tract infections, 76
Urination
  caffeine and, 38–39
  fetal, 63
  frequent, 155, 171
  painful, postpartum, 215
  in pregnancy testing, 19
  as symptom of pregnancy, 18
  at term, 171
Urine, leakage of, 150, 155
Uterus
  breastfeeding and, 161
  breathing problems and, 139
  in constipation, 120
  in fertilization, 13, 14f
  heartburn and, 103
  placenta in, 15f
  in second trimester, 65
  size of, 96f, 97
  in vaginal birth after cesarean delivery, 48

V

Vaccine(s)
  flu, 52, 99, 393
  hepatitis B, 390
  human papillomavirus, 99
  infections and, 379–380
  measles, mumps, rubella, 99
  tuberculosis, 99
  varicella, 99
Vacuum extraction, 181, 199–200
Vagina, 14f
Vaginal birth after cesarean (VBAC)
  delivery, 48–50
Vaginal discharge, 76–77
Vaginosis, bacterial, 77, 388–389
Varenicline, 30
Vas deferens, 236
Vasectomy, 134, 236
VBAC. See Vaginal birth after cesarean delivery
Vegans, 256
Vegetables, 249, 252t
Vegetarianism, 255–257
Veins
  in hemorrhoids, 139–140
  spider, 66
  varicose, 140
Velocimetry, Doppler, 404
Violence, domestic, 58–60
Vitamin(s)
  in diet, 246–248
  prenatal, 23–24, 255
  vitamin A, 243t, 244t
  vitamin B, 104–105
  vitamin B$_6$, 21, 243t
  vitamin B$_{12}$, 243t
  vitamin C, 157, 243t, 244t
  vitamin D, 134–135, 243t, 244t, 248, 261
  vitamin E, 243t, 244t
  vitamin K, 212–213, 243t
Volume, blood, 307, 320
Vomiting
  in morning sickness, 20–21
  as symptom of pregnancy, 18